Basic Biology of New Developments in Biotechnology

BASIC LIFE SCIENCES

Alexander Hollaender, General Editor

Associated Universities, Inc., Washington, D.C.

Recent volumes in the series:

Volume 16 • DEVELOPMENT AND NEUROBIOLOGY OF DROSOPHILA
Edited by O. Siddiqi, P. Babu, Linda M. Hall, and Jeffrey C. Hall

Volume 17 • GENETIC ENGINEERING OF SYMBIOTIC NITROGEN FIXATION
Edited by J. M. Lyons, R. C. Valentine, D. A. Phillips, D. W. Rains, and R. C. Huffaker

Volume 18 • TRENDS IN THE BIOLOGY OF FERMENTATIONS FOR FUELS AND CHEMICALS
Edited by Alexander Hollaender, Robert Rabson, Palmer Rogers, Anthony San Pietro, Raymond Valentine, and Ralph Wolfe

Volume 19 • GENETIC ENGINEERING OF MICROORGANISMS FOR CHEMICALS
Edited by Alexander Hollaender, Ralph D. DeMoss, Samuel Kaplan, Jordan Konisky, Dwayne Savage, and Ralph S. Wolfe

Volume 20 • MOLECULAR AND CELLULAR MECHANISMS OF MUTAGENESIS
Edited by J. F. Lemontt and W. M. Generoso

Volume 21 • GENETIC TOXICOLOGY: An Agricultural Perspective
Edited by Raymond A. Fleck and Alexander Hollaender

Volume 22 • PLANT CELL CULTURE IN CROP IMPROVEMENT
Edited by Kenneth L. Giles and S. K. Sen

Volume 23 • INDUCED MUTAGENESIS: Molecular Mechanisms and Their Implications for Environmental Protection
Edited by Christopher W. Lawrence

Volume 24 • ORGAN AND SPECIES SPECIFICITY IN CHEMICAL CARCINOGENESIS
Edited by Robert Langenbach, Stephen Nesnow, and Jerry M. Rice

Volume 25 • BASIC BIOLOGY OF NEW DEVELOPMENTS IN BIOTECHNOLOGY
Edited by Alexander Hollaender, Allen I. Laskin, and Palmer Rogers

---

Basic Biology of New Developments in Biotechnology

Edited by

Alexander Hollaender

Associated Universities, Inc.
Washington, D.C.

Allen I. Laskin

Exxon Research and Engineering Co.
Linden, New Jersey

Palmer Rogers

University of Minnesota Medical School
Minneapolis, Minnesota

and

Stanley Dagley, Richard Hanson, Lawrence McKay, and Joachim Messing

Claire M. Wilson, Technical Editor

PLENUM PRESS · NEW YORK AND LONDON

Library of Congress Cataloging in Publication Data

Main entry under title:

Basic biology of new developments in biotechnology.

(Basic life sciences; v. 25)
Proceedings of a symposium held May 25 – 28, 1982 at the University of Minnesota, Minneapolis.
Includes bibliographical references and index.
1. Bioengineering—Congresses. 2. Biology—Technique—Congresses. I. Hollaender, Alexander, 1898- . II. Series. [DNLM: 1. Bioelectric energy sources—Congresses. 2. Biological products—Congresses. 3. Fermentation– Congresses. W3 BA255 v. 25 / QW 75 B311 1982]
TA164.B37 1983 660'.6 82-22301
ISBN 0-306-41244-6

Proceedings of a symposium on the Biological Basis of New Developments in Biotechnology, held May 25-28, 1982, at the University of Minnesota, Minneapolis, Minnesota

A Division of Plenum Publishing Corporation
233 Spring Street, New York, N.Y. 10013

Printed in the United States of America

ACKNOWLEDGEMENTS

The success of this symposium on "The Biological Basis of New Developments in Biotechnology" was made possible by the fortunate conjunction of support, cooperation, and the vision of many institutions and individuals. First, we are grateful for general financial support from the U.S. Department of Energy's Division of Biological Energy Research, from the Office of Naval Research, and from the Minnesota Agricultural Experiment Station. We also acknowledge the augmenting grants made by five visionary Minnesota based industries: Control Data Corporation; Economics Laboratory, Inc; General Mills, James Ford Bell Technical Center; Molecular Genetics, Inc.; and Minnesota Mining & Manufacturing, Inc. The facilities for the conference and additional funds were generously contributed by our hosts at the University of Minnesota, which included: the Medical School - Departments of Biochemistry and Microbiology; the Departments of Biochemistry and Genetics-Cell Biology, College of Biological Sciences; the Institute of Technology; and the College of Agriculture.

Most significant were the conception, imagination, and planning efforts for the conference lead by our symposium organizer, Allen Laskin and supported by our Scientific Advisory Committee, consisting of Victor Bloomfield, Stanley Dagley, Richard Hanson, Harry Hogenkamp, and Alexander Hollaender. We appreciatively acknowledge the valuable consultation and expertise of the Local Organizing Committee and the Office of Continuing Medical Education.

This symposium forms the third in a series of conferences including "Trends in the Biology of Fermentations for Fuels and Chemicals" held in December, 1980, and "Genetic Engineering of Microorganisms for Chemicals" held in May, 1981; both of which have also been published by Plenum Publishing Corp., New York. Taken together, these three volumes describe the interfacing of basic knowledge of genetics, biochemistry, and microbiology with the new advances in fermentation technology, drug design, agricultural plant development, and medicine, that will assist in opening new directions in the biotechnology of the future.

I express thanks to my fellow associate editors, Allen Laskin and Alexander Hollaender assisted by our editorial team of Stanley Dagley, Richard Hanson, Larry McKay, and Joachim Messing. We appreciate the conscientious and exceptionally competent job of our Technical Editor, Claire M. Wilson and her associates in assembling the manuscripts.

Most importantly, the success of this symposium rested squarely upon the creativity, vitality, and cooperation of the speakers, conveners, and authors whose efforts we enthusiastically acknowledge in composing this fine volume.

Palmer Rogers

CONTENTS

BIOTECHNOLOGY FOR AGRICULTURE

DRUGS AND ANTIBIOTICS

FUELS AND CHEMICALS

INDUSTRIAL AND APPLIED MICROBIOLOGY

BIODEGRADATION AND ENZYME TECHNOLOGY

INTRODUCTION

Allen I. Laskin
Biosciences Research
Exxon Research and Engineering Company
Linden, New Jersey

I was contacted in the Fall of 1981 by Professors Martin Dworkin and Palmer Rogers, of the University of Minnesota and asked to participate in the orgnization of the 1983 conference in the series, "Interface Between Biology and Medicine". They and the other members of the advisory committee had the vision to realize that this was a time to depart somewhat from the traditional theme, since one of the major areas of interest in the biological and related sciences these days is that of biotechnology in a broader sense than its impact on medicine alone. In designing the format of the Conference, we considered another factor. There has been a plethora of conferences, symposia, and meetings on biotechnology over the past few years, and the faces and topics have become rather familiar. There has been a strong emphasis on the development of the technology and the "biotechnology industry"; less attention has been paid to the science behind it. One might get the impression from some of these meetings and from the popular press that biotechnology has just recently sprung up, apparently full blown; the very fundamental scientific discoveries and the great body of continuing research that forms that basis for the technology is often obscured.

Thus, those of you who have been attending biotechnology conferences will recognize from this program that the mix of people is quite different. An attempt was made to touch upon points across the entire spectrum, from fundamental biological, biochemical, or genetic research on one end, to bioengineering, perhaps, on the other. We were faced, however, with some constraints and conflicting goals: carrying out the mission of spanning that entire spectrum, but limiting the number of speakers and providing enough time for effective communication and discussion, covering as many areas as possible upon which biotechnology impacts, and doing it all in the space of two and a half days. I hope we have succeeded in our major goal -- to emphasize the great importance of the fact that the new developments in biotechnology have depended upon, and continue to depend upon basic research in a large number of biological and related science disciplines.

At this point, since the theme of this conference is the basic biology of new developments in biotechnology, we should attempt to define what we think biotechnology is. Again, if one reads the popular and semi-popular press, one might get some rather distorted impressions. One, for example, is that biotechnology and recombinant DNA are the same thing; I have seen the two terms used synonymously. I think each of us readily recognizes that biotechnology is not recombinant DNA; neither is it "genetic engineering". Genetic engineering, of course, includes recombinant DNA technologies plus a number of other technologies for manipulating genetic material, but all of that together still represents only one aspect of biotechnology. Another area to be considered is "enzyme engineering". Last Fall, I was invited to a conference in Tokyo, the title of which was, "Biomolecular Technology". The Japanese scientists involved in that conference were putting together a discipline that they propose to call "biomolecular technology", which is a marriage of genetic engineering and enzyme engineering. That is certainly a valid concept, but it still represents only a part of what I like to think is biotechnology.

Others have wrestled with a definition of biotechnology. A working party of the European Federation of Biotechnology came up with the following in 1980:

> "Biotechnology is the application of biological systems or processes to manufacturing and service industries."

At first glance that seems OK, but after pondering over it, I wondered if that definition also included the horses that pulled the Budweiser beer wagons in the television commericals! The Federation didn't accept that definition, and in 1982 a new definition was promulgated:

> "Biotechnology is the integrated use of biochemistry, microbiology, and engineering sciences in order to achieve the technological application of the capacities of microorganisms, cultured tissue cells, and parts thereof."

Other terms are used in the context of biotechnology: applied microbiology, industrial microbiology, applied biochemistry, biochemical technology, and the previously discussed biomolecular technology. And relatively recently, the scope of the field has been broadened significantly by the inclusion of hybridoma technology. It is clear that a simple, generally acceptable definition of biotechnology is elusive. It is an integrated multidisciplinary field that utilizes many different technologies and impacts on a wide variety of areas. Let me detail some of these.

As a microbiologist, I place microbiology in the center, among the other core disciplines -- biochemistry, enzymology, and molecular genetics. Surrounding this core are the broader areas of molecular and cell biology, immunology (which, especially with the advent of monoclonal antibodies, may well be considered a core discipline), organic chemistry in many of its manifestations, and some more applied disciplines such as agricultural science, food and fermentation science, and special technologies such as animal and plant tissue culture. One can undoubtedly think of others; the point is clear, i.e., that biotechnology involves and is intimately connected with a large number of scientific disciplines and technologies.

And what of the impact areas for biotechnology? A few of the key areas that have received the most attention are pharmaceuticals and human/veterinary health care, chemicals, energy, food, agriculture, and environment. Most of these are touched upon in this conference, but there are other areas, such as microbe/metal interactions and marine science, which have received considerable attention. Indeed, there are few areas of human endeavor which have not received consideration with respect to biotechnology.

Let me return to the theme of the conference, the importance of fundamental science as related to biotechnology. As an example, I've selected what is perhaps the most widely known and popular "breakthrough" that relates to biotechnology -- recombinant DNA. Some think that recombinant DNA is a phenomenon that burst forth suddenly a few years ago. I think most of us recognize that this development represented a series of interdependent breakthroughs, all in turn dependent on a huge body of research in molecular biology, genetics, microbiology, and biochemistry. Examples include the discovery of Class II restriction enzymes by Smith and colleagues; methods of ligating DNA molecules, including the Khorana and Sgaramella work on blunt end ligation with T_4 ligase and the work of two Stanford groups (Lobban and Kaiser; Jackson, Symons, and Berg) on ligating molecules with complimentary cohesive ends; additional work at Stanford on Eco Rl (Mertz and Davis; Sgaramella); rapid DNA sequencing (Maxam and Gilbert; Sanger); gel methods for analyzing DNA fragments (Sharp). All of these and many more were necessary before Cohen, Chang, Boyer, and Helling produced their well known biologically functional recombinant DNA molecules.

For the Conference, we selected several of the more important impact areas of biotechnology, and have attempted to provide some feeling of the inter-relationship between fundamental research in various disciplines and the development of the related biotechnology. In some areas, there has been a more-or-less orderly progression from fundamental research through technology and on towards commercialization; in others, attempts to develop technology have have proceeded much faster than has been warranted by the science background, and they are languishing, waiting for the science to catch up.

For decades in the drug and antibiotic field, brute screening methods were used for new drug discovery or for the improvement of production. In the past few years, fundamental new understanding in biochemistry and genetics of the antibiotic-producing streptomycetes has opened new pathways for new compounds and for improvements in their production. New approaches to drug design are also based on fundamental new knowledge, e.g., of enzyme mechanisms.

Biotechnology in agriculture has vast and multiple ramifications. In one area, plant genetics is an example where the fundamental work of Barbara McClintock at Cold Spring Harbor Laboratory over several years went practically unnoticed, or more accurately, not understood. Only recently has it been fully appreciated that she was working with the first reported system of movable genetic elements; one of the presentations in this volume addresses this system. Similarly, decades of work on the microbially-caused tumors of plants, known as crown galls, have led to the development of a most promising vector for gene transfer in plants, the Ti plasmid.

The special lecture by Professor Whittenbury deals with organisms, the methane-oxidizing bacteria, that have been known since 1905. In the past decade, basic studies on microbiology, biochemistry, and enzymology carried out in Prof. Whittenbury's lab in Warwick; by a group at the University of Kent; by Prof. Hanson, now director of the Freshwater Institute here in Minnesota; and in our own laboratories at Exxon have led to a very great interest in these methane-oxidizing and related microbes as important biotechnological organisms.

Several papers deal with one of those areas where attempts to develop biotechnology have perhaps been several steps ahead of the required fundamental knowledge in biochemistry and genetics. This relates to the anaerobic bacteria, which carry out many interesting reactions. One of the most famous biotechnological processes is the acetone/butanol fermentation, developed during World War I, and carried on through the Second World War. Work here in Professor Roger's laboratory is now going on in an attempt to better understand these organisms, and another paper in this volume discusses these and other anaerobes. Almost nothing is known about the genetics of anaerobic bacteria, and there is a lot of catching up to do in genetics as well as biochemistry before we can fully exploit their capabilities.

I'll just mention one other area -- that of biodegradation of pesticides, herbicides, and other potential environmental pollutants. While many of these are readily biodegradable, others have proved to be recalcitrant and are persistent in soil and water. In recent years, a great deal of research has been done on the biochemistry and genetics of pesticide-degrading organisms; much important work has been done by Professors Chapman and Dagley, here at Minnesota. Based on this new knowledge, it is now possible to construct new strains that are able to attack substances previously thought to be quite resistant to biodegradation.

Although these proceedings range widely, it can only begin to scratch the surface. What is clear is that there is a great deal to be done in fundamental biology, in biotechnology, and at the interface between the two.

IN VITRO DNA SYNTHESIS AS A TOOL TO ANALYZE AND ALTER GENES

Joachim Messing
Department of Biochemistry
University of Minnesota
St. Paul, Minnesota 55108

This overview describes some of the biochemical procedures which are used to analyze the primary structure of genetic information. This is one of the first steps in engineering genetic material so that it can be used for the production of materials in the medical, agricultural, and chemical industries. Another important step is the design and construction of synthetic genetic alterations either to explore function or to alter function in the sense of making a better product, e.g., yield, stability, higher activity, or specificity.

The biochemical procedure which is used for both steps involves the synthesis of DNA *in vitro*. DNA, which is normally double-stranded, is converted into single-stranded DNA. One of the two DNA strands, in some cases both strands, is then copied into a newly synthesized DNA strand. The part of the template which is copied into the complementary information is defined by the 3' end of a DNA strand complementary to the template. This piece of complementary DNA can be very short and is named a primer, since DNA polymerase *in vivo* as well as *in vitro* cannot initiate DNA synthesis on a DNA template with deoxynucleotidetriphosphates, the precursor of DNA.

Therefore, every DNA synthesis can be considered as a gap filling mechanism.

With the advent of molecular cloning, any DNA can be purified and reproduced in large quantities. The molecular cloning procedure involves a cloning vector in which the desired DNA is introduced enzymatically so that a chimeric DNA molecule is formed. Such a molecule which is recovered from an individually transformed *E. coli* cell and is therefore a clone, consists out of the vector DNA and the desired DNA, also called the passenger DNA. In terms of *in vitro* DNA synthesis, a primer can be used to initiate DNA synthesis to the 3' or 5' site of the inserted DNA or within the cloned DNA as shown in Fig. 1. Two of these primers are subject to our discussion on the analysis of the primary structure of DNA and the production of synthetic variants of the analyzed gene. A more detailed discussion of the use of primers is given in another article [6].

It can be seen at this stage that an important component in the described biochemical procedure is the cloning vector. The vector is a replicon which carries useful markers like one to detect a transformed cell, the most important step for the cloning process, or a marker useful for the insertion of the passenger DNA. One may argue here in a similar way as with automobiles. Certainly transportation is the key thing, but there is not a universal automobile, and everybody will have a different interest in using a vehicle. In DNA manipulation, a number of vectors have been developed, and they can be viewed to fall into three different classes. Lambda phage derivatives are used to clone large DNA fragments because of their packaging mechanism, plasmids to clone medium or small DNA fragments, M13 phage derivatives to convert double-stranded DNA into single-stranded DNA. For *in vitro* DNA synthesis, the latter class seems to be appropriate, and the viral DNA of such a phage has been the first one which has been reproduced in the test tube [2].

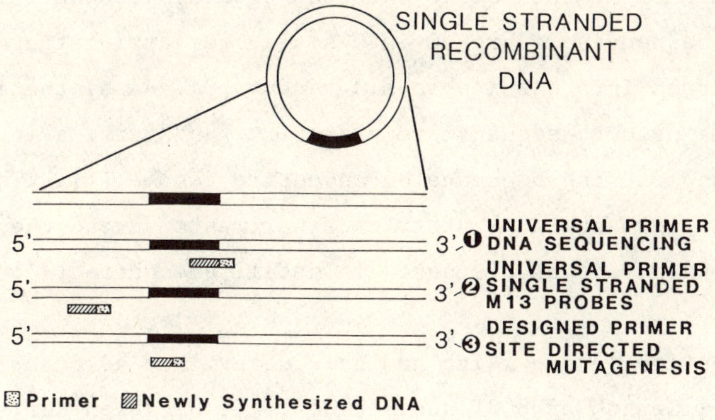

Fig. 1. In vitro DNA synthesis of recombinant DNA with different classes of primers.

The same single-stranded DNA phage system has also been used to develop a fast method of determining the DNA sequence [10] and a method to alter the DNA sequence by designing the change with an oligonucleotide [4]. At the same time, another single-stranded DNA phage, phage M13, has been used to separate the two strands of a double-stranded DNA by molecular cloning techniques [9].

The DNA sequencing method has to be conducted in a discontinuous manner. The DNA synthesis which is carried out in the presence of base specific chain terminating inhibitors permits the deduction of a DNA sequence by determining the length of those chains by a one dimensional gel electrophoresis system. The enzymatic reaction as well as the resolution of the gel system limit the amount of sequence determined at a time. Consequently, the reaction has to be repeated for a long stretch of DNA in a manner such that overlap can be used to reconstruct a continuous stretch of DNA sequence. With every enzymatic reaction, the starting point of DNA synthesis has to be reset to ensure the generation of overlapping information. A rapid form of accumulating data is the use of an approach which allows the reuse of the same primer over and over again [3]. The reset mechanism is then built into the cloning procedure itself. DNA to be sequenced is broken into small overlapping fragments and shotgun cloned into a suitable M13 vector [8]. A synthetic oligonucleotide is used to sequence templates at random and a few selected ones to complete the sequence of an entire genome [1]. The impact of this DNA sequencing strategy on experiments beyond the first structural analysis is discussed in detail elsewhere [7].

The entire genome which has been determined as described above has a total length of 8031 nucleotides. It has been derived from 175 different templates. This large amount of information, which accumulates in a short time, requires the use of a computer program for storage, assembly, and evaluation of overlapping sequences [5]. Dr. Modelevsky's presentation in this volume discusses this in more detail presenting how the computer, in general, can aid in recombinant DNA research.

Even if the primary structure of an isolated gene has been determined, its borders and its important regulatory features mapped, the structure can only, ultimately, be related to its function by carefully designed changes in the primary structure. Random mutagenesis induced by chemicals or UV light, the characterization of mutant sequences, and the functional analysis of mutants help to design very specific changes in the DNA sequence. These changes do not occur by the use of the agents mentioned above, but require the chemical synthesis of the DNA sequence. This is the most versatile approach to relate gene structure to gene function. The understanding of gene function, however, is an important prerequisite in order to apply genetic engineering to industrial purposes.

Although the chemical synthesis of DNA is much slower than the enzymatic <u>in vitro</u> DNA synthesis, its most important feature is the building of an oligonucleotide of defined sequence in the absence of a DNA template. Since changes in a DNA sequence usually involve only a few nucleotides, the remainder of sequences are added to the synthetic oligonucleotide by the faster enzymatic reaction. This scheme, again, involves the same components as the DNA sequencing procedure. The addition of sequences to the synthetic oligonucleotide are done in the presence of a DNA template, the one which carries the wildtype sequence information. Different from DNA sequencing, this procedure uses an oligonucleotide as a primer which is only partially complementary to the template. Despite this difference, a primer elongation reaction can be carried out if the reaction temperature is lowered to ice temperature to allow the addition of the first nucleotides. Although a double-stranded DNA is now produced which has a number of mispairing bases, the two strands can be separately inherited by transforming a competent cell. With this step the synthetically altered sequence becomes a clone, can be reproduced, analyzed, and tested for function. Since the alteration is usually not phenotypically visible in the transformed cell, a strategy is necessary to enhance mutagenesis and to use a simple physical detection test. If a single-stranded cloning vector is used, then repair or reproduction is reduced to one template strand. Since the binding of the synthetic oligonucleotide to the template is critical with rising temperature (this actually depends on its length and the mispairing bases), wildtype and mutant sequences can be differentiated by using the oligonucleotide as a hybridization probe. The flow of steps is summarized in Fig. 2.

We have seen a few important biochemical procedures which are playing an important role in the development of Biotechnology. Cloning vectors, DNA sequencing methods, and oligonucleotide synthesis are essential components in some of the work that is described in these chapters.

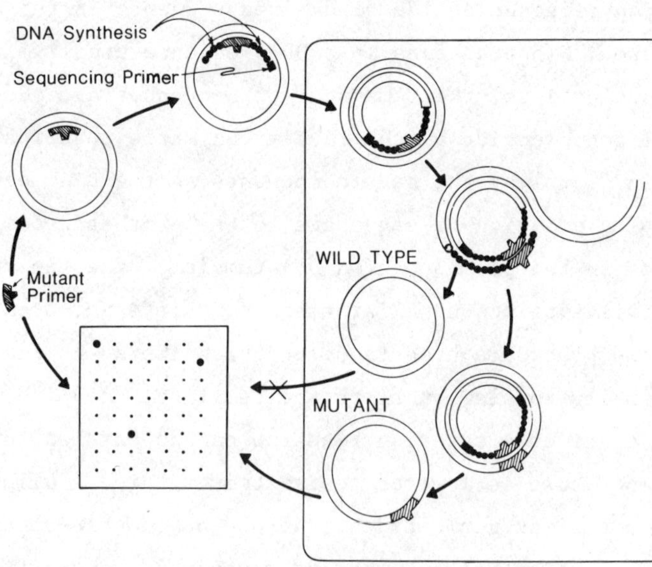

Fig. 2. Flow of site directed mutagenesis using bacteriophage M13.

REFERENCES

1. Gardner, R.C., A.J. Howarth, P. Hahan, M. Brown-Luedi, R.J. Shepherd, and J. Messing. The complete nucleotide sequence of an infectious clone of cauliflower mosaic virus by M13mp7 shotgun sequencing. Nucl. Acids Res. 9:2871-2888 (1981).
2. Goulian, M., A. Kornberg, and R.L. Sinsheimer. Enzymatic synthesis of DNA. XXIV. Synthesis of infectious phage ϕX174 DNA. Proc. Natl. Acad. Sci., U.S.A., 58:2321-2328 (1967).
3. Heidecker, G., J. Messing, and B. Gronenborn. A versatile primer for DNA sequencing in the M13mp2 cloning system. Gene 10:69-73 (1980).
4. Hutchinson, C.A., III, S. Phillips, M.H. Edgell, S. Gillam, P. Jahnke, and M. Smith. Mutagenesis at a specific position in a DNA sequence. J. Biol. Chem., 253:6551-6560 (1978).
5. Larson, R. and J. Messing. Apple II software for M13 shotgun DNA sequencing. Nucl. Acids Res. 10:39-49 (1982).
6. Messing, J. An integrative strategy of DNA sequencing and

experiments beyond. In Genetic Engineering: Principles and Methods (J. Setlow and A. Hollaender, eds), Vol 4, Plenum Press, New York, pp 19-36 (1982).

7. Messing, J. New M13 vectors for cloning, In Methods in Enzymology (R. Wu, ed). Academic Press, New York (in press, 1982).

8. Messing, J. R. Crea, and P.H. Seeburg. A system for shotgun DNA sequencing. Nucl. Acids Res., 9:309-321 (1981).

9. Messing, J., B. Gronenborn, B. Müller-Hill, and P.H. Hofschneider. Filamentous coliphage M13 as a cloning vehicle: Insertion of a Hind II fragment of the lac regulatory region into M13 replicative form *in vitro*. Proc. Natl. Acad. Sci., U.S.A., 74:3642-3646 (1977).

10. Sanger, F., S. Nicklen, and A.R. Coulson. DNA sequencing with chain terminating inhibitors. Proc. Natl. Acad. Sci., U.S.A., 74:5463-5467 (1977).

COMPUTER APPLICATIONS IN RECOMBINANT DNA RESEARCH

Joseph L. Modelevsky
Lilly Research Laboratories
A Division of Eli Lilly and Company
307 East McCarty Street
Indianapolis, Indiana 46285

INTRODUCTION

I would like to present an "audience-friendly" introduction to computer applications in recombinant DNA research. For those who wish to rapidly learn more about computer applications in general, I recommend the February 12, 1982, issue of Science [1]. For an in-depth look at some specific programming efforts in nucleic acids research, I recommend the January 11, 1982, issue of Nucleic Acids Research [2].

We have all noticed that the computer is rapidly becoming an essential tool for the molecular biologist. Computers can save labor, increase productivity, and permit instantaneous exchange and analysis of information. Clever applications of the computer can assist in data acquisition and analysis, in the modeling of test systems, and can provide rapid solutions to complex theoretical problems. I would like to describe how the computer can assist the molecular biologist. The examples I present will be documented by output from programs developed at Lilly Research Laboratories.

Recombinant DNA research relies heavily upon sequence analysis at the nucleotide and amino acid levels. Such analyses, for the most part, are based upon complex algorithms which are unmanageable for the researcher, but are routine for the computer. These facts prompted our division to independently develop a set of computer programs to perform a variety of nucleic acid and amino acid sequence manipulations and analyses.

Under the direction of Dr. Richard Douthart, and through the programming efforts of Mr. Frank Norris, a set of 35 programs was developed which can manipulate, analyze, display, and store nucleic acid and amino acid sequences; hence, the title, the MAD sets [3]. These programs can simulate a wide variety of relevant molecular biological manipulations and can perform a large number of analyses relevant to recombinant DNA research.

In addition to the MAD sets, we have a variety of programs of general utility for the molecular biology laboratory. These programs carry out routine calculations, plot data, etc. In each program we have tried to translate molecular biological problems into a programmable sequence of logical steps with input and output formats designed for the molecular biologist. Such programs can be great, objective timesavers and provide a reproducible, orderly method for repeated handling of extremely difficult or confusing analyses.

Anyone can collaborate with the computer to provide research support through routine or theoretical analyses. Through a CRT (a television with alpha-numeric display and a typewriter-like keyboard) at the bench, each laboratory has access to a system which provides text editors, file sharing, analytical programs, databases, electronic mail, and bulletin boards. Now, let us examine some specific examples of computer applications for the recombinant DNA scientist at the bench.

Information Storage and Management

Information storage is a problem scientists have dealt with throughout history. We have all maintained laboratory notes, recipes, data, and such. We are beginning to store such information in computer files and build knowledge and data bases. Using key words, we can easily search such data bases. In addition, our data bases are dynamic; our entire group can update and add to or alter protocols, product information, data, and so on. Local interactive user networks are developing, linking our laboratories together, allowing access to the latest developments from our colleagues.

Figure 1 is a simple example of the kind of information our laboratories might wish to share. This figure contains the output from a file entitled 32PROBE. This file contains instructions for preparing a nick-translated DNA probe for use in colony hybridization. Anyone in our group may simply call up this file to find out how we currently prepare probes. If a hard copy of this protocol is desired, one merely requests a printout. Should this file be edited in any way, we can easily notify the entire user network, via electronic mail, that changes have been introduced.

The following contains instructions for preparing a 32P-probe for colony hybridization.

1 μg (200-750bp) DNA to be labelled
+76 μl H_2O
+10 μl 10X Buffer 0
+10 μl dNTP mix (600μM dG, dA, dTTP; 60 μM dCTP)
+ 4 μl 100pg DNAseI/ μl

One minute at RT, then to ice.
Transfer to a tube containing 200 μCi dry 32P-dCTP (hi sp. act.).

+100 Units ENZO polI

---

150 minutes at 14C

Extract with phenol:CHC_{13}:isoamyl (25:24:1)
Re-extract organic phase with 20μl 20mM NaCl.
Pool aqueous phases.
Extract aqueous phase twice with 20μl CHC_{13}.
Take two 2μl samples to TCA ppt'ion.
Calculate TCA ppt'able cpm per μl·μg.

Fig. 1. Computer file 32PROBE.

```
This program will either calculate the number of G's or C's tailed
onto a template DNA population or will predict the counts to be
incorporated for a given tail length under given experimental
conditions.
The number—R—is the number of residues added per DNA end.
That is, R = tail length.
NOTICE: You MUST answer all questions!
You may answer questions with the FIRST LETTER of the answer.
Have fun, you tailer, you!
Do you want to calculate a decay correction? Y
This program will determine remaining activity of 32P, assuming a
half-life of 14.22 days.
Input original activity (note units)? 4
No. days of decay? 4
Decay Correction = .822999

Will we calculate tail length (R), estimate counts in a given tail (E) or
quit (Q)?? R
All new variables? Yes or No? Y
T = TCA ppt'able DPM per μl Reaction Mix
N = Nucleotide concentration (μMolar)
M = MW of DNA template (DAL)
D = DNA concentration in RX mix (μg/μl)
H = Label present in RX mix (μCi/μl)
Enter decay correction (decimal fraction less than 1.0)? .82
Enter sample volume (μl)? 20
Enter N (μMolar)? 20
Enter M (dal)? 2.6E6
Enter D (μg/μl)? .025
Enter H (μCi/μl)? 0.1
Enter T (DPM/μL)? 54000
R = 15.7522
Don't you think that's a long enough tail?
I hope you appreciate the complexity of the calculations I just made.
(Jan probably doesn't't!)
```

Fig. 2. Sample program with demonstrating desirable program attributes.

Routine Calculations

The computer is used to carry out routine calculations at speeds beyond human ability. In addition to the obvious statistical analyses available for years, we take advantage of programs designed for the molecular biology laboratory. For example, we have programs which help us calculate radioactive decay corrections, calculate efficiencies of cDNA synthesis, calculate the length of tailed fragments, etc.

The program represented in Figure 2 displays many of the program attributes desired by the molecular biologist. The program carries out a simple, routine calculation related to terminal transferase tailing reactions in a fraction of a second. The program is "user-friendly" in that the language used is familiar to the molecular biologist. All the variables are defined and are requested in a logical order, documenting the essential factors in the reaction. Once the program has completed a round of calculations, a hint of artificial intelligence is presented. We simply decided that ten to fifteen residues per DNA end was optimal, informed the computer, and it now shares our opinion. Imagine the time savings such a program can provide during repeated analytical runs in the development of specific protocols.

Sequence Manipulation

Sequence manipulating programs are extremely valuable in nearly every thought and design process that the recombinant DNA scientist goes through. The computer can store any number of DNA, RNA, or amino acid sequences. These sequences may be accessed instantaneously, regardless of the size of the data base. More importantly, the computer does not forget entered information; it's data base grows and grows.

Using the computer, we can manipulate stored sequences and simulate nearly every manipulation we might carry out in the test tube. The main DNA editor in the MAD sets, EDMAIN, carries out 22 such sequence manipulations (Fig. 3). Stringing together a series of these manipulations, one can construct model recombinant DNA molecules and examine the characteristics of the DNA, the RNA from a constructed transcription unit, the recombinant protein which would be synthesized, and so on. One must keep in mind that each of these computerized manipulations is 100 percent efficient, which is often uncharacteristic of their real-world counterparts.

DNA > HELP

Command	Action	Abbreviation
Amino Acids	—Convert DNA to AA	(A, AA)
Base Comp	—Compute GC comp.	(BASE, BA)
CF	—Change from file	(CHGF)
Change	—Change	(C, CH, CHG)
Delete	—Delete a segment	(DE)
Enzyme	—Restriction enzyme	(EZ)
Find	—Find a sequence	(F, FI, FIN, ALLFIND, EVERY)
Input	—Create a new seq.	(I, IN, INP)
Insert	—Insert a sequence	(IS)
IF	—Insert from file	(INSF)
List	—List a sequence	(LI)
Allchange	—Change every occur.	(AL, ALLC, PAS, PAST)
Palindromes	—Find palindromes	(PL)
Print	—List to line print.	(P, PR, PRI)
Randomize	—Randomize sequences	(RAN)
Read	—Read from file	(RE)
Renumber	—Set starting number	(RN)
Reverse	—Reverse a sequence	(RV)
Save	—Temporary save seq.	(SA)
Shift	—Shift seq. rt or lt	(SH)
Statistics	—Summary statistics	(ST)
Stop	—Exit the program	($$)
Symbols	—To see the DNA symb.	(SYMB)
Transform	—Convert DNA<=> RNA	(TR)
Unsave	—Get saved sequence	(UN, UNS)
Write	—Write to perm. file	(WR)

Fig. 3. Operations available in EDMAIN, the main sequence of the MAD sets.

Sequence Analysis and Display

The computer can be used to analyze sequences. In a matter of seconds, we can generate complete restriction maps, find symmetrical elements, locate regions of homology, reverse translate, and so on. Reverse translation (translating back from amino acid sequence to all possible coding DNA sequences) is an excellent example of an analytical process managed most efficiently by a computer. The genetic code is redundant. For a given amino acid, there may be from one to six possible codon choices. Reverse translation must take into account each codon possiblity. There are twelve possible coding sequences for the short chemotactic peptide, f-met-leu-phe (Fig. 4). Let us examine the application of a computer's ability to rapidly reverse translate in a hypothetical, medically important cloning project.

```
CHEMOTAXIS PEPTIDE F-MET-LEU-PHE

1      Fixed =    6    GC = 0.29630   Chains = 12
1 MET LEU PHE
1 ATG CTA TTC
      CTC TTT
      CTG
      CTT
      TTA
      TTG
```

Fig. 4. Reverse translation of the chemotactic peptide, f-met-leu-phe.

Let us imagine that we would like to clone the imaginary PANACEA gene. The PANACEA gene product, excreted from human pituitary in infinitely small quantities, has been studied in some detail. There may be a variety of potentially worthwhile medical applications for PANACEA protein - if only we can produce enough material for study. The protein has been sequenced and found to contain 125 amino acids (Fig. 5). Starting from the amino acid sequence, we will design a DNA probe which will hybridize to PANACEA coding sequence.

```
  1 HIS SER GLU GLY THR PHE THR SER ASP TYR SER LYS TYR LEU ASP
    --- --- --- --- --- --- --- --- --- --- --- --- --- --- ---
  1 CAC AGC GAA GGA ACA TTC ACA AGC GAC TAC AGC AAA TAC CTA GAC
    CAT AGT GAG GGC ACC TTT ACC AGT GAT TAT AGT AAG TAT CTC GAT
        TCA     GGG ACG     ACG TCA         TCA         CTG
        TCC     GGT ACT     ACT TCC         TCC         CTT
        TCG                     TCG         TCG         TTA
        TCT                     TCT         TCT         TTG


 15 ASP SER ARG ARG ALA GLU ASP PHE VAL GLU TRP LEU MET ASN THR
    --- --- --- --- --- --- --- --- --- --- --- --- --- --- ---
 43 GAC AGC AGA AGA GCA GAA GAC TTC GTA GAA TGG CTA ATG AAC ACA
    GAT AGT AGG AGG GCC GAG GAT TTT GTC GAG     CTC     AAT ACC
        TCA CGA CGA GCG             GTG         CTG         ACG
        TCC CGC CGC GCT             GTT         CTT         ACT
        TCG CGG CGG                             TTA
        TCT CGT CGT                             TTG
```

Fig. 5. Reverse translation of glucagon.

At this point, let me digress to tell you how I created the PANACEA gene. In a matter of three or four minutes, I sat down at the computer and called up the DNA sequence of pBR322 (a plasmid used as a cloning vector). I deleted all but 1000 bases of the sequence. The sequence was randomized and I searched for the longest open reading frame. The longest open reading frame was translated into protein, and this computer-generated protein was designated the PANACEA protein (Fig. 6). This sequence is the basis for all of the manipulations described below.

```
PANACEA PROTEIN

----- Amino acid sequence   Starting point    1.
  1 MET SER VAL VAL ALA -- CYS VAL MET LEU LEU -- ASP PRO GLY LEU TRP
    --- --- --- --- --- -- --- --- --- --- --- -- --- --- --- --- ---
 16 LYS ALA PRO ALA HIS -- GLY PRO LEU TRP LEU -- ARG LEU CYS GLY ILE
    --- --- --- --- --- -- --- --- --- --- --- -- --- --- --- --- ---
 31 VAL PHE ASN GLU MET -- PRO MET ASP TRP PRO -- PRO ILE SER VAL ALA
    --- --- --- --- --- -- --- --- --- --- --- -- --- --- --- --- ---
 46 CYS ASN ASN ILE SER -- GLY CYS LEU GLN SER -- ARG LEU ALA GLN CYS
    --- --- --- --- --- -- --- --- --- --- --- -- --- --- --- --- ---
 61 GLU CYS ALA VAL LEU -- ARG ASP LEU HIS SER -- PRO ILE ASN ARG LEU
    --- --- --- --- --- -- --- --- --- --- --- -- --- --- --- --- ---
 76 TYR ILE SER GLY ARG -- VAL ILE SER ASN HIS -- ALA ALA ASP GLY LEU
    --- --- --- --- --- -- --- --- --- --- --- -- --- --- --- --- ---
 91 SER LEU ASP LEU LYS -- VAL ARG GLY ARG THR -- SER PRO THR PRO CYS
    --- --- --- --- --- -- --- --- --- --- --- -- --- --- --- --- ---
106 ILE ILE ILE LEU VAL -- CYS VAL ASN VAL GLY -- ALA ASP THR ILE PHE
    --- --- --- --- --- -- --- --- --- --- --- -- --- --- --- --- ---
121 PRO MET ARG PRO THR --
    --- --- --- --- --- --
```

Fig. 6. The amino acid sequence of the hypothetical PANACEA protein. This amino acid sequence was generated by randomization of a 1,000-base pair region of pBR322. The randomized nucleotide sequence was searched for open reading frames. The protein coded for by one of these frames was designated to be PANACEA protein. This PANACEA protein sequence was then used as the starting point for the analyses described in the text.

The PANACEA amino acid sequence has been entered into the computer. Using the computer's ability to reverse translate, we will project all possible coding sequences for this protein. We will

```
Enter the low amino acid location, length of segment: 33,10

   33     Fixed =  23         GC = 0.51111    Chains =         1536

   32 PHE ASN GLU MET PRO MET ASP TRP PRO PRO ILE SER
      --- --- --- --- --- --- --- --- --- --- --- ---
   94 TTC AAC GAA ATG CCA ATG GAC TGG CCA CCA ATA AGC
      TTT AAT GAG     CCC     GAT     CCC CCC ATC AGT
                      CCG             CCG CCG ATT TCA
                      CCT             CCT CCT     TCC
                                                  TCG
                                                  TCT
```

Fig. 7. Least redundant PANACEA coding region located by reverse tranlation.

then examine the hypothetical coding sequences for minimal redundancy (degeneracy), and hopefully find a stretch of coding region which could be accounted for by as few different oligonucleotide chains as possible.

As shown in Figure 7, the computer has located a three amino acid region of the PANACEA protein sequence which may be coded for by a maximum of two oligonucleotide chains. This region may be coded for by a pair of 11-mers containing 10 fixed bases. If we synthesize a pair of oligonucleotide chains which are complementary to the identified coding regions, we may use these chains to probe for the presence of cloned PANACEA cDNA by colony hybridization, as probes for PANACEA transcripts in a pool of polyA RNA or as primers in a cDNA synthesis reaction, depending upon the stage we are at in the cloning project.

If we decide to use the synthetic oligonucleotides as colony hybridization probes, we must first be certain there will be little or no hybridization of probe to vector. To test this, we use a routine which searches for homologies between two strings of DNA based upon thermodynamic considerations. By examining the family of homologous, potentially hybridizable regions found in the computer search, we may assess the probability that a high background of false positives will arise. As shown in Fig. 8, the PANACEA probes do not share any significant homologies with our vector, pBR322.

```
From 1731 to 1741.
From   16 to   25.  Pct 0.81818 Len 11.
TGGCATTGACC
TGGATTGGCC← Probe No. 2

From 2146 to 2156.
From    1 to   11.  Pct 0.81818 Len 11.
ATGGCTGCGCC
ATGGACTGGCC← Probe No. 1
```

Fig. 8. Homology between hypothetical PANACEA DNA probes and pBR322.

Let us assume that we have identified a PANACEA cDNA clone and confirmed the sequence of the PANACEA coding region. Using the computer, we can examine the gene sequence to develop strategies for gene editing and vector construction (Fig. 9). The sequences of useful cloning and expression vectors at our disposal are in the computer data base. All the known restriction enzyme recognition and cut sites are also stored in the computer. We can therefore assemble any DNA combinations we desire in the computer and search for problems or advantages - before the actual labor ensues. We may insert the PANACEA sequence into a vector of our choice and predict many of the characteristics of the resultant molecule.

One characteristic used for confirmation of a construction is a restriction pattern. Cutting a piece of DNA with a restriction enzyme generates a family of DNA fragments of varying lengths. The length of a DNA fragment is often the only differentiating characteristic we can employ in separation procedures. It is very helpful to know ahead of time the size and number of fragments to expect in a restriction pattern (Fig. 10).

Computer-User Interaction

A major barrier between the molecular biologist and the computer is the fact that they now communicate through a typewriter-like keyboard. To lower this barrier, we are incorporating a voice-recognition unit into our system which allows the scientist to

```
                                                MET SER VAL VAL
 AG CTT ACA ATT CTT GGG GAA CTA GAG CGT GCC TCC ATG AGT GTA GTA
             10           20            30           40

5                   10                  15                  20
ALA CYS VAL MET LEU LEU ASP PRO GLY LEU TRP LYS ALA PRO ALA HIS
GCT TGT GTC ATG CTC TTG GAC CCC GGT CTG TGG AAA GCT CCT GCC CAT
  50            60           70           80            90

                25                  30                  35
GLY PRO LEU TRP LEU ARG LEU CYS GLY ILE VAL PHE ASN GLU MET PRO
GGG CCA CTC TGG TTG AGA CTC TGC GGA ATC GTT TTC AAC GAG ATG CCT
     100          110           120          130          140

            40                  45                  50
MET ASP TRP PRO PRO ILE SER VAL ALA CYS ASN ASN ILE SER GLY CYS
ATG GAC TGG CCT CCT ATT TCC GTC GCA TGC AAC AAT ATA TCC GGA TGC
        150          160          170           180          190

        55                  60                  65
LEU GLN SER ARG LEU ALA GLN CYS GLU CYS ALA VAL LEU ARG ASP LEU
CTT CAG TCC CGG CTA GCC CAA TGT GAA TGC GCC GTT CTA CGA GAT CTC
          200           210          220          230

    70                  75                  80
HIS SER PRO ILE ASN ARG LEU TYR ILE SER GLY ARG VAL ILE SER ASN
CAT TCA CCC ATT AAC AGA CTA TAC ATT TCC GGG CGT GTG ATA TCG AAT
240          250          260           270          280

85                  90                  95                  100
HIS ALA ALA ASP GLY LEU SER LEU ASP LEU LYS VAL ARG GLY ARG THR
CAC GCG GCC GAT GGT CTT TCG TTG GAT CTG AAG GTT AGG GGG AGA ACC
  290           300          310          320           330

                105                 110                 115
SER PRO THR PRO CYS ILE ILE ILE LEU VAL CYS VAL ASN VAL GLY ALA
TCG CCG ACG CCA TGT ATC ATC ATC CTT GTT TGT GTG AAC GTT GGC GCT
     340          350           360          370          380

            120                 125
ASP THR ILE PHE PRO MET ARG PRO THR ?1?
GAT ACC ATT TTC CCG ATG CGT CCC ACA TAA CTT TCA
        390          400          410
```

Fig. 9. Translation of hypothetical PANACEA cDNA contained on a HindIII fragment.

simply talk to the computer. With a voice synthesizer, we could enable the computer to talk back to the scientist.

Computer input is not limited to alpha-numeric or audio input. Video input capabilities are rapidly improving. Soon we will have computers routinely reading our gels and autoradiographs. It will not be long before an image analyzer will read a set of sequencing gels, enter the sequences, analyze reading frames, and locate promoters and other DNA elements in a matter of seconds in a single session.

```
Tic marks occur every  500 bases.
The DNA segment is  4781 bases long (    1 to  4781)
ACC.I       ______._______.!____.______.______.__!___.______.______._______.____ 2
ACC.II      ____!_.___!__.!_!!!!!!_!!!.!___!!_!___!.______!___!_.____!_._!__ 24
ACY.I       ____!_.___!!!.______._!____.______.______.______.______.___!__._!__ 7
ALU.I       !!___!._______.!____!______.____!!!___!_.!_!__!.______!!!____.____ 19
AOS.I       ______._!____.______.___!!_.______.______.______.____!______.____ 4
ASU.I       _!____.!____!.__!!_.!_!_!!._!__!.______.______.___!!._!____.__!_ 17
ATU.I       ______.!_____.______!____!_.______.______!.!_____._____.______.____ 6
AVA.I       ______._______.______.____!_.______.______.______.______.______.____ 1
AVA.II      _!____._______.__!!_.!___!!._!___.______.______.____!._!____.____ 9
BAL.I       ______._______.______.____!_.______.______.______.______.______.____ 1
BAM.HI      ______.___!__.______.______.______.______.______.___.______.____ 1
BBRS.I      ______._!____!_!___.____!_!!____!!!_!!_.__!!__!___!_.!_!___.____ 21
BGL.I       ______._______.___!_.!_____.______.______.______.____!.______.____ 3
^O

HHA.I       ___!_!!_!_!!!.!!!!_._!_!!_.!!___!_!_!__.!!!_!_!____!!____!_._!__ 33
HINC.II     ______._______.!____.______.______.______.______.____.___!__.____ 2
HIND.III    !____!._______.______.______.______.______.______.______.______.____ 2
HINF.I      _!__!_._______!__!_!.__!__!.______!___!!_.____!__.__!_.______.____ 13

XMA.III     ____!_._______.___!_.______.______.______.______.______.______.____ 2
XMN.I       ______._______.______.______.______!______.______.______.____!_.____ 2
XOR.II      ______._______.______.______.______.______.______.______._!____.____ 1

Noncutters:
  ASU.II        AVA.III       AVR.II        BCL.I         ECA.I         HPA.I
  KPN.I         SAU.I         SMA.I         SST.I         SST.II        STU.I
  XBA.I         XHO.I         XMA.I
```

Fig. 10. Restriction map of pBR322/PANACEA cDNA construction.

The day of the intelligent, dedicated molecular biology computer is not far away. As data and knowledge bases grow, the adaptation of general problem-solving programs to specific molecular biology problems will occur. We must actively input expert knowledge to develop machines which can reason through strategies for gene synthesis, cloning, expression vector design, and so on.

SUMMARY

I have tried to describe why the computer is an essential tool for the recombinant DNA scientist. As our data bases grow, we will require information storage and communication systems unlike the paper based record systems with which we currently work. Molecular biological data is being generated so rapidly that I believe electronic data exchange will soon be the only way we will be able to keep each other up to date.

We have seen some specific computer applications which provide assistance to the researcher at the bench. Sequence manipulation, analysis, and display are too difficult for the unaided molecular biologist to accomplish readily. The computer, being able to provide intelligence at speeds unmatchable by humans, will continue to be used as a tool in recombinant DNA research and will rapidly grow to be an essential tool for all scientists.

REFERENCES

1. Abelson, P.H. and M. Dorfman, Eds. Computers and electronics, Science 215:4534, February 12, 1982.
2. Nucleic Acids Research 10 (1), pp. 1-457, January 11, 1982.
3. Douthart, R.J. and F.H. Norris. The MAD sets: Interactive computer programs for the manipulation, analysis and display of DNA sequences. Presented at Second ASM Conference on Genetics and Molecular Biology of Industrial Microorganisms, Bloomington, Indiana (October, 1980).

DISCUSSION

Q. BLOOMFIELD (Minnesota): When you have a number of people sharing the same data base, able to update protocols and that kind of thing, how do you keep - either by by accident or design - people from putting in wrong information and erasing the previous correct protocol?

A. MODELEVSKY: Most systems have designed in them what are called "privileges" and "protections", and one can set the protection on any file to allow reading privileges, writing privileges, executing privileges, deleting privileges, editing privileges, etc. If you have something that is valuable to you and you want to keep control of it so that no mistakes can be added or so you can be the only one to edit that file, it's very easy to accomplish.

Q. H. GINSBERG (University of Minnesota): I have two questions. The first one, do you have any optical scanners set up to read a sequence from a paper, not so much from a gel, but rather an optical scanner that would automatically read the sequences from a piece of paper?

A. MODELEVSKY: First of all, we recently found out that there is a company in Indianapolis that manufactures an optical scanner that will read print. We don't have it yet. The fact is, all of this technology costs a lot of money. It took Dick and Frank a long time to develop these programs, and you have to weigh whether or not it would be worth your while to develop or buy the programs, to buy the hardware, or to send jobs out and have some of the work done for you by the people who do have the equipment. So, the question is still standing, whether we will send out pieces of paper with sequences on them and let someone else use their reader, or not. But the technology exists, and we'll get our hands on it.

Q. GINSBERG: My second question is one that you alluded to without discussing. I'm going to try to make you discuss it. You alluded to the differences between data bases and knowledge bases; knowledge bases being a term from artificial intelligence, especially in regard to types of programs known as expert systems. The most elaborate expert systems to my knowledge that have been constructed for use in molecular biology are the MOLGEN systems, and I say "to my knowledge" because I don't know what is going on at Lilly or elsewhere. The MOLGEN systems which were called GENESIS, GEL, and MAXIMIZE (at least the parts that they published in Nucleic Acid Research), are from Stanford. The technical reports that came out of Stanford, from a computer science standpoint, implied a lot of limitations in terms of the ability of those programs to deal with some of the more complex problems in planning; essentially, here's the problem, give me the cloning protocol. Do you see that these problems will be surmountable in the future?

A. MODELEVSKY: First of all, we have examined that system and we do not have it at Lilly. Secondly, I do not see a great deal of intelligence in the system to which you just referred. Artificial intelligence in the field of recombinant DNA research must be developed. There are general problem-solving routines which may be adapted as specific molecular biological problem-solving routines. For example, you may tell the computer to begin at point A and ask how to get to point Z; you let the computer filter through a maze of intelligent options, each option having a specified point value. A tally of points is kept for each attempted pathway through the maze, and the computer determines which pathway is the cheapest to follow. All of the options must be programmed in. I am not aware of any molecular biology system that is working like that. That's something we would like to develop at Lilly.

The most intelligent program of which I am aware is one called "Doctor" by Joseph Weisenbaum. It's an artificial intelligence program which was designed to simulate a psychiatrist. As I understand it, you tell the computer what's bothering you and it makes you feel better. I was told that it got to the point where an attempt was made to introduce this kind of program to the hospitals throughout the country so that people could have a psychiatrist to talk to for nothing! Another program called "Perry", developed by Kenneth Mark Colbey, was designed to simulate a paranoid schizophrenic's behavior. At one computer meeting, they had two such machines talking to each other!

Q. STARLINGER: When we hired post-docs 10 or 15 years ago, it took about three weeks until they received their first salaries; they were mad, and rightly so. If we hire a post-doc today, it takes about 4 months until he gets his first salary and he cannot even try to get mad because the administration simply says, "Well, you know, everything is on computer now and you must understand that it takes longer." So, what I would like to know is, has anybody tried to really work out the time economics of using computers for something like, let's say, having protocols in the computer that are displayed on the screen? Obviously, once everything is set up, you just push a button and you get the result. But somebody has to initially take time to set up the program and my question is, has anybody seriously investigated whether any time was really saved, taking into account the time that the graduate student, for example, needs to master the system?

A. MODELEVSKY: That's a very good point. First of all, the time that it takes for the calculation of the program to run is very often dependent on a couple of things. First of all, how well the program was written. Good programmers can take a lot of short-cuts and save a lot of time. That's a problem that we've seen in programs that people are attempting to sell on the market that are developed in DNA laboratories; they are programmed by a graduate student or by the scientist who gets a personal computer or something like that. There are programming problems, and a lot of time is lost just because the expertise in programming might not be there. The other thing is the machine you use. We are using a VAX 11/780. This machine is very fast. We have a molecular modeling system at Lilly, as well, that's on the same computer and it absorbs an enormous amount of processing time. Even with that system going and supporting half a dozen to a dozen users, the system is still incredibly fast. The slowness comes in with the design of the machine. The problem of learning to use the system should be very short if the programs are written in a very "friendly" fashion, such that the molecular biologist can understand it and all of the manipulations that the machine is going to do. He can then sit down at the keyboard and "speak his own vernacular". If the programs are designed in this manner, no formal introduction to the computer is needed.

Q. BUXTON (Minnesota): Has there been any attempt to centralize information to put it on-line, like MED-LAR or anything like that?

A. MODELEVSKY: Yes, there are a number of networks that are developing. For example, there is a sequence bank in Europe called the "European Molecular Biology Organization". Margaret Dayhoff has an extensive data base into which we can tap and the network that MOLGEN or INTELLIGENETICS offers has some information as well. There are others, and again, you've got to realize that not everybody is going to share every sequence that is put into the system. While you may get into a network, you may or may not be able to get all of the sequences.

Q. BUXTON: What about public sequences, more specifically?

A. MODELEVSKY: There are a number of sequence repositories, but networks linking these computers have to be developed to allow easy access to the information contained in these repositories. We have sequence data bases at Lilly. Lots of people have sequence information on disks or tape, but not all of this information is compatible from system to system. I do know that such networks are developing and Indianapolis may be the first city to have such a network.

C. J. MESSING (Minnesota): One problem with such network systems is, of course, time sharing. The more users you have, the more difficult it is to get on line. We had a bad experience in using the Stanford program, for example, because it's always backed up and more users are getting into the system. Therefore I think one important concern in the application of computers for recombinant DNA is certainly the costs. What about the prices, the interchangeability of software, and compatibility? A very important concern is that some of the items now developed for a few privileged laboratories become more generally available to university laboratories as well as industrial laboratories.

A. MODELEVSKY: We want to update our entire system at Lilly. Each electronic station is going to cost about $2,000 per laboratory. There will be a terminal with a keyboard, a telephone coupler, and perhaps a printer. We already have a central processor. Manufacturers have lines of computer models that, much like the automobile industry, are available with a variety of features so that, for a few thousand dollars, a workable set- up can be purchased to accommodate the work of the molecular biologist. A laboratory could conceivably save one human-year per year for each computer installed.

HUMAN IMMUNE INTERFERON (IFN-γ)

GENE SEQUENCE AND STRUCTURE

Patrick W. Gray and David V. Goeddel

Department of Molecular Biology
Genentech, Inc.
460 Point San Bruno Boulevard
South San Francisco, California 94080

ABSTRACT

Human IFN-γ is encoded by a single gene which, in contrast to the IFN-α and IFN-β genes, contains three introns. This gene has been isolated from a recombinant human-λ gene library, and the entire gene and 5' and 3' flanking regions have been sequenced. Southern hybridizations failed to show any polymorphism of the gene or its flanking regions. The first intron contains a repetitive element which is unrelated to the Alu family repeat.

INTRODUCTION

Interferons (IFNs) are proteins which induce an antiviral state in target cells [1]. Three classes of human interferon have been distinguished on the basis of antigenic, biological, and biochemical properties [2]. IFN-α (leukocyte IFN) and IFN-β (fibroblast IFN) are proteins which are stable to treatment with acid (pH 2), detergent (0.1 percent SDS), and heat [1]. IFN-γ (immune IFN) is labile to these treatments but insensitive to reducing agents such as β-mercaptoethanol [10,20,36,54,58,62]. IFN-α and IFN-β are rapidly induced within 1-8 hours following treatment with virus (IFN-α and IFN-β) or synthetic polynucleotides (IFN-β) [1]. Alternatively, IFN-γ is more slowly induced (12-24 hours) in T-lymphocytes by treatment with mitogens [10,20,36,54,58,62].

DNA sequence determination of cloned cDNAs and genes has revealed more than a dozen members of the human IFN-α gene family [15,17,22,25,29,32,46,55]. These genes code for mature polypeptides of 165 or 166 amino acids which differ from each other in about 10 to 25 percent of their residues. Similar analyses have demonstrated the existence of a single gene for IFN-β [9,10,17,18,24,26,39,53] coding for a mature protein of 166 amino acids and having about 25 percent amino acid homology to the IFN-α [52]. The genes for human IFN-α and IFN-β are found on chromosome 9 [40] and do not contain any introns [9,24,26,35,39,60].

We recently reported the isolation, sequence, and heterologous expression of a cloned cDNA for human IFN-γ [20]. This cDNA codes for a protein of 166 amino acids, the first 20 of which comprise a signal sequence. The polypeptide produced by expression of this DNA sequence in _E. coli_ or cultured monkey cells had characteristic properties of authentic human IFN-γ. A single human gene was observed in Southern hybridizations of human genomic DNA using IFN-γ cDNA as a probe. This gene has been localized to human chromosome 12 [37]. We report here the isolation and DNA structure of the human IFN-γ gene.

Materials and Methods

IFN-γ Gene Isolation. The human IFN-γ gene was isolated from the recombinant human-λ library described by Lawn *et al* [27]. Approximately 10^6 phage were plated on ten 15-cm plates and screened by the method of Maniatis *et al*. [31] with $3x10^7$ cpm of ^{32}P-labelled [55] cDNA probe (the 887 bp *Sau*3A fragment described in ref. 8). Hybridizing plaques were subjected to another round of plaque purification [31]. Individual plaques were isolated and phage DNA was prepared [14,31] from 500 ml cultures. Each phage DNA was mapped with *Eco*RI, *Bam*HI, *Hind*III, *Kpn*I, and *Xba*I (New England Biolabs) by analysis of 1.0 percent agarose gel electrophoresis. Gels were blotted onto nitrocellulose [48] and hybridized with the ^{32}P-labelled IFN-γ cDNA probe to determine which bands contained IFN-γ sequences. The sizes of fragments were determined by comparison with *Hind*III digested λ molecular weight standards. The 8.6 kbp *Bam*HI fragment of λG9 was isolated by electrophoresis through 1.0 percent agarose, electroeluted, and ligated into the *Bam*HI site of pBR322 [3]. Recombinant clones were identified by sensitivity to tetracycline and one, pB9KB-1, was mapped extensively with restriction endonucleases.

DNA Sequence Determination. The entire IFN-γ gene sequence was determined by a combination of the chemical degradation technique of Maxam and Gilbert [33] and the dideoxy chain termination method of Sanger and colleagues [47]. Synthetic single stranded DNA primers, synthesized by the modified solid phase phosphotriester method [7], were utilized for dideoxy sequencing. The sequences of the primers were designed from the cDNA sequence [20]: dCTCTCGGAAACG (found at nucleotides 97-109 of the cDNA), dGGTCATTCAGATG (229-241 of the cDNA), dAATGCAGAGCCAA (309-321 of the cDNA), and dCGAAAAGCTGACT (453-465 of the cDNA). The reverse complements of the above primers were also utilized for sequencing in the 3' to 5' direction. Two other synthetic DNA primers, in addition to the M13 lac primer [34], were also used: dCTGCCAGGACCCA (174-186 of the cDNA) and dAAATATT-GCAGGC (complementary to 620-632 of the cDNA). The templates for dideoxy sequencing were four restriction fragments (*Hpa*I-*Hind*III,

HindIII-PvuII, PvuII-EcoRI, and PstI-HincII) which were subcloned in both orientations of the M13 vector mp7 [34].

Hybridization Analysis. Human genomic lymphocyte DNA was isolated by the method of Blin and Stafford [2]. DNA was separated on 1.0 percent agarose gels and transferred to nitrocellulose (Scheicher and Schuell) by the method of Southern [48]. ^{32}P-labelled probes were prepared by the calf thymus primer method [55] from restriction fragments isolated from 5 percent acrylamide gels. The hybridization solution [14] was 50 percent formamide, 5X SSC, 0.05 M sodium phosphate pH 6.5, 5X Denhardt's solution, 0.1 mg/ml sonicated salmon sperm DNA, 10 percent dextran sulfate, and 10^6 to 10^7 cpm of heat-denatured probe. Blots were prehybridized for 2 hours at 42°C without probe or dextran sulfate prior to overnight incubation. Approximately 20 ml hybridization solution was used per blot. Blots were washed twice in 0.2X SSC, 0.1 percent SDS for 30 minutes at 50°C (approximately 500 ml per blot per wash). Blots were then rinsed in approximately 200 ml 2X SSC, dried, and exposed to X-ray film with intensifying screens at -70°C. The Alu family repeat probe was prepared from a 300 bp BamHI fragment of pBLUR8 (kindly provided by C. Houck and R. Lawn) which contains Alu family repeat DNA [45].

RESULTS

A Single IFN-γ Gene. In order to estimate the number of IFN-γ genes in the human genome, human lymphocyte DNA was digested with various restriction endonucleases, electrophoresed through agarose gels, transferred to nitroculluloser [48], and hybridized to a ^{32}P-labelled probe isolated from the coding region of IFN-γ cDNA (Fig. 1). HincII was the only endonuclease used which cleaves the IFN-γ cDNA sequence, but this HincII site cleaves outside of the DNA fragment used as a probe. A unique gene without introns would have appeared as a single hybridizing band in each lane of the Southern blot. Instead, two hybridizing bands were observed in the PvuII,

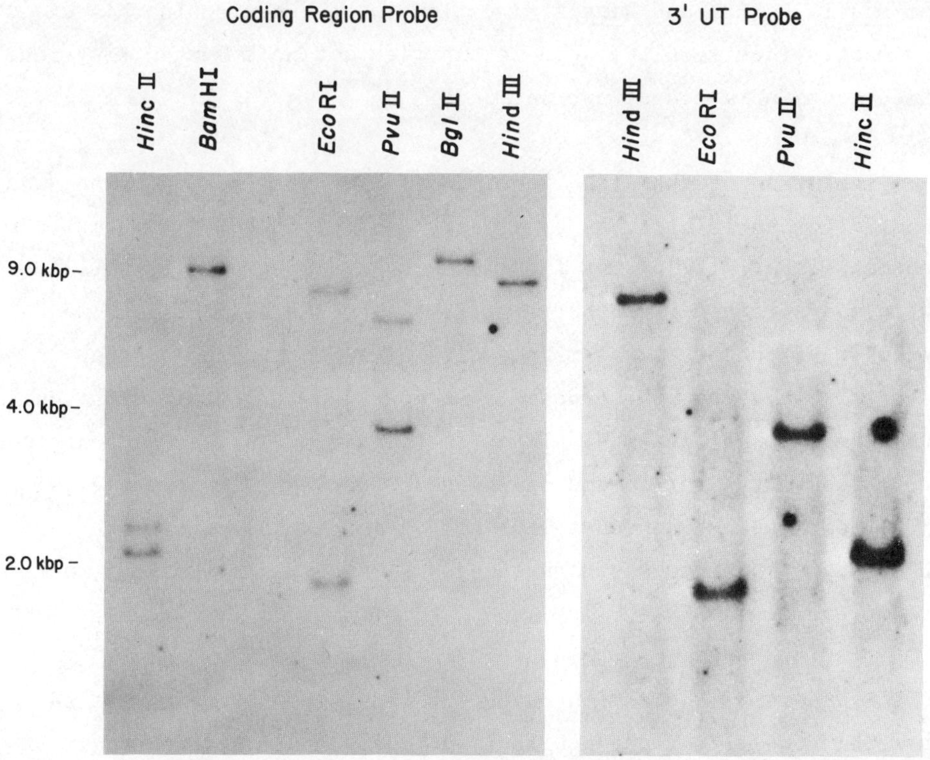

Fig. 1. Southern hybridization of human genomic DNA with two different IFN-γ cDNA probes. On the left, a coding region probe (594 bp DdeI fragment, ref. 20) hybridizes with two bands in the PvuII, EcoRI, and HincII digestions. On the right, a probe from the 3' untranslated region (120 bp DdeI fragment, ref. 20) hybridizes with single bands in the PvuII, EcoRI, and HincII digestions.

EcoRI, and HincII digested DNAs and single bands were observed for the other digestions (HindIII, BglII, and BamHI). These results could be due to two homologous and closely linked IFN-γ genes (which are separated by PvuII, EcoRI, and HincII sites), or these results may be explained by a single IFN-γ gene which contains one or more more introns with internal PvuII, EcoRI, and HincII sites. As shown in Fig. 1, the latter possibility was supported by repeating the hybridizations with a ^{32}P-labelled probe prepared from the 3' untranslated region of IFN-γ cDNA. Only single hybridizing bands in the PvuII, EcoRI, and HincII digestions were observed in this experiment. This result is consistent with a single human IFN-γ gene which contains at least one intron.

Isolation of the IFN-γ Gene. An IFN-γ specific cDNA probe was used to screen 10^6 plaques of a bacteriophage λ Charon 4A/human genomic library [27]. Six individual hybridizing plaques were isolated and purified from the library. As presented in Fig. 2, each recombinant phage DNA was mapped with five restriction endonucleases. Only two of the phage DNAs appeared to contain identical human genomic DNA inserts. Three of the human DNA inserts contained sequences to the far 5' end of the gene, while a single phage DNA (λG5) contained sequences to the far 3' end of the gene. The insert DNAs span a contiguous region of 33.5 kilobasepairs (kbp) of the human genome.

Southern hybridizations with the IFN-γ cDNA probe suggested that only two of the phage DNAs (λG9, γG10) contained the entire IFN-γ gene, as illustrated in Fig. 2. The IFN-γ cDNA probe hybridized specifically to an 8.6 kbp BamHI fragment. This fragment was electrophoretically isolated from λG9 on a 1.0 percent agarose gel, electroeluted, and ligated into the BamHI site of pBR322 [3]. One of the resultant recombinants, pB9KB-1, was extensively mapped with restriction endonucleases to facilitate DNA sequence analysis.

Sequence Analysis of the IFN-γ Gene. The entire IFN-γ gene was sequenced by a combination of the chemical degradation technique of Maxam and Gilbert [33] and the dideoxy chain termination method of Sanger and colleagues [47] after subcloning fragments into the M13 vector mp7 [34]. Nearly 6,000 contiguous base pairs of the IFN-γ gene region were determined by sequencing the majority of both strands and are presented in Fig. 3. The IFN-γ cDNA sequence previously determined [20] was aligned with the gene sequence and matches completely except for a single base pair transition (4712 of

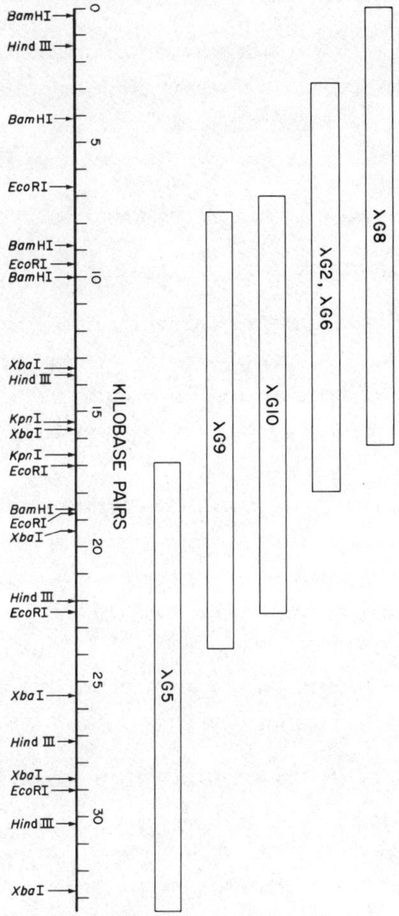

Fig. 2. Restriction endonuclease map of the human IFN-γ gene region. The limits of each phage DNA insert are shown above. Positions of EcoRI, BamHI, HindIII, KpnI, and XbaI sites were determined by digestions of the inidividual phage DNAs. The BamHI sites used in subcloning are positioned at 10.0 and 18.6 kbp. The orientation of the map is 5' → 3' (left to right).

Fig. 3; postion 588 of ref. 20) which changes the glutamine codon found at position 140 in the cDNA sequence to an arginine. We have subsequently sequenced five additional IFN-γ cDNAs which all contained arginine codons at this position [12]. This single nucleotide difference may be due to a transcription error during in vitro

```
                                       HincII
1    AGCAAATGATCAATGTGCTTTGTGAATGAAGAGTCAACATTTTACCAGGGCGAAGTGGGGAGGTACAAAAAAATTTCCAGTCCTTGAATGGTGTGAAGTA
101  AAAGTGCCTCAAAGAATCCCACCAGAATGGCACAGGTGGGCATAATGGGTCTGTCTCATCGTCAAAGGACCCAAGGAGTCTAAAGGAAACTCTAACTACA
201  ACACCCAAATGCCACAAAACCTTAGTTATTAATACAAACTATCATCCCTGCCTATCTGTCACCATCTCATCTTAAAAAACTTGTGAAAATACGTAATCCT
     MstII                                         *
301  CAGGAGACTTCAATTAGGTATAAATACCAGCAGCCAGAGGAGGTGCAGCACATTGTTCTGATCATCTGAAGATCAGCTATTAGAAGAGAAAGATCAGTTA

                                                                                   Met Lys Tyr Thr Ser Tyr
401  AGTCCTTTGGACCTGATCAGCTTGATACAAGAACTACTGATTTCAACTTCTTTGGCTTAATTCTCTCGGAAACG    ATG AAA TAT ACA AGT TAT

     Ile Leu Ala Phe Gln Leu Cys Ile Val Leu Gly Ser Leu Gly Cys Tyr Cys Gln Asp Pro Tyr Val Lys Glu Ala
493  ATC TTG GCT TTT CAG CTC TGC ATC GTT TTG GGT TCT CTT GGC TGT TAC TGC CAG GAC CCA TAT GTA AAA GAA GCA

     Glu Asn Leu Lys Lys Tyr Phe
568  GAA AAC CTT AAG AAA TAT TTT  GTAAGTATGACTTTTTAATAGTACTTGTTTGTGGTTGAAAATGACTGAATATCGACTTGCTGTAGCATCTC
                                                                                                  XbaI
660  TGATAGGCTGTCATCTCTTGTAGGCAGTCATTTTGAGATTTGGTGTTATTTTGTTAATTATTGACTAGATGAGTTCCTTGACTAAATAATCTAGATATTG
760  TTTTAACCTTCTGCTCAGTTTGTATAGAGACTTAAAAGGGATTTATGAATTTTCCAAAAGATGGGCATAATATGGGTATGAAGCATAATGATGTTAATAA
860  TTTTGTGGTGGGAACTCATTCAGTTGTGATAGTCAAGGAGTATGCAGATTGAAAAAAATGATTGGTTATTAGTTTTTGACTTCTCAGACTCTAAGGTCAA
                                                                       HindIII
960  GATTAGCATTAAAAAGGTAATAGGAAATGTTTACAAATTAAAGTCAAAAAGGTCCTTAAAGCTTTGGCTTAAAAAAATAACTGATAGGTGATTTTCTCCA
                                                                HpaII
1060 AAAAGTGATTTCAACATTCTGCTTCTCTATCTATATTACTTGTGAAGTATTCCGGAACTTCGTTGCTCACTGGGATTTTGGAAGAATTATGATTCTGGCT
1160 AAGGAATGTTTAAAAATTTTAAGTGAATTTTTTGAGTTTCTTTTAAAATTTTATTGATGGTTAATGAAAAGTTTTTACATTTTAAATATTTCATTATTTG
1260 TTTAAAACTTAGCTGTTATAATTATAGCTGTCATAATAATATTCAGACATTCACAATTGATTTTATTCTTACAACACAAAATCAAATCTCACACACACAC
1360 ACACACACACACACTCGCACATGTTTGGAACTATCTTTTAAAGCTCGTATAATAATACCCTACAGGAAGGCACAGTAGATGTAATAGAAACCTGTACCAT
1460 TGGGGGGCAGTATTTTATAGTGGGGTGGCTTTGCTGTTTTTTGTTTTTGTATTTTTTAGCCTAGCTTGAAAATACTTTCTTTAGCTTACTATAGTTTTTG
                                  SacI
1560 GGACCTTTGGAGTATCAGCTTTGTTGAGCTCATTTGTGACATTGCAATTTAATGGTTATATTGGGAAATAAAAAAGCTAAAAGAACATAATAGTCTTTGT
1660 CTATATCTCACATAAGCCTTTTGGGAATACTTATTGTTAGAACTAAGCAGAAGAGTTGAAAAGGAAATCAGTGAATATTGTCACATCTGAGTTCAATGAA

                                                                         Asn Ala Gly His Ser Asp Val Ala
1760 ACTTGAAATATATTTTTAAGGCAATTTATGGGCTAATTGTAAACCAATTTTTTCTTTTTTTTTTTTAG AAT GCA GGT CAT TCA GAT GTA GCG

     Asp Asn Gly Thr Leu Phe Leu Gly Ile Leu Lys Asn Trp Lys Glu
1852 GAT AAT GGA ACT CTT TTC TTA GGC ATT TTG AAG AAT TGG AAA GAG  GTAAGCTGAATATTCCCATTTGGCTAATTTTCCTGTTGC

                                                          Glu Ser Asp Arg Lys Ile Met Gln Ser Gln Ile
1936 TTGCTTTCTGATGGATAAATTCACATCATCCTCTGTTTGTGCTCTTTCCTTCCAAG GAG AGT GAC AGA AAA ATA ATG CAG AGC CAA ATT

     Val Ser Phe Tyr Phe Lys Leu Phe Lys Asn Phe Lys Asp Asp Gln Ser Ile Gln Lys Ser Val Glu Thr Ile Lys
2025 GTC TCC TTT TAC TTC AAA CTT TTT AAA AAC TTT AAA GAT GAC CAG AGC ATC CAA AAG AGT GTG GAG ACC ATC AAG

2100 Glu Asp Met Asn Val Lys Phe Phe Asn Ser Asn Lys Lys Lys Arg Asp Asp Phe Glu Lys Leu Thr Asn Tyr Ser
     GAA GAC ATG AAT GTC AAG TTT TTC AAT AGC AAC AAA AAG AAA CGA GAT GAC TTC GAA AAG CTG ACT AAT TAT TCG
                                                                            AccI
2175 GTGAGGCTATTTAAATTCTTTCTTTGGTTTCATTGCCGAGGGTCTTGCAAAGCATTTATTCTCCAGAAAGTAGACATTAGCTATTTAACAGTTGCTAAAG
2275 CTATGAACTCAACTCATGGCTGAAACTCTACCTTACTATTTCCATTCGTGTTTGGGTGACTTTGCAAAGCCAGTAAGAGAATCGCTGAAGTATGTAATGT
                                          HincII
2375 AGAGAAATGCTGGCATTGTAACTATTGCGTAAAGACAGGTGAGTTGACAAATTCCAGTGAAGAGGAAGTAGGTGAGGAAGAAGCAGGGAGTACTGAGAAG
2475 CAGTTCTCTCATTGTCCCTTGCTCATATGATGGAAATTCTCTTACTTTGAATGAGAGGCTGTCTGTCTTAATGGAAAGAGCAGTGGGAGGAGCTGAGAAG
2575 ATGTGTGTTCTCCTCCCAACTCAGCCACCAAGGAACTGTGATGAATCACATGGCTGGCTGGGCTCAGTTTCCTCATCTTAAAAGGAAACTGTTAGGTTCA
                                                                                                    KpnI
2675 CTGTATAAGTTTGATGACCTTCTTTGCTCCAAAACTCTACAATGCAAAGAATAGAAAATGAGAATGAGATAGAAGAAAGCTACAGTCTTTGAATAGGTAC
2775 CAGGGACACCCCACTGCAAGTCTCTAGCCAACCTATCAGATTGTACTGCCCAATTAGAAGCAAGAATGGTTGCTGTTTGTTTGTTTTTAGGGAAAAATAG
```

Fig. 3. Human IFN-γ gene sequence. Only the sense strand is presented. Coding sequences have been translated and the start of RNA transcription is marked with an asterisk as is the position of polyadenylation. The CCAAT box ($GG^{C}_{T}CAATCT$ consensus sequence, 1), Goldberg-Hogness box

```
                                                                           PvuII
2875 ATAGAATTTATACCTTATGAAAAGATTGTTCTATCAACTCTCTATCAACTTTCAGAATATCTCAGCTGGAGAACTCCTTAGACTCCTAAGTCTTACCTCA
                                                                                               XbaI
2975 TGAACTTGTATCTTTAAGTTATGGCTTCTATAAACAGAAAGATAACGTTGAGGCATAAAGACAAATCATGTTTTTCAGAATGTTTTCTAGAAGACAAAGG
       XbaI        HincII
3075 CCTCTAGATTCCTTTGGGGTTGACTTTGATATAAATGGGCTCAAATGAGAGGGACCAGGGTCTTCAAGCTAGCATTTGTGTTCTTAGGATATGTGCTCAG

3175 CTTTCACTATTGCTGGGCCTGCCTCTCACTCCTCTCATGTAAGCCCCCAGAAACAGAAAGGAGAGACATGGCAACAGGTCTCCTTTGGTTATAAACTAGA

3275 CACTCAGCACTTGTTTCTAATCCAGTGGTGCCCCTGGCTTACTGTTCAGTCCTGGATAAGTCTCTTAGTTTCTTGGTGATGATTTGAACATTGGAAAGTA
                                                  PstI
3375 AAATCTGTCACTTGCAAACACACAGCTTGTCGAAAATTTTTTCTACTCTGCAGGAACTGGGCCTTAAAAAAATGAAAAAAAATCTGTGGTTTCTTCCTTC
                                             SacI
3475 TGGAAGCTACAAACCTCCTGTTTCTTGATGGGCAATCTTGAGTGAGCTCTATTAATTATTATTCTCTTTGGCTCAGTTGCTAAGCTATTTTATGCATGTT

3575 ATGCCCTTTGACAATTAGTCTTTAGCTGTAATCCCCCAGCCATCCTCAGAAATGTGGTGAGGTAGCCATAGTGTTCCCAAGATTAGAAAAATGTAATGGC

3675 AGAGCCAAGAGGAAGGTAAATGGTCCACATCTTATGAAGCATCATCTAAATGGCCCTATTGGTTAGAGTGAGGAGATGCAAGTAGTTCAATTTGCTTGCC
     BglI
3775 TAGAAGGCAGGGTACTGGAAAAGTTGTTGCAATTCTTAATTTTAAACTTTATATATCAGTAAGCCATATATAAATATGATTGGGGGTGTTTATTTTAAAA
                                                                                                 KpnI
3875 TCTATTATGGAAATTGAGAGACTGACCTAATCTGGGAGAAATTAAAAATTACAGTTTTCACTCGTTTTGGATTTGGTGTTTTCTAGGGTACCTAACCTAG

3975 ATCAGTGGTTCTCAAACTTAGGTGGATGTCAGAATCACCTGGGGAGCTTAGTGAATGCACAGGGCACAGTCCTTCCACTTCATGCACCTGGATCTCTGAG
                   HpaII
4075 GTCTTTGACAGGTTTCCGGATTAATCTGCTATGCACAACAGTGAGAATCATTGACCTATAGTTACTCATTTGATGCATACAGGAAAGACTGAAGTATAAA

4175 GTGATATAATTGGTAGATTGATGATAGAGAGGTCATAGAAACAGTCTCATCCTCCTTTAGATGAGAAAATAGAAGTTCAGAGAGGTTAAGTAGCTGGCTC
                                                                                                  EcoRI
4275 AAGGTCAGAATTATTGCATGCATGAGATTCAAACCCACCTTTTTATGCTGACTCCACAACCAGGAGTCTTTTCACTATATAATTTCAAGAATTCTATAGA

4375 AGTAGATTTAAAGATATGTGATGGACTCCACCACATTATAGCACAACTAGAAATGTAATTGTAATTTTTAGCTTCAACTGCTGAAGAAGTAAATATTGTA

4475 TATTAAGGTAATACGGTCCATTTTTTAAAGGAATACTTTTATTTTCACTGACCATCATGACATTAGCAGAATATCCTGATGGCTTATATGCCTGAAATTA

                                Val Thr Asp Leu Asn Val Gln Arg Lys Ala Ile His Glu Leu Ile Gln Val Met
4575 ATTTGCTCTTTTCTTTCCCGATAG   GTA ACT GAC TTG AAT GTC CAA CGC AAA GCA ATA CAT GAA CTC ATC CAA GTG ATG

     Ala Glu Leu Ser Pro Ala Ala Lys Thr Gly Lys Arg Lys Arg Ser Gln Met Leu Phe Arg Gly Arg Arg Ala Ser
4654 GCT GAA CTG TCG CCA GCA GCT AAA ACA GGG AAG CGA AAA AGG AGT CAG ATG CTG TTT CGA GGT CGA AGA GCA TCC

     Gln STOP
4729 CAG TAA  TGGTTGTCCTGCCTGCAATATTTGAATTTTAAATCTAAATCTATTTATTAATATTTAACATTATTTATATGGGGAATATATTTTTAGACTC

4826 ATCAATCAAATAAGTATTTATAATAGCAACTTTTGTGTAATGAAAATGAATATCTATTAATATATGTATTATTTATAATTCCTATATCCTGTGACTGTCT
                                                                            BglI
4926 CACTTAATCCTTTGTTTTCTGACTAATTAGGCAAGGCTATGTGATTACAAGGCTTTATCTCAGGGGCCAACTAGGCAGCCAACCTAAGCAAGATCCCATG
                                                                                HpaII
5026 GGTTGTGTGTTTATTTCACTTGATGATACAATGAACACTTATAAGTGAAGTGATACTATCCAGTTACTGCCGGTTTGAAAATATGCCTGCAATCTGAGCC

5126 AGTGCTTTAATGGCATGTCAGACAGAACTTGAATGTGTCAGGTGACCCTGATGAAAACATAGCATCTCAGGAGATTTCATGCCTGGTGCTTCCAAATATT
     HincII                                                                                       *
5226 GTTGACAACTGTGACTGTACCCAAATGGAAAGTAACTCATTTGTTAAAATTATCAATATCTAATATATATGAATAAAGTGTAAGTTCACAACTACTTATG

5326 CTGTGTTGGACTTTTTCTAAGTGAGACCTGGAGTGAAAGAACTACCTATTAATGAATTAGTAGGGAGGGGAGTCTTCTTAGCTGTGAAAATTTTAGAGTT

5426 GCATTTGGTTCCATTAAATGTGGTATTTCTTTCCACTAGCATTTTGTTGGCTTTCGCTTTTCCAGTTAGCAGCTCTTTGAATTATCTTTCTAAGATACAG

5526 ATTTAATTATGTCACTATTCAATTCAGAGGTTCTGCTATGGAATGTAGTTTAAACTGCTTAGCTTGGCACACAGAGATTTATTTCTAGCCCCTTCTCCAC

5626 CTTCCTATTTCCTCCTTCGTTTCAGAATCTTCCTCTCCCTCATCCAATGCTGGCAAACACCAGTGGGGGTGGAGTAGTGGGTGTAAGCTCTAGGGAGAAG

5726 GCTTGGATTGGAATCCAAGTTATTCCATTACAAGTAGTGTGACCTTTAATACATTATGTATATTGTCTAAGTTTCAGCTTTATTGTCTGAAAAAGAAAAA
                                                                                                  AccI
5826 TAATTGTGTGTTCCTCATAATATTGTGGTACGAATTGATTCTTTCACTCAAGAAATATTTACTGGAGTACCTACTACATGCCTGGTGCTGTTGTAGACCT
                                   BamHI
5926 TGAGATACCTTACTCAAGCAAAACAGCCAAGGATCC(5961)
```

[15,41], and polyadenylation recognition sequence (ATAAAA)[42] have been underlined. Also presented are cleavage positions of common restriction endonucleases which recognize hexameric sequences and HpaII sites.

cDNA synthesis; alternatively, the originally isolated cDNA may be an allelic variant of this gene and the other sequenced cDNAs.

There are clearly three introns in the coding region of the gene. The introns are quite variable in length: intron 1 is 1238 bp, intron 2 is 95 bp, and intron 3 is 2422 bp. The four exons are less variable, coding for 38, 23, 61, and 44 amino acids, respectively. This arrangement is depicted schematically in Fig. 4A. Each intron interrupts the reading frame precisely between codons. Although the first and third introns are quite large, they have a relatively small coding potential due to a large number of stop codons in all phases. Only two proteins larger than 50 amino acids could be encoded by these introns (73 amino acids in intron 1 and 62 amino acids in intron 3).

Southern Analysis of the IFN-γ Gene. As shown in Fig. 1, the IFN-γ cDNA hybridizes with unique, single copy DNA. To determine if introns or adjacent flanking regions of the IFN-γ gene contain repetitive DNA sequences, probes were prepared from individual regions of the gene used for the hybridization with Southern blots of human genomic DNA. All but one of five probes hybridized to unique human DNA fragments, as shown in Fig. 4. The sizes of the hybridizing fragments correspond to the lengths predicted from the map derived from the phage DNAs (Fig. 2). The first intron contains DNA which hybridizes to DNA throughout the blot, characteristic of repetitive sequences. This same probe was also hybridized with a Southern blot of the five different IFN-γ phage DNAs to determine if this repetitive element was present in the mapped 33.5 kbp IFN-γ gene region. As shown in Fig. 5, hybridization was observed only to DNA fragments containing the first intron, suggesting only a single copy of this repetitive element in the IFN-γ gene region.

The human genome contains more than 300,000 copies of a family of related sequences termed *Alu* sequences [23] which are about 300

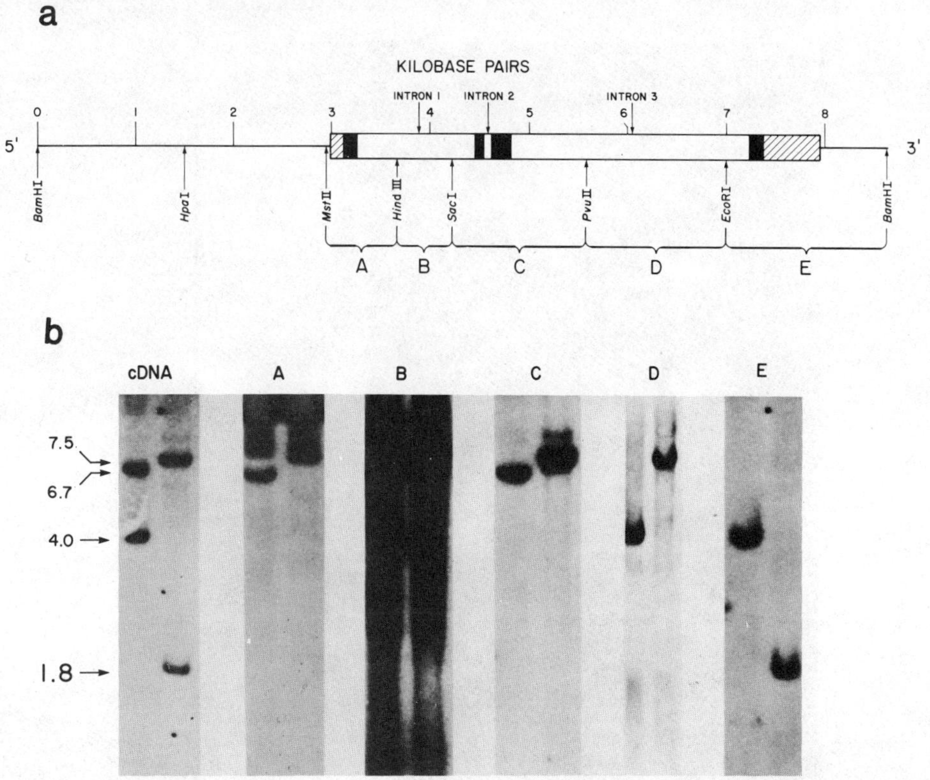

Fig. 4. The IFN-γ gene region contains a repetitive element in the first intron. The cloned IFN-γ gene was fragmented with the restriction endonucleases shown below and ^{32}P-labelled probes were prepared from regions A to E. Four of the probes hybridize to unique copy DNA, while the B probe hybridizes throughout the blot. The 5' and 3' untranslated regions of the IFN-γ gene are shown as cross-hatched boxes, while coding regions of exons are presented as solid boxes.

base pairs long and for which no known function has been demonstrated, although these sequences have homology with viral DNA replication origins. Comparison of the IFN-γ gene sequence (Fig. 3) with the Alu family repeat consensus sequence [45] failed to show significant homology. Furthermore, an Alu family repeat probe (BLUR8, ref. 45) failed to hybridize with DNA fragments containing

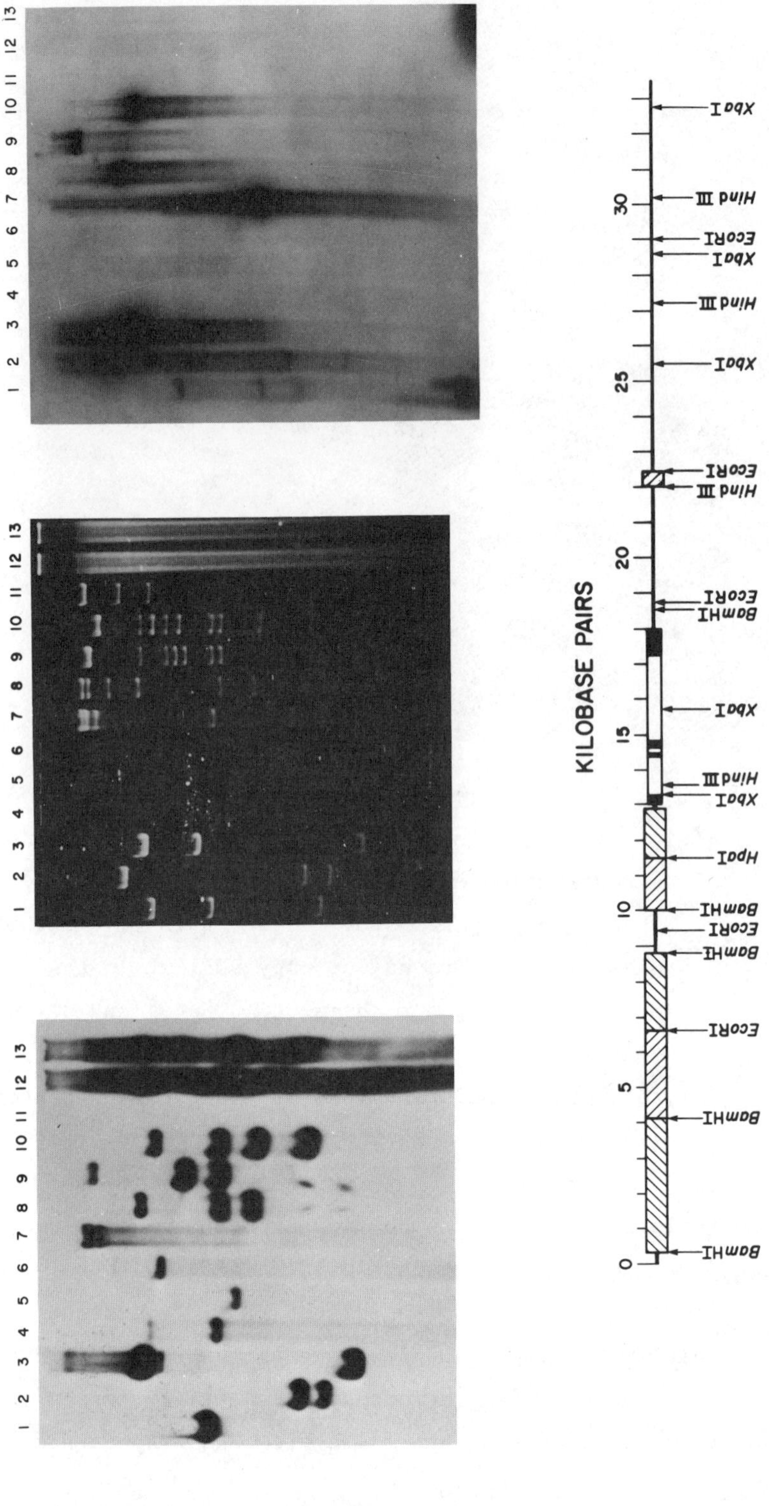
KILOBASE PAIRS
0
5
10
15
20
25
30
BamHI
BamHI
EcoRI
BamHI
EcoRI
BamHI
HpaI
XbaI
HindIII
XbaI
BamHI
EcoRI
HindIII
EcoRI
XbaI
HindIII
XbaI
EcoRI
HindIII
XbaI

Fig. 5. Hybridization of repeated DNA to the IFN-γ gene region. The ^{32}P-labelled Alu family repeat probe was prepared from a 300 bp fragment of pBLUR8 and hybridized to a blot of the gel shown in the center (Southern results presented to the left). The ^{32}P-labelled intron 1 probe (B of Figure 4) was hybridized to a blot of an identical gel and the results are presented to the right. Lane 1, HindIII + SacI digest of pB9KB-1; 2, HindIII + HpaI digest of pB9KB-1; 3, BamHI + HpaI digest of pB9KB-1; 4, EcoRI digest of λG5; 5, XbaI + HindIII digest of λG5; 6, XbaI digest of λG5; 7, XbaI digest of λG9; 8, EcoRI digest of λG6; 9, BamHI digest of λG8; 10, EcoRI + BamHI digest of λG8; 11, HindIII digest of λDNA (size markers); 12, PvuII digest of human genomic DNA; 13, EcoRI digest of human genomic DNA. Mapping of the six different hybridizing signals (cross-hatched) of the Alu family repeat is presented above. The IFN-γ gene region is shown as a smaller box with solid bars for exons and open bars for introns.

the first intron, as shown in Fig. 5. This probe did hybridize with six different regions of the 33.5 kbp IFN-γ gene region. Five hybridizing regions are "clustered" in 13 kbp upstream from the start of the IFN-γ gene. Such a clustering of Alu family repeats has been observed in other human DNA regions [6]. IFN-α genomic clones also contain Alu family repeats [28].

We previously have sequenced six different IFN-γ cDNA clones [12,20] from four different individuals and observed only a single nucleotide variation. This suggests that the mRNA sequence of IFN-γ may be relatively consistent throughout individuals. To determine if the IFNγ gene sequence is conserved in a broader segment of the human population, a limited search for restriction fragment length polymorphisms was undertaken. Genomic DNA was isolated from lymphocytes of nine different individuals of various ethnic backgrounds, cleaved with a series of restriction endonucleases, and analyzed by Southern blotting using the IFN-γ cDNA probe. As shown in Fig. 6, no detectable differences in mobility of hybridizing fragments were seen when the DNA was digested with PvuII, HincII, or XbaI. Similar results were observed when the DNA was digested with PstI, HinfI, EcoRI, or RsaI (data not shown). These results suggest that the IFN-γ gene and surrounding DNA sequences are relatively conserved.

Methylation of the IFN-γ Gene. Many genes which are actively transcribed appear to be less methylated or methylated at different positions than when they are dormant (reviewed in refs. 13 and 43). In animals, the site of methylation is usually the cytosine residue of the sequence CpG [37]. The nucleases HpaII and MspI, which recognize the sequence CCGG, are useful analytical tools for such studies [57]. HpaII will cleave this sequence only if the internal C is not methylated, whereas MspI cleaves whether the internal C is methylated or not. Differences in methylation patterns between active and inactive genes have been observed in the chicken ovalbumin gene [30], the human globin genes, and mouse metallothionein-1 gene [8].

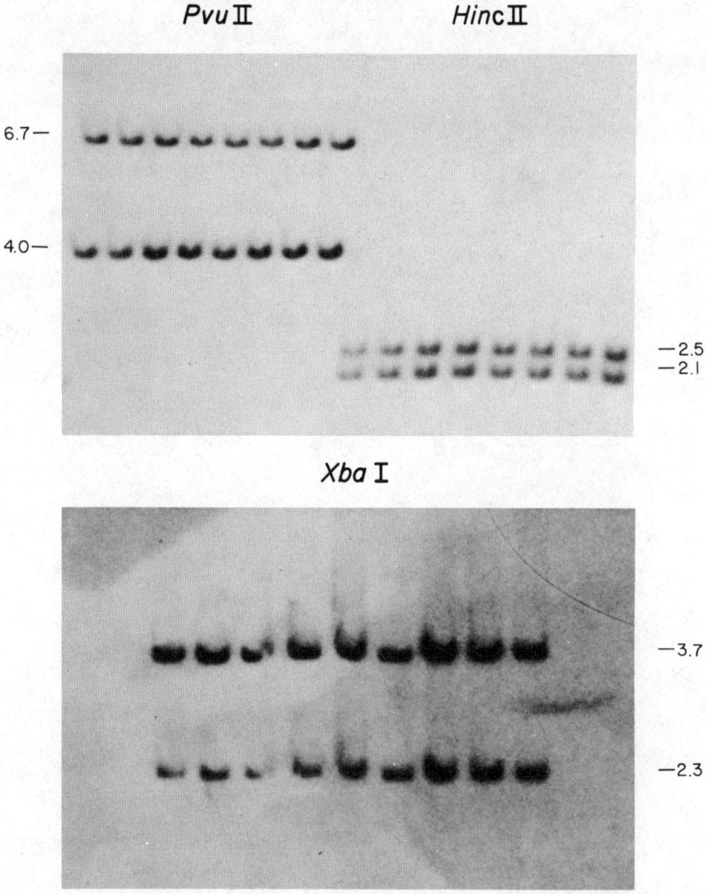

Fig. 6. The IFN-γ region is not highly polymorphic. Nine different human genomic lymphocyte DNAs were digested with a variety of restriction endonucleases, separated by electrophoresis through 1 percent agarose, transferred to nitrocellulose [48], and hybridized with a ^{32}P-labelled IFN-γ cDNA probe (887 bp <u>Sau</u>3A fragment, ref. 20). The Southern hybridization results shown indicate no detectable size differences between restriction fragments of different individuals (sizes shown to the side in kbp). Only eight different DNAs are presented in the <u>Pvu</u>II and <u>Hin</u>II digestion patterns.

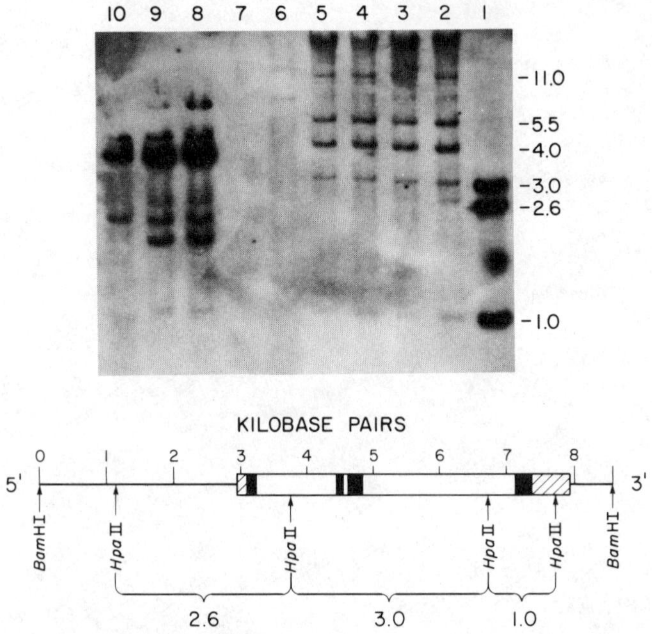

Fig. 7. Methylation of HpaII sites sites within the IFN-γ gene region. 10 υg of human genomic DNA from different sources was separated 1 percent agarose gel electrophoresis, transferred to nitrocellulose [48], and hybridized with 10^7 cpm of ^{32}P-labelled IFN-γ cDNA probe (887 bp Sau3A fragment, ref. 20). Mitogen-stimulated (induced) lymphocyte cultures (20) were harvested 24 hours after induction for DNA preparation. Lane 1, MspI digest of sperm DNA. Lane 2, HpaII digest of induced lymphocyte DNA (individual 1). Lane 3, HpaII digest of induced lymphocyte DNA (individual 1). Lane 4, HpaII digest of uninduced lymphocyte DNA (individual 2). Lane 5, HpaII digest of induced lymphocyte DNA (individual 2). Lane 6, HpaII digest of sperm DNA. Lane 7, HindIII digest of λDNA. Lane 8, PvuII and HpaII digest of uninduced lymphocyte DNA (individual 1). Lane 9, PvuII and HpaII digest of uninduced lymphocyte DNA (individual 1). 10, PvuII and HpaII digest of sperm DNA. MspI patterns were identical for sperm and lymphocyte DNAs (not shown). Positions of HpaII sites

(unmethylated) are shown on the IFN-γ gene map below. Introns are represented on the map as open boxes, exons as solid boxes, and 5' and 3' untranslated regions as cross-hatched boxes.

We have investigated the methylation patterns of the IFN-γ gene in DNA isolated from mitogen-stimulated (induced) lymphocytes, normal (uninduced) lymphocytes, and sperm. Figure 7 shows the results of Southern hybridizations of a cDNA probe to *Hpa*II digested or *Msp*I digested DNAs. As expected from the gene sequence, three *Msp*I hybridizing fragments (1.0, 2.6 and 3.0 kb) are observed in all the DNAs. The *Hpa*II patterns, five hybridizing bands (3.0, 4.0, 5.5, 11 kb and a large amount of higher molecular weight DNA) are identical for the induced and uninduced lymphocyte DNAs. The sperm DNA, in contrast, gives a single hybridizing HpaII fragment of 7.0 kb, consistent with complete methylation of the two *Hpa*II sites within the IFN-γ gene introns. These results suggest that IFN-γ genes which are capable of being expressed have a particular methylation pattern and that the induction of IFN-γ synthesis is probably not due to a gross change in the methylation pattern of the IFN-γ gene after mitogen stimulation. However, if the percentage of lymphocytes responsive to induction is low, then physiologically significant changes in methylation patterns in those cells could be missed by this analysis.

DISCUSSION

Southern analysis clearly indicated that the single human IFN-γ gene contained at least one intron. The number and size of introns were determined directly by DNA sequencing of the isolated gene.

Gilbert has proposed [16] that eukaryotic genes may have evolved by exon shuffling, the rearrangement of various coding sequences to form functional proteins. Although there is no obvious overall amino acid homology between IFN-γ and IFNα [20], the first exon of IFN-γ codes for two groups of amino acids which are homologous with IFN-α. Four homologous amino acids are found at the signal/mature sequence junction (ser-leu-gly-cys, where cys is the first mature amino acid). Another homology with the first exon of IFN-γ is found nearer the carboxyl terminus of IFN-α2:

	130	131	132	133					134	135	136
IFN-α	tyr-	leu-	lys-	glu-					lys-	lys-	tyr
IFN-γ	tyr-	val-	lys-	glu-	ala-	glu-	asn-	leu-	lys-	lys-	tyr
	7	8	9	10	11	12	13	14	15	16	17

Neglecting the four amino acid insertions of IFN-γ, six of seven amino acids are homologous (17 of 21 at the nucleotide level). This homology may be significant considering that the IFN-α sequence is highly conserved in this region when 11 different IFN-α sequences are compared [17]. Furthermore, this region is proposed to be highly α-helical in both IFN-α and IFN-γ [63]; the insertion of four amino acids would increase the length of the helix by one turn, but would not disturb the position of amino acids on the helix.

The comparison of a large number of intron splice site sequences has suggested that for correct RNA splicing, introns must begin with a GT dinucleotide and end with an AG [4,29]. These dinucleotides and their adjacent consensus intron sequences [29,44, 46] exhibit a high degree of complementarity to the 5' end of the small nuclear U1 RNA, which has been proposed to be involved in the splicing of introns from mRNA precursors [24,44]. The sequences in the IFN-γ gene conform well with the consensus sequences found in other eukaryotic genes. The 3' ends of each intron are particularly rich in pyrimidine residues; for example, the end of the first intron contains 19 contiguous pyrimidines, 18 of which are T residues.

Both the introns (64 percent A+T) and the coding region of the gene (61 percent A+T) are overall rich in A+T content. This is in contrast to many genes, such as the chicken pro α2(I) collagen gene [61], which contain G+C rich coding regions embedded in A+T rich introns.

The identification of the complete nucleotide sequence of the IFN-γ gene allows comparison of sequences proposed to be important in gene regulation. Such a sequence is the Goldberg-Hogness box [15,41], or TATA box, located approximately 30 bp upstream from the 5' end of the site of RNA initiation. This sequence, 5' $\mathrm{TATA}^{T}_{A}\mathrm{A}^{T}_{A}$3', is thought to be necessary for the correct positioning of the start of RNA synthesis [22]. Such a sequence, TATAAATA, is found in the IFN-γ gene 29 bp upstream from the 5' end of the mRNA which we previously determined [12]. This same sequence is positioned 30 bp upstream from the 5' end of the IFN-β mRNA [9,39] although there is little further homology in the 5' extragenic region with IFN-β. Seven different members of the IFN-α gene family contain a sequence [28], TATTTAA, which is significantly different from IFN-γ.

Another sequence which is conserved in the 5' end of many (but not all) genes is the consensus sequence $\mathrm{GG}^{C}_{T}\mathrm{CAATCT}$ [1], located approximately 80 bp upstream of the cap site. This sequence is thought to modulate transcription by RNA polymerase II and, furthermore, has been shown to be necessary for efficient transcription of rabbit β-globin gene <u>in vivo</u> [21]. A similar sequence containing one extra nucleotide, GTCACCATCT, is found 89 bp upstream from the 5' end of the IFN-γ mRNA. This sequence or the consensus sequence is not found in either the IFN-α genes or IFN-β gene [9,28,39].

Although IFN-α and IFN-β have extensive homology in 5' flanking regions [2,39], IFN-γ does not share this homology. Perhaps it is not surprising that sequences important for the initiation of RNA synthesis are different when IFN-γ and the other IFNs are compared. These IFNs are induced by different agents and the kinetics of induction are much slower for IFN-γ. Consequently, the molecular mechanisms of induction may be different in these systems.

An interesting sequence was observed in the first intron at position 1349-1374. This sequence consists of 25 alternating C-A residues. This alternating pyrmidine-purine structure has a potential for forming left-handed Z-DNA [59]. Z-DNA hs been found in the interband regions of Drosophila polytene chromosomes [38]. Z-DNA sequences are capable of reversible structural conformations (Z-DNA to B-DNA transition) and may play a significant role in gene regulation.

Southern analysis of the IFN-γ gene suggests that the first intron contains a repetitive DNA element. This element is unrelated to the Alu family repeat, as shown by hybridization and sequence comparison studies. This repetitive DNA element is probably not as frequently represented in the human genome as the Alu family repeat, since only a single copy was observed in the 33.5 kbp IFN-γ gene region. In addition, the hybridization intensity of this probe appeared to be less when qualitatively compared with the Alu family repeat probe in Southern hybridizations of human genomic DNA (Fig. 5).

Hybridization of the IFN-γ cDNA probe to HpaII or MspI digested human genomic DNA suggests that a particular methylation pattern may be a consequence of differentiation; induction of the IFN-γ gene does not seem to alter the methylation pattern.

The observed incomplete digestion of lymphocyte DNA by HpaII could be due to a general partial methylation of the IFN-γ gene in mixed lymphocyte cultures. Alternatively, it is possible that individual classes of lymphocytes have IFN-γ genes with different extents of methylation and that only those cells with a particular methylation pattern can be induced to synthesize IFN-γ. This question can be addressed by experiments on homogeneous classes of lymphocytes which correlate the ability of those cells to produce IFN-γ with their pattern of IFN-γ gene methylation.

ACKNOWLEDGEMENT

We thank Mark Vasser for deoxyoligonucleotide synthesis and Dr. Ellson Chen for preparation of templates for dideoxy sequencing.

REFERENCES

1. Benoist, C., K. O'Hare, R. Breathnach, and P. Chambon. 1980. The ovalbumin gene-sequence of putative control regions. Nucleic Acids Res. 8:127-142.
2. Blin, N. and D.W. Stafford. 1976. A general method for isolation of high molecular weight DNA from eukaryotes. Nucleic Acids Res. 3:2303-2308.
3. Bolivar, F., R. Rodriquez, P. J. Greene, M. Betlach, H. L. Heyneker, H.W. Boyer, J. Crosa, and S. Falkow. 1977. Construction and characterization of new cloning vehicles. Gene 2:95-113.
4. Brenthrach, R., C. Benoist, K. O'Hare, F. Gannon, and P. Chambon. 1978. Ovalbumin gene evidence for a leader sequence in mRNA and DNA sequences at the exon-intron boundaries. Proc. Natl. Acad. Sci. U.S.A. 75:4853-4857.
5. Brenthrach, R. and P. Chambon. 1981. Organization and expression of eukaryotic split genes coding for proteins. Ann. Review Biochem. 50:349-383.
6. Calabretta, B., D.L. Robberson, H.A. Barrera-Saldana, T.P. Lambron, and G.F. Saunders. 1982. Genome instability in a region of human DNA enriched in Alu repeat sequences. Nature 296:219-225.
7. Crea, R. and T. Horn. 1980. Synthesis of oligonucleotides on

cellulose by a phosphotriester method. Nucleic Acids Res. 8:2331-2348.

8. Compere, S.J. and R.D. Palmiter. 1981. DNA methylation controls the inducibility of the mouse metallothionein-I gene in lymphoid cells. Cell 25:233-240.

9. DeGrave, W., R. Derynck, J. Tavernier, G. Haegeman, and W. Fiers. 1981. Nucleotide sequence of the chromosomal gene for human Fibroblast (B_1) interferon and of the flanking regions. Gene 14:137-143.

10. deLey, M., J. van Damme, H. Claeys, H. Weening, J.W. Heine, A. Billiau, C. Vermylen, and P. de Somer. 1980. Interferon induced in human leukocytes by mitogens: production, partial purification and characterization. Eur. J. Immunol. 10:877-883.

11. Derynck, R., J. Content, E. DeClereq, G. Volckaert, J. Tavernier, R. Devos, and W. Fiers. 1980. Isolation and structure of a human fibroblast interferon gene. Nature 285:542-547.

12. Derynck, R., D.W. Leung, P.W. Gray, and D.V. Goeddel, 1982. Human interferon γ is encoded by a single class of mRNA. Nucleic Acids Res. (in press).

13. Felsenfeld, G. and J. McGhee. 1982. Methylation and gene control. Nature 296:602-603.

14. Fritsch, E.F., R. M. Lawn, and T. Maniatis. 1980. Molecular cloning and characterization of the human β-like globin gene cluster. Cell 19:959-972.

15. Gannon, F., K. O'Hare, F. Perrin, J.P. LePennec, (Benoist, M. Cochet, R. Breathnach, A. Royal, A. Garapin, B. Cami, and P. Chambon. 1979. Organization and sequences at the 5' end of a cloned complete ovalbuimin gene. Nature 278:428-434.

16. Gilbert, W. 1978. Why genes in pieces. Nature 271:501.

17. Goeddel, D.V., D.W. Leung, T.J. Dull, M. Gross, R.M. Lawn, R. McCandliss, P.H. Seeburg, A. Ullrich, E. Yelverton, and P.W. Gray. 1981. The structure of eight distinct cloned human leukocyte interferon cDNAs. Nature 290:20-26.

18. Goeddel, D.V., H.M. Shepard, E. Yelverton, D. Leung, and R.

Crea. 1980. Synthesis of human fibroblast interferon by E. coli. Nucleic Acids Res. 8:4057-4074.

19. Goeddel, D.V., E. Yelverton, A. Ullrich, H.L. Heyneker, G. Miozzari, W. Holmes, P.H. Seeburg, T. Dull, L. May, N. Stebbing, R. Crea, S. Maeda, R. McCandliss, A. Sloma, J.M. Tabor, M. Gross, P.C. Familletti, and S. Pestka. 1980. A human leukocyte interferon produced by E. coli is biologically active. Nature 287:411-416.

20. Gray, P.W., D.W. Leung, D. Pennica, E. Yelverton, R. Najarian, C. Simonsen, R. Derylnck, P.J. Sherwood, D.M. Wallace, S.L. Berger, A.D. Levinson, and D.V. Goeddel. 1982. Expression of human immune interferon in E. coli and monkey cells. Nature 295:503-508.

21. Grosveld, G.C., E. de Boer, C.K. Shewmaker, and R.A. Flavell. 1982. DNA sequences necessary for transcription of the rabbit β-globin gene in vivo. Nature 295:120-126.

22. Grosveld, G.C., C.K. Shewmaker, P. Jat, and R.A. Flavell. 1981. Localization of DNA sequences necessary for transcription of the rabbit β-globin gene in vitro. Cell 25:215-226.

23. Houck, C.M., F.P. Rinehart, and C.W. Schmidt. 1979. A ubiquitous family of repeated DNA sequences in the human genome. J. Molec. Biol. 132:289-306.

24. Houghton, M., I.J. Jackson, A.G. Porter, S.M. Doel, G.H. Catlin, C. Barber, and N.H. Carey. 1981.

25. Lawn, R.M., J. Adelman, T. J. Dull, M. Gross, D. Goeddel, and A. Ullrich. 1981. DNA sequence of two closely linked human leukocyte interferon genes. Science 212:1159-1162.

26. Lawn, R.M., J. Adelman, A.E. Franke, C.M. Houck, M. Gross, R. Najarian, and D.V. Goeddel. 1981. Human fibroblast gene lacks introns. Nucleic Acids Res. 9:1045-1052.

27. Lawn, R.M., E.F. Fritsch, R.C. Parker, G. Blake, T. Maniatis, 1978. The isolation and characterization of linked γ and β-globin genes from a cloned library of human DNA. Cell 15:1157-1174.

28. Lawn, R.M., M. Gross, C.M. Houck, A.E. Franke, P.W. Gray, and D. V. Goeddel. 1981. DNA sequence of a major human leukocyte interferon gene. Proc. Natl. Acad. Sci. U.S.A. 78:5435-5439.

29. Lerner, M.R., J.A. Boyle, S.M. Mount, S.L. Wolin, and J.A. Steitz. 1980. Are snRNPs involved in splicing. Nature 283:220-224.

30. Mandel, J.L. and P. Chambon. 1979. DNA methylation: organ specific variations in the methylation pattern within and around ovalbumin and other chicken genes. Nucleic Acids Res. 7:2082-2103.

31. Maniatis, T., R.C. Hardison, E.Lacy, J. Lauer, C. O'Connell, D. Quon, G.K. Sim, and A. Efstratiadis. 1978. The isolation of structural genes from libraries of eukaryotic DNA. Cell 15:687-701.

32. Mantei, N., M. Schwarzstein, M. Streuli, S. Panem, S. Nagata, and C. Weissman. 1980. The nucleotide sequence of a cloned human leukocyte interferon cDNA. Gene 10:1-10.

33. Maxam, A.M. and W. Gilbert. 1980. Sequencing end-labeled DNA with base-specific chemical cleavages. Methods in Enzymno. 65:499-560.

34. Messing, J., R. Crea, and P.H. Seeburg. 1981. A system for shotgun DNA sequencing. Nucleic Acids Res. 9:309-321.

35. Nagata, S., N. Mlantei, and C. Weissman. 1980. The structure of one of the eight or more distinct chromosomal genes for human interferon-α. Nature 287-401-408.

36. Nathan, I., J.E. Groopman, S.G. Quan, N. Bersch, and D.W. Golde. 1981. Immune (γ) interferon produced by a human T-lymphoblast cell line. Nature 292:842-844.

37. Naylor, S.L., A.Y. Sakaguchi, T.B. Shows, M.L. Law, D.V. Goeddel, and P.W. Gray. 1982. Human immune interferon (IFN-γ) gene is located on chromosome 12. Nature (in press).

38. Nordheim, A., M.L. Pardue, E.M. Lafer, A. Moller, B.D. Stoller, and A. Rich. 1981. Antibodies to left-handed Z-DNA bind to interband regions of _Drosophila_ polytene chromosomes. Nature 294:417-422.

39. Ohno, S. and T. Taniguchi, 1981. Sructure of a chromosomal gene for human interferon β. Proc. Natl. Acad. Sci. U.S.A. 78:5305-5309.

40. Owerbach, D., W.J. Rutter, T.B. Shows, P. Gray, D.V. Goeddel, and R.M. Lawn. 1981. Leukocyte and fibroblast genes are located on human chromosome 9. Proc. Natl. Acad. Sci. U.S.A. 78:3123-3127.

41. Proudfoot, N.J. 1979. Eukaryotic promoters. Nature 279:376.

42. Proudfoot, N.J. and G.G. Brownlee. 1976. 3' non-coding region sequences in eukaryotic messenger RNA. Nature 263:211-214.

43. Razin, A. and A.D. Riggs. 1980. DNA methylation and gene function. Science 210:604-610.

44. Rogers, J. and R. Wall. 1980. A mechanism for RNA splicing. Proc. Natl. Acad. Sci. U.S.A. 77:1877-1879.

45. Rubin, C.M., C.M. Houck, P.L. Deininger, T. Friedmann, and C.W. Schmid. 1980. Partial nucleotide sequence of the 300-nucleotide interspersed repeated human DNA sequences. Nature 284:372-374.

46. Sharp, P.A. 1981. Speculations on RNA splicing. Cell 23:643-646.

47. Smith, A.J.H. 1980. DNA sequence analysis by primed synthesis. Methods in Enzymo. 65:560-580.

48. Southern, E.M. 1975. Detection of specific sequences among DNA fragments separated by gel electrophoresis. J. Molec. Biol. 98:503-517.

49. Stewart, W.E. II 1979. The Interferon System. Springer, Berlin.

50. Stewart, W.E. II, J.E. Blalock, D.C. Burke, C. Chany, J.K. Dunnick, E. Falcoff, R.M. Friedman, G.J. Galasso, W.K. Joklik, J.T. Vilcek, J.S. Younger, and K.C. Zoon. 1980. Interferon nomenclature. Nature 286:110.

51. Streuli, M., S. Nagata, and C. Weissman. 1980. At least three human type α interferons: structure of α2. Science 209:1343-1347.

52. Taniguchi, T., N. Mantei, M. Schwarzstein, S. Nagata, M.

Muramatasu and C. Weissman. 1980. Human leukocyte and fibroblast interferons are structurally related. Nature 285:547-549.

53. Taniguchi, T., S. Ohno, Y. Fujii-Kuriyama, and M. Muramatsu., 1980. The nucleotide sequence of human fibroblast interferon cDNA. Gene 10:11-15.

54. Taniguchi, T., R.H.L. Pang, Y.K. Yip, D.Henriksen, and J. Vilcek. 1981. Partial characterization of γ (immune) interferon mRNA extracted from human lymphocytes. Proc. Natl. Acad. Sci. U.S.A. 78:3469-3472.

55. Taylor, J.M., R. Illmensee, and S. Summers. 1976. Efficient transcription of RNA into DNA by avian sarcoma virus polymease. Biochim. Biophys. Acta 442:324-330.

56. van der Ploeg, L.H.T. and R.A. Flavell. 1980. DNA methylation in the human γαβ-globin locus in erythroid and nonerythroid tissues. Cell 19:447-958.

57. Waalwijk, C. and R.A. Flavell. 1978. MspI, an isoschizimer of HpaII which cleaves both unmethylated and methylated HpaII sites. Nucleic Acids Res. 5:3231-3236.

58. Wallace, D.M., M.J.M. Hitchcock, S.B. Reber, and S.L. Berger. 1981. Translation of human immune interferon messenger RNA in Xenopus laevis oocytes. Biochem. Biophys. Res. Comm. 100:865-871.

59. Wang, A. H.-J., G.J. Quigley, F.J. Kolpak, J.L. Crawford, J.H. van Boom, G. van der Marel, and A. Rich. 1979. Molecular structure of a left-handed double helical DNA fragment at atomic resolution. Nature 282:680-686.

60. Weissman, C. 1981. The cloning of interferon and other mis-takes. Interferon 3:101-134.

61. Wozney, J., D. Hanahan, V. Tate, H. Boedtker, and P. Doty. 1981. Structure of the proα2(I) collagen gene. Nature 294:129-135.

62. Yip, Y.K., R.H.L. Pang, C. Urban, and J. Vilcek. 1981. Partial purification and characterization of human γ (immune) interferon. Proc. Natl. Acad. Sci. U.S.A. 78:1601-1605.

63. Zoon, K.C. and R. Wetzel. 1982. Comparative structures of mammalian interferons. In P.E. Came and W.A. Carter (eds.) Handbook of Experimental Pharmacology, Springer, New York.

CORRECTION OF INBORN ERRORS OF METABOLISM BY BONE MARROW TRANSPLANT

William Krivit
Department of Pediatrics
University of Minnesota
Minneapolis, Minnesota 55455

A new development in medicine is the utilization of bone marrow transplantation for correction of inborn errors of metabolism. In the past, bone marrow transplantation had been utilized for the curative treatment of aplastic anemia, leukemia, neuroblastoma, and congenital immune and hematologic deficiencies. The fullest explanation of the potential for bone marrow transplant in the correction of inborn errors of metabolism has been outlined by Hobbs [8]. The final indication of the usefulness of this new development awaits case by case analysis. This review will illustrate the biological basis for the use of bone marrow transplant for correction of inborn errors of metabolism.

ENZYME CHANGES INDUCED IN ANIMALS BY BONE MARROW TRANSPLANTATION

Three sets of animal experiments have proved that bone marrow transplantation can replace peripheral blood enzymes. The enzymes that have been changed due to bone marrow transplantation have been beta glucuronidase [13,18], catalase [14], and lipase [9] (Table 1). An interesting aspect of the beta glucuronidase experiment was that the enzyme activity in the liver of the chimera was greater than that found in the donor (Table 2). Furthermore, a bone marrow trans-

Table 1

Correction of Plasma Enzyme Defects in Animal Experiments By Bone Marrow Transplantation

	Beta Glucuronidase[+] (Ref. #2)	Catalase[++] (Ref. #3)	Lipase[+++] (Ref. #4)
DONOR (Normal)	20.4	153	1.0
RECIPIENT (Abnormal)	9.5	20	2.5
CHIMERA (Recipient After BMT from Donor)	16.5	168	1.0

[+] nm/hr/ml
[++] PU/ml
[+++] DMPTu $x/10^4$

plant protected acatalasemic mice against H_2O_2 challenge (Table 3). These experiments suggest the hypothesis that bone marrow cells were able to transfer regulatory capacity for synthesis and/or activity of certain enzymes. The data noted below and in above experiments indicated that bone marrow derived cells such as monocytes - macrophages are probably responsible for a change of enzyme levels and for protection against challenge.

THE RETICULOENDOTHELIAL SYSTEM

The reticuloendothelial system (r.e.s.) is derived mainly from bone marrow monocytes. The r.e.s. is composed of hepatic macrophages (Kupffer cells), pulmonary macrophages, and the lymphoid and monocyte macrophages of the lymphoid system. These data indicate

Table 2

Correction of Liver Enzyme Defects in Animal Experiments By Bone Marrow Transplantation

	Beta Glucuronidase[+]
DONOR (Normal)	135
REICIPIENT (Abnormal)	23
CHIMERA (Recipient After BMT from Donor)	207

[+]nm/hr/mg protein

that bone marrow from a donor will repopulate the r.e.s. of the recipient with new cells. These new r.e.s. cells as well as the new bone marrow cells would participate in providing new enzymes or normal amounts of enzyme for the recipient.

Origin of Hepatic Macrophages

After bone marrow transplant, the sex chromatin of hepatic macrophages in two male patients were identified as being totally female [5]. The methods used included fluorescent Y body for male after staining with quinacrine and/or Barr body observations (Table 4).

Hepatic macrophages (Kupffer cells) in a recipient were shown previously in animal experiments to be derived from the bone marrow cells of the donor after completion of a bone marrow transplant [4].

Also the reverse experiment has been done. Orthotopic transplantation of donor liver into recipient has been done. The Kupffer cells of the liver in the recipient are of recipient origin,

Table 3

Protection of Animals from H_2O_2 Challenge
After Bone Marrow Transplantation

	H2O2 Challenge
DONOR	100% Survival
RECIPIENT	0% "
CHIMERA	64% "

i.e., from a circulating cell from marrow. This again demonstrates the marrow origin of Kupffer cells.

Bone Marrow Origin of Monocytes - Osteoclasts

Walker demonstrated in his brilliant experiments that bone marrow transplantation completely corrected bone defects in congenital osteopetrotic mice [16]. (Indeed, the reverse was also accomplished by Walker in that he made normal mice into osteopetrotic mice by bone marrow transplant.)

In the human, osteopetrosis has been corrected by bone marrow transplant [3]. The abnormal osteoclast, incapable of removing osteoid tissue, proliferates and replaces normal marrow elements. The monocyte is also abnormal in the human osteopetrotic patient as tested by bactericidal ability and chemotactic movement. This defect in monocyte function was also corrected by bone marrow transplant.

Origin of Pulmonary Macrophages

The pulmonary macrophages are another important aspect of the

Table 4

Hepatic Macrophages from Two Males Who Had Received Bone Marrow Transplantation from Females*

	% of Cells with	
	Y Body	Sex X Chromatin
NORMAL MALE	16	0
NORMAL FEMALE	0	21
PATIENT (559 days after BMT)	0	16
PATIENT (104 days after BMT)	0	16

*Ref.#5

r.e.s. Alveolar macrophages are repopulated from bone marrow derived donor cells in rodents and dogs [17]. The results derived from bone marrow transplantation in humans demonstrated that the alveolar macrophages do come from bone marrow [15].

Origin of Brain Macrophages

Circulating monocytes do penetrate the central nervous system and are present in the brain macrophage system. This experiment has been done in animal models. Normal circulating monocytes tagged with radioactive labels and injected into the peripheral vein were noted in brain tissue surrounding artificially induced inflammation by trauma or allergic encephalitis [1,10,11].

This experimental datum will most likely be confirmed in humans following bone marrow transplant. Much like the pulmonary and hepatic macrophages, the use of sex markers in the brain reticulo-endothelial system cells will probably demonstrate that the latter cells are of donor origin. An equally convincing confirmation would be presented if the acatalasemic mice were used to detect catalase positive cells in brain tissue after bone marrow transplant.

BONE MARROW TRANSPLANTATION IN THE HUMAN FOR THE CORRECTION OF INBORN ERRORS OF METABOLISM

There are several inborn errors of metabolism of the host defense mechanism of lymphocytes and neutrophils which have been corrected by bone marrow transplantation. These include Wiskott-Aldrich syndrome; Chediak-Higashi; chronic granulomatous disease; severe, combined immune deficiency; and several other entities whose cellular aberrations would be expected to be controlled because bone marrow derived cells are abnormal.

The new concept espoused here is that inborn errors of metabolism of enzyme deficiency can be effectively treated with bone marrow transplant. The report by Hobbs in the Hurler patients and mucopolysaccharidosis cases indicated that their patients have developed normal levels of enzyme in plasma and urine and in leukocytes. This, therefore, is evidence of a bone marrow "take" from the donor in the bone marrow transplant process. This was to be anticipated and provides another method of proving that recipient cells are derived from the donor.

However, the data from Hobbs indicate more than that there is a bone marrow "take". The enzyme must have accumulated in sufficient amount to produce clinical changes and improvement in symptoms. The disappearance of hepatosplenomegaly and the clearing of the cornea indicate that enzyme has penetrated the tissues [6,7]. The establishment of this specific type of gradient is a prerequisite for improvement at the cellular level. Clearly, this has been accomplished (Table 5).

Table 5

Bone Marrow Transplant for Hurler's Syndrome

	Days of Graft	Resolved Hepatosplenomegaly	Corneal Clouding
Patient #1	7623	Yes (4-8 wks.)	Yes (6 mos.)
Patient #2	7340	Yes (4-8 wks.)	Yes (6 mos.)
Patient #3	7196	Yes (4-8 wks.)	Yes (6 mos.)

Ref. #16

UNIVERSITY OF MINNESOTA EXPERIENCE

We have had experience with osteopetrosis and with Maroteaux-Lamy syndrome (Mucopolysaccharidosis VI).

The first patient with osteopetrosis that we herein cite has been reported ref. 3. The second patient with osteopetrosis had a bone marrow "take" and had evidence of regeneration of normal osteoclasts and resolution of hepatosplenomegaly.

The patient with Maroteaux-Lamy syndrome (mucopolysaccharidosis VI) has been following the course quite similar to that reported by Hobbs in his Hurler-type patients. The patient who was transplanted at the University of Minnesota Hospitals had enzymes measured and reported in an earlier paper [2].

At the University of Minnesota we, in 1982, have evidence of a "take" by the fact that enzyme levels in the recipient (patient) have returned to normal. This has been measured as an activity of the Arylsulfatase B. Of even greater physiologic meaning has been the clearing of the cloudy cornea. Before the bone marrow transplant there had been significant impenetrable cloudiness so that vision was nil. Within several weeks after evidence of "take" as measured by a rise of the peripheral blood leukocyte count, there was improvement in visual acuity. This included decreasing pressures secondary to glaucoma and decreasing corneal cloudiness. There has also been a marked decrease in hepatosplenomegaly. The spleen is no longer palpable and shows normal on a scan. There has been a general improvement in, or a loss of stiffness of the joints.

GENERAL COMMENTS

Observations during the next several years will indicate what the long-term role of the bone marrow transplant procedure will be in the treatment of inborn errors of metabolism. We specifically should indicate that these diseases so treated must have no other accepted therapy available.

The risks of bone marrow transplant procedures have decreased greatly in the past several years. The problem of graft versus host disease is becoming less frequent with our present methodology [12]. And there is a very low incidence of failure of bone marrow engraftment.

The significance of these studies lies in whether or not any of the enzymes will be able to develop a sufficient gradient to cross into parenchymal cells. We have reduced size of liver and spleen in osteopetrosis and in mucopolysaccharidosis. The clearest data to indicate a gradient is that of disappearance of corneal clouding. This theoretically would develop through lysosomal enzymes which are known to be present in tears.

The final problem that will need to be reviewed is that of the potential passage of enzyme into brain cells. The blood-brain barrier is usually noted as an impediment to utilizing bone marrow transplant when central nervous system disease is present. Yet, if the r.e.s. cells of the brain indeed do have their origins from bone marrow derived cells, then there is potential for the enzymes to pass into the brain and prevent further damage.

There are several caveats which must be taken into consideration. These consist of the fact that the parents and physicians caring for these child patients must be fully cognizant of the risks and gains to be obtained.

Informed consent in the fullest sense is absolutely mandatory if we are to proceed with these trials in the treatment of inborn errors of metabolism. We must also realize that allogeneic match from a normal sibling is most desirable. We should then be able to provide quite adequate enzyme from donor marrow and also reduce the incidence of graft versus host disease.

Some disease entities which we might contemplate treating in this manner include Glycogen Storage Disease IV, alpha-1-antitrypsin deficiency, and potentially Krabbe's disease. Each has its own conceptual problems and each will need to be reviewed on an individual basis.

REFERENCES

1. Adrian, E.K., Jr., and B.E. Walker. Incorporation of thymidine-H^3 by cells in normal and injured mouse spinal cord. J. Neuropathol. and Exp. Neurol. 21:597 (1962).
2. Beates, N.G., B.M. Turner, B. Weiss, and K. Hirschhorn. Arylsulfatase B deficiency in Maroteaux-Lamy syndrome cellular studies and carrier identification. Ped. Res. 9:475-480 (1975).
3. Coccia, P.F., W. Krivit, J. Cervenka, C. Clawson, J.H. Kersey, T.H. Kim, M.E. Nesbit, N.K.C. Ramsay, P. Warkentin, S.I. Teitelbaum, A.J. Kahn, and D.W. Brown. Successful bone marrow

transplantation for infantile malignant osteopetrosis. NEJM 302:701-708 (1980).

4. Bone Marrow Origin of Kupffer Cells. (editorial) Lancet, p 130 (Jan. 19, 1980).

5. Gale, R.P., R.S. Sparkes, and D.W. Golde. Bone marrow origin of hepatic macrophages (Kupffer cells) in humans. Science 201:937 (1978).

6. Hobbs, J.R., et al. Bone marrow transplantation correction of systemic disease in three patients with Hurler's, mucopolysaccharidosis, Sanfillipo B disease and mitochromatic leukodystrophy. Eighth Annual Meeting of the European Bone Marrow Transplantation Group. International Society for Experimental Hematology Vol. 10, Suppl. 10. Allen Press, Lawrence, KS, 48-52 (1982).

7. Hobbs, J.R., et al. Reverse of clinical features of Hurler's disease and biochemical improvement after treatment by bone marrow transplantation. Lancet, p 709 (Oct. 3, 1981).

8. Hobbs, J.R. Bone marrow transplantation for inborn errors. Lancet, p 735 (Oct. 3, 1981).

9. Jyonouchi, H., J.C. Cyong, F.W. Shen, G. Fernandes, N.K. Day, and R.A. Good. Alteration of murine serum lipase activity after allogeneic bone marrow transplantation. Clin. Immunol. and Immunopathol. 22:94 (1982).

10. Konigsmark, B.W., and R.L. Sidman. Origin of brain macrophages in mouse. J. Neuropathol. and Exp. Neurol. 22:643 (1963).

11. Kosunen, T.U., B.H. Wahsman, and I.K. Samuelsson. Radioautograph study of cellular mechanisms in delayed hypersensitivity. J. Neuropathol. and Exp. Neurol. 22:367 (1963).

12. Krivit, W., et al. Bone marrow transplant in pediatrics. Adv. in Ped. (in press, 1983).

13. Slavin, S., and S. Yatziv. Correction of enzyme deficiency in mice by allogeneic bone marrow transplantation with total lymphoid irradiation. Science 210:1150 (1980).

14. Sutherland, D., E.R. David, C. Hong, and J.S. Najarian.

Cellular transplantation for enzymatic and metabolic deficiencies. _In_ Enzyme Therapy in Genetic Diseases: 2. Birth Defects: Original Article Series (R.J. Desnick, Ed.) Vol. XVI, pp 207-217. Alan R. Liss Co., New York (1981).

15. Thomas, E.D., R.E. Ramberg, G.E. Sale, R.S. Sparkes, and D.W. Golde. Direct evidence for a bone marrow origin of the alveolar macrophage in man. _Science_ 192:1016-1017 (1976).
16. Walker, D.G. Bone resorption restored in osteopetrotic mice by transplant of normal bone marrow and spleen cells. _Science_ 190:784 (1975).
17. Weiden, P.L., R. Storb, and M.S. Tsoi. Marrow origin of canine alveolar macrophages. _J. Reticuloendothelial Soc._ 17:6:342-345 (1975).
18. Yatziv, S., L. Weiss, S. Morechi, Z. Fuks, and S. Slavin. Long term enzyme replacement therapy in B glucuronidase-deficient mice by allogeneic bone marrow transplantation. _J. Lab. Clin. Med._ 99:792.

DISCUSSION

Q. ROGERS (Minnesota): What are the management problems once you have completed a bone marrow transplantation?

A. KRIVIT: Thank you, Dr. Rogers. There are several immediate problems that face the bone marrow transplant recipient. These would be a failure of a "take," rejection of "take", graft versus host disease (acute and chronic) and infectious complications. Most recently all of these problems have been reduced in magnitude and frequency. The methods of preparation of donor by immunosuppression and radiation have reduced failure of recipient marrow to "take" to a new low percentage of 1.2% or less. The recipient engrafted marrow will be lost or rejected in only a rather small number. However, on the other hand, graft versus host disease both acute and chronic, is to be anticipated in many of the patients. This can consist of skin, gastrointestinal, liver, and other organ destruction by graft. Graft versus host disease, however, is changing in severity and frequency due to treatment and preventive methodology. (Ramsey, N.K.C., J. Kersey, L. Robison, P. McGlave, W. Woods, W. Krivit, T. Kim, A. Goldman, and M. Nesbit, 1982. A randomized study for prevention of acute graft versus host disease. NEJM 306:392-397). Infectious complications of opportunistic bacteria, aspergillosis, viruses, and other assorted infectious problems are being studied. All together these complications must be considered serious and devastating and life threatening. Mortality may be as high as 15-25% from these undesirable effects.

The balancing act begins when considering this potential against the certainty of death from malignant processes being treated by utilization of bone marrow transplant process. When considered in the light that approximately 85-75% of patients will not have a mortality from bone marrow transplant process and when one understands the 100% mortality consequences of doing nothing, bone marrow transplant has become the primary choice of treatment in many diseases (severe aplastic anemia and relapsed leukemia). We are now intending to study the use of bone marrow transplant in the inborn errors of metabolism and believe we will have just as good if not potentially better clinical results than obtained so far to date in aplastic anemia and leukemia.

These patients who have once passed the 100-day post bone marrow transplant critical period are free to return to school, participate in all social and athletic events, and are not on any specific medication.

Q. CLINE (UCLA): We need to be aware that a specific allogeneic donor will be needed for the bone marrow transplant process that is projected. So, therefore, that is an inherent limitation at the moment for the majority of patients.

A. KRIVIT: Yes, at present we are limited to perfect allogeneic matches. Although chances of a sibling being identical is only 1:4 of siblings, there are matches of 1/3 of families in whom we do complete testing.

However, maternal and paternal bone marrow transplants have been frequently successful. And, in addition, the team of the University of Minnesota (Dr. Lisa Filipovich and others) are working on lectin treated marrows to remove graft versus host cells and just transplant with normal hematologic stem cells. If that comes to pass, then we will have a significant increase in the number of potential donors. But for the moment, Dr. Cline is correct. We are limited to perfect allogeneic sibling matches.

Q. GINSBURG (Minnesota): How long is the longest life span for someone with a bone marrow transplant?

A. KRIVIT: The longest living marrow transplant was done here at the University of Minnesota by Dr. Robert Good and colleagues for an infant with immune deficiency. This was over 18 years ago. The patient is alive, well and growing and is normal. Patients who had had bone marrow transplants over a decade ago have been noted by Dr. D. Thomas in Seattle who has several patients who had had leukemia and then received bone marrow transplant. The same concept, therefore, also applies to the non-immune deficient patients (i.e., leukemia, aplastic anemia).

Q. GINSBURG: What is the average lifespan with a bone marrow transplant?

A. KRIVIT: The average longevity following bone marrow transplant is a relatively meaningless figure. Certainly most of these patients will live many more years in the future. There is no reason to expect them to die now. And, of course, the relapse of leukemia would also reduce the average survival found subsequent to bone marrow transplant. This later problem -

i.e., relapse of original disease - should not be a problem when inborn errors of metabolism are studied.

I have developed a list of specific types of disease in which criteria for undertaking bone marrow transplant are met. The criteria include:

1) Replacement of normal marrow of enzyme deficient recipient;

2) Certainty of demise or incapacitation in recipient in very near future;

3) A perfect allogeneic match; and

4) Truly informed consent.

Some of the diseases which could be so treated would include: chronic orthopaedic Gaucher's disease, Krabbe's disease, and Type IV Glycogen Storage disease.

RESEARCH ON GENE THERAPY

Martin J. Cline
University of California School of Medicine
Center for the Health Sciences
Los Angeles, California 90024

I would like to begin by describing the methods that are currently available for introducing new genes into mammalian cells. These techniques have generally been applied to cells in tissue culture. Historically, the oldest method for insertion of genes into cells utilizes chromosomes as the mechanism of gene transfer. A variety of chromosomal techniques have been described [1]. Recipient and donor cells can be fused together; chromosomes can be isolated and incubated with target cells for endocytosis; and finally, chromosomes can be entrapped within a nuclear membrane and the membrane can then be fused to the target cell. None of the chromosomal techniques are very efficient at gene transfer; and, in general, only about one cell in ten million is transformed. By transformed, I mean that the target cell acquires new genetic information and expresses that information for some period of time.

The chromosome techniques are also non-specific in the sense that they introduce a great many genes in addition to the gene of interest. The major advantage of chromosomal techniques is that the genes inserted are, presumably, in their native configuration with the upstream promoters as well as all of the remote control sequences that influence gene expression. The main limitation of this type of gene insertion technique is its inefficiency, and transferred genes are frequently unstable.

Currently, the most commonly used method of gene transfer is often referred to as DNA mediated gene transfer [1]. It involves precipitation either of high molecular weight DNA or purified genes with calcium phosphate to produce a very fine amorphous precipitate. The precipitate is internalized or endocytosed by the target cells whether these are tissue culture cells or the mouse bone marrow cells shown in Fig. 1. Some of the internalized DNA traverses the cytoplasm and makes its way to the nucleus where it may be integrated into a variety of sites. DNA mediated gene transfer is also inefficient. Roughly one cell in a million is transformed. The advantage of this technique is that one can use highly purified gene sequences such as, for example, isolated insulin genes or beta globin genes.

A little over a year ago, another gene transfer technique was described. It is designated spheroplast fusion [1]. With this technique, one takes a bacterium such as *E. coli* and introduces recombinant plasmids containing the gene of interest. These plasmids may be amplified so that each *E. coli* contains perhaps 1 to 3,000 plasmid copies. The cell wall of the *E. coli* is removed with lysozyme to produce a spheroplast or protoplast. The bacterial membranes are fused to the mammalian target cells by appropriate chemical techniques and the recombinant plasmids are introduced into the target cells. Since 1,000 or 10,000 spheroplasts can be used for each target cell, the transfer of genetic information is potentially very efficient and, indeed, in several laboratories the transformation efficiency is between 1 and 3 transformants per 1,000 target cells.

The disadvantages of spheroplast fusion are that we do not yet know much about the stability of the newly inserted genes and the

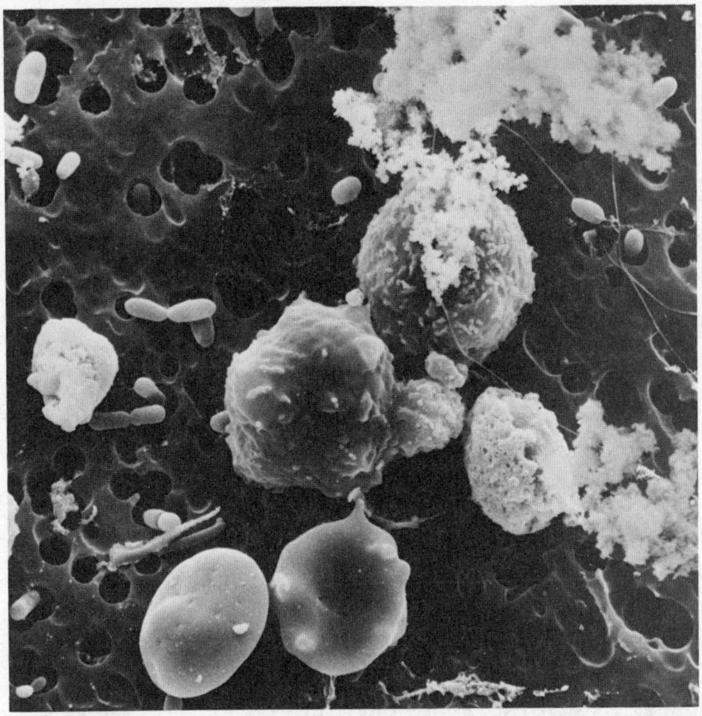

Fig. 1. Scanning electron micrograph of mouse bone marrow cells and a calcium phosphate microprecipitate of high molecular weight DNA.

potential adverse effects of introducing a good deal of genetic information from the *E. coli*.

Another technique of gene transfer is to directly inject cells with DNA. One can conveniently inject between 20 and 2,000 DNA molecules. This is a very efficient technique and, as a generalization, about 10% of the cells may be transformed. The disadvantages are obvious. Only a limited number of cells can be injected per unit of time. Fairly sophisticated equipment is required with a highly trained operator. For cells such as hematopoietic stem cells, this technique cannot readily be used because the cells are too small and cannot readily be identified in a heterogeneous population of cells. Nevertheless, for embryos and embryo transfer work, DNA injection seems to be a very useful technique.

Still another method of gene transfer uses recombinant DNA viruses [1]. The most commonly used virus is SV-40. A portion of the virus nucleic acid is removed and a gene of interest is spliced in. Generally the viral promoter is left intact and another gene such as the insulin gene, a β-globin gene or a growth hormone gene is spliced in. The SV-40 virus is a rather simple virus. Its DNA contains between 4,000 and 5,000 nucleotides. When a piece of the virus is removed and a new gene is inserted, the virus is defective for replication. To circumvent this problem, one can use a variety of strategies. A common one is to use a helper virus to coinfect the target cells along with the engineered recombinant virus. This is a very efficient technique for gene transfer since nearly 100% of the cells are infected. The viruses replicate to high copy numbers, usually several thousand copies per cell. And as they replicate, the inserted genes within the virus are also replicated. The limitations of this technique are that all the action is over within a day or two because viral replication results in lysis of the target cells. Therefore, although this technique is useful for the monkey kidney cells in culture, it has some obvious limitations for use in living animals.

I shall later consider still another approach which I believe may be "the ultimate technique for gene transfer". Certainly it will be extensively utilized for gene transfer over the next few years.

Because of the diverse backgrounds of our readers, I would like to introduce a concept which I'm sure is familiar to many; the concept of selectability. If one is dealing with a gene insertion technique which is of low efficiency, then in order to ensure the spread of the newly introduced gene throughout the target cell population, a gene and culture condition must be chosen which provide the transformed cells with some proliferative advantage. If a gene can then be introduced into only one cell in a million, and if the gene doesn't offer any advantage in cell proliferation, then this cell and its progeny will never be detected among the large number of untransformed cells. For that reason, there has been concern with choosing a variety of selectable genes as dominant selectable markers.

The dominant selectable markers most commonly used have been drug resistance genes. For example, one can use the strategy of introducing a gene for drug resistance and then use drugs to exert selection pressure. The drug inhibits proliferation of all but that one cell in a million which has been transformed by the resistance gene. The prototypic experiment which illustrates this concept of selectability was described by Bacchetti and Graham in 1978. They used human cells that were thymidine kinase (TK) deficient, and which would not grow under conditions of inhibition of *de novo* DNA synthesis. These cells were exposed to DNA from herpes virus by the calcium phosphate technique and were then exposed to selective pressure by "HAT" medium which inhibits the *de novo* DNA synthesis but provides thymidine for DNA synthesis by the "salvage pathway". Any cell surviving in this medium is dependent upon the existence of the TK enzyme. What these investigators observed was that about one cell in a hundred thousand survived and began to proliferate to form a clone of cells. The clones were of variable stability. The important point was that the TK enzyme expressed in these cloned cells was always the viral-type enzyme rather than the human enzyme. In other words, under selective conditions, one cell in 10^5 to 10^6 cells had incorporated and expressed the viral gene and had a proliferative advantage over nontransformed cells.

One other concept is important in understanding gene transfer.

Although a selectable gene (a dominant selectable marker) is needed to introduce genetic information by low efficiency techniques, you can nevertheless simultaneously introduce other important genes which do not themselves provide a proliferative advantage. Insulin, beta globin, and growth hormone all come to mind as useful, but not selectable, genes. One either covalently links the non-selectable gene to the selectable gene or, in some cases, one can merely co-precipitate the two genes. With high efficiency, the genes are carried into the recipient cells together.

I would like to consider a particular system for introducing new genetic information into living animals. One of the objectives of our work was to introduce genes into the hematopoietic cells of mice with the ultimate aim of developing models for treating human genetic diseases of the bone marrow. The gene transfer system we decided upon involved a drug resistance gene with methotrexate (MTX) as the drug of interest. Methotrexate is an inhibitor of the enzyme dihydrofolate reductase (DHFR), a critical enzyme in folate and one carbon metabolism. DHFR is necessary for both DNA synthesis and synthesis of glycine. Inhibition of dihydrofolate reductase interrupts folate metabolism and stops DNA synthesis. We sought a source of genes for resistance to this drug and obtained several cell lines which grew at high concentrations of MTX. There are several mechanisms for resistance to this drug, a point which becomes important later in interpreting the results of our experiments. Cell lines can grow at high levels of methotrexate because: 1) they develop altered transport systems so that MTX no longer gets inside the cell to the active site of the enzyme; 2) they develop a mutant dihydrofolate reductase which no longer binds the drug; or, and most commonly, (3) they develop amplification or reduplication of the gene which codes for the enzyme that is inhibited. Normally, all higher animals have a single copy of the DHFR gene. When mouse or human cell lines grow in the presence of increasing concentrations of methotrexate, the cell line eventually becomes drug resistant. The typical mechanism of resistance is an increase in the number of copies of the DHFR gene. Instead of one copy, the cells may develop one hundred or even three hundred copies of the dihydrofolate reductase gene.

In seeking a source of drug resistance genes, we examined a variety of mouse and hamster cell lines which could grow at very high levels of methotrexate. We selected one for detailed study which continued to grow at 4×10^{-4} M methotrexate. This concentration is between one thousand and ten thousand times the concentration of drug that is used clinically and which will inhibit wild-type cells. Thus, the cells that provided the source of MTX-resistance genes are exceedingly drug resistant.

At the time we obtained this cell line from scientists at Stanford, it was thought that the principal mechanism of cellular resistance to MTX was based on a 30-fold amplification of the DHFR gene, with a corresponding 30-fold increase in the enzyme synthesis. As time would tell, this wasn't the whole story [1,3]. In addition to gene amplification, this cell line had a mutant dihydrofolate reductase with a reduced affinity for methotrexate. This mutation was to be critically important in the success of the transformation experiments in animals. In introducing drug resistance genes into hematopoietic cells, it is likely that genes are introduced at a low copy number. Therefore, if it is to be effective, the introduced gene had better code for an exceedingly effective drug resistant enzyme.

The evidence that this MTX-resistant cell line (3T6R1 cells) [1-4] contained a mutant dihydrofolate reductase can be briefly summarized. The isolated enzyme from wild-type MTX-sensitive cells is readily inhibited at increasing concentrations of methotrexate, and at about 10^{-8} M MTX the wild-type mouse enzyme is about 50 percent inhibited. DHFR enzyme from the resistant 3T6R1 cell line containing a mutant enzyme is highly resistant to the inhibitory effects of methotrexate and functions at 10^{-5} M drug concentration. The mutant DHFR has altered heat stability and electro- phoretic mobility [2,3].

To recapitulate, the source of drug resistance genes for our experiments was a mouse cell line which grows at very high levels of concentration of methotrexate which has amplification of the DHFR genes and also has mutant DHFR genes. Our target tissues for gene transfer in mice were hematopoietic cells. Why hematopoietic cells? Considering potential target organs in adult animals, there are very few tissues which maintain proliferating pools of stem cells throughout adult life. The bone marrow is one that does; skin and gut are others. Only the bone marrow has stem cells that are readily accessible and can be manipulated by gene transfer techniques. Furthermore, one would presume that if one were successful in introducing genes into the early precursor cells, then these genes would ultimately be expressed in all the mature differentiated cells of the blood system - the red cells, granulocytes, macrophages, and so forth. To date, genes have been introduced into intact animals in only two systems, the hematopoietic system and into mouse embryos. In the embryo system, fertilized embryos at the one cell stage have been injected with a variety of genes - interferon, thymidine kinase, and rabbit beta-globin. These embryos have been transferred to foster mothers and grown up to adult animals. In a reasonably high percentage of the cases they have retained the genes that have been injected at the one cell stage.

The CBA mouse was our test system [3,4]. It is a highly inbred strain of mouse which comes in two genetically identical varieties - the T6 variety, which contains a distinctive chromosome marker, and the Ca variety, which is genetically identical to the T6 but lacks the chromosomal marker. Otherwise, T6 and Ca can exchange skin grafts, marrow grafts, kidney grafts, and others. The T6 marker is an easily recognized chromosomal translocation. The reason for utilizing this animal in the initial experiments was the necessity for analyzing the success or failure of gene insertion by indirect means. We could introduce genes into bone marrow cells which were chromosomally marked and, after transfer of these cells to irradiated recipients, we could ask whether or not there was a predominance of the chromosomally marked cell in bone marrow population. The initial outline of the studies was reasonably straightforward [4]. Bone marrow was taken from T6 animals. The isolated bone marrow cells were in proliferative cycle and were exposed to DNA by the calcium phosphate technique. The DNA was obtained from the methotrexate resistant mouse 3T6R1 cell line. We presumed that perhaps one in one hundred thousand or one in a million of the marrow cells would incorporate the DNA containing drug resistance genes. Then the bone marrow was transferred to recipient animals of the same strain but which lacked the chromosomal marker (i.e., CBA/Ca mice). They had been irradiated to destroy their own bone marrow. The newly injected bone marrow then "homed" and began to proliferate to restore blood cell formation. During the time of proliferation, we exerted selective pressure by treating the animals with methotrexate with the expectation that we would inhibit proliferation of any cells which hadn't incorporated the MTX-resistance genes.

If we used the karyotype marker in marrow cells as evidence of transformation, then about 70% of the mice had evidence of gene expression [3,4]. Expression was time-dependent and would take about one month to appear after bone marrow injection. Expression required methotrexate selection. If we failed to treat the animals with methotrexate, then we did not observe the T6 karyotype dominance. The hematopoietic tissues of these animals were generally resistant to methotrexate and instead of observing the normal suppression of hematopoiesis (anemia, low white count), the transformed animals had normal marrow cellularity. In general, the karyotype of the transformed marrow, once established, was stable. Furthermore, the mutant DHFR of the methotrexate resistant cell line was expressed in the recipient mice - it was only expressed in hematopoietic tissues and was not expressed in other somatic tissues such as the liver. As one would anticipate, when a gene is placed into bone marrow cells, it stays there and is not transferred to other cells. Mice have now carried these mutant genes for periods of up to sixteen months - a significant portion of their life span. At the time of sacrifice, they were clinically well. At the time of autopsy, we detected no abnormalities. There were no obvious adverse side effects in several hundred mice.

Although we were successful with our studies utilizing a mutant dihydrofolate reductase gene, we were unsuccessful when we substituted DNA from methotrexate resistance cell lines which were resistant on the basis of amplification of the normal DHFR genes. This observation suggests that one probably transforms with only a very limited number of gene copies and that in order to be successful, the inserted genes must code for a highly drug resistant protein. Similar points have been observed in Bertino's laboratory, doing essentially identical experiments. Our preliminary conclusions on this are that one needs effective, probably mutant drug resistance genes to successfully achieve bone marrow transformation *in vivo*. For this reason, over the past many months we have set out to clone this mutant gene. Our strategy has been to isolate messenger RNA from the resistant 3T6R1 cell line which contains the mutant gene. The cDNA copies that were made from the mRNA clones containing the DHFR gene could be identified because the normal mouse dihydrofolate reductase cDNA probe was available to determine whether we were dealing with the mutant DHFR or wild-type DHFR in these clones.

We can put them into plasmids and into *E. coli* and then determine if the bacteria are resistant to trimethoprim (TMP). The bacterial dihydrofolate reductase is sensitive to TMP, whereas the mammalian enzyme is resistant. Therefore, any bacteria that can grow in TMP presumably have the mammalian enzyme. These bacteria can be grown up and then selected once more; this time at a very high level of methotrexate. Methotrexate doesn't get into bacteria cells very readily, but above 10^{-3} M does enter and does inhibit the bacterial enzyme. Therefore, any bacteria which could then grow at these very high levels of methotrexate can be presumed to have inserted copies of the mutant DHFR cDNA. Extracts can be made, and the isolated DHFR tested for its resistance to methotrexate. In this manner, one can clone and identify the mutant DHFR.

I would now like to return to the subject of the methods of gene insertion and describe one which I think will be of importance for the future. It involves what I would call encapsudated recombinant retroviruses. The retroviruses, as you know, are a class of RNA tumor viruses which, as part of their life cycle, reverse transcribed their RNA by viral enzymes to yield a DNA copy. This DNA transcript integrates into the DNA of the host genome. The DNA form, the virus , is called a provirus. Some of these retroviruses contain malignant transforming gene sequences, usually at the 3' end of the viral genome. For our purposes, these "oncogenes" can be eliminated. Because of this life history, the virus behaves as an insertion element. In theory at least, they are ideal vectors for introducing new genes into mammalian cells, provided certain conditions can be met. One must eliminate the malignant transforming region of the viral genome. Ideally a strategy should be devised for reducing viral replication within the target cell so that only a limited number of copies of virus are introduced. Drs. Shimotohno and Temin at the University of Wisconsin developed such a strategy utilizing the spleen necrosis virus (SNV) of chickens [5].

The engineered retrovirus is defective. It lacks much of the genetic information necessary for its replication. It is introduced into a permissive cell along with a helper virus. The permissive cell in this case is a chicken cell, which allows viral replication.

The recombinant virus and the helper virus complement each other and produce progeny. The important progeny viruses in this case are those which contain an introduced gene such as the TK gene of herpes virus. The SNV virus containing the TK insert is packaged by the chicken cells. This virus can then be introduced into a non-permissive cell, such as a rat cell, which does not permit viral replication. The recombinant virus enters and presumably integrates into host DNA, bringing with it the inserted TK gene. Now, how can we test this system to see if it really works?

This system of gene insertion is very efficient and nearly 100% of the rat cells can be transformed to TK^+ status. The potentialities of this type of system are, I think, enormous. If one had viruses with particular tissue tropism for muscle cells or neurologic tissues, one could, in theory, target genes to the specific tissues of interest. It then becomes conceivable to introduce new genes into the nervous system and into the muscle cells, as well as into bone marrow cells.

I would like to outline potential scenarios for treating genetic diseases of man. I shall take sickle cell as my model system. Sickle Cell Disease is a genetic disease based on a single nucleotide substitution in the beta-globin gene, resulting in a single amino acid substitution in the beta chain of globin. This substitution changes the physiology of the globin molecules so that they form a semi-crystalloid structure under reduced oxygen tensions. The crystalloid distorts the shape of the red cells from normal biconcave discs to sickled cells, and makes these cells relatively inflexible. When the sickled cells attempt to traverse the microcirculation, they do not bend and fold as do normal red cells. They become impacted and obstruct the microcirculation, depriving the tissues of oxygen so that they die. A vicious cycle ensues - reduced blood flow, more oxygen deprivation, more sickling, more obstruction - which result in the death of tissues in the kidney, brain, lung, and bone. These result in the typical crises and infarcts of sickle cell disease. This is a genetic disease in which a single base substitution in DNA results in this very complex clinical syndrome with a great deal of morbidity and early death. Can one conceive of correcting such a disorder? I shall present some alternative strategies.

One strategy would be to remove a small amount of the patient's own bone marrow and insert normal globin genes into these cells. One could use one of the techniques which I have described, for example, the calcium phosphate technique. In this strategy, one would presumably have to introduce a selectable gene, such as a drug resistance gene as well as a normally functioning, but non-selectable, beta-globin gene. The marrow containing a few transformed cells would then be reinfused. In some circumstances, some of the cells would home to the marrow and begin proliferating. During that period of time, one would exert selective pressure in the form of a drug, favoring those cells which had incorporated the new genes. If one had designed the beta-globin gene correctly, one would achieve gene expression and normal beta-globin production. One can develop a long list of genetic diseases of the bone marrow which should, in theory, be approachable by this type of technique.

In a different scenario, one might use an engineered retrovirus to introduce the beta-globin gene into bone marrow cells *in vitro*. The beta-globin gene would presumably be in a form where it had a promoter and would be expressed in a high proportion of the target cells. This is a much simpler strategy than our first scenario and does not require any selective pressure in the form of drugs.

A question often asked is how one is going to control the expression of newly inserted genes. Several strategies are being considered at the present time. The most commonly considered strategy is to insert, upstream of the gene of interest, a hormone responsive gene sequence. Such sequences have already been cloned from mouse mammary tumor viruses. Then, when transformed cells are exposed to steroids, the rate of production of messenger RNA of the insert is increased 6- to 10-fold. When steroid exposure is stopped, transcription falls again to baseline levels. This is one way of switching a gene on and then switching it off.

REFERENCES

1. Cline, M.J. Genetic engineering of mammalian cells: Its potential application to genetic diseases of man. J. Lab. Clin. Med. 99:299-308 (1982).
2. Salser, W., B.D.Tong, H.D. Stang, J. Browne, K. Mercola, M. Bar-Eli, and M.J. Cline. Gene therapy techniques: Use of drug resistance selections in intact animals to insert human globin genes into bone marrow cells in living mice. In Molecular Mechanisms of Hemoglobin Switching (G. Stamatoyannopoulos and A.W. Nienhuis, Eds.) New York, Grune & Stratton (1981).
3. Bar-Eli, M., K.E. Mercola, D.J. Slamon, N. Mauritzson, H.D. Stang, and M.J. Cline. Insertion of drug resistance genes in animals. J. Cell. Physiol. (suppl.) 1:213-217 (1982).
4. Cline, M.J., H. Stang, K.E. Mercola, L. Morse, R. Ruprecht, J. Browne, and W. Salser. Gene transfer in intact animals. Nature 284:422-425 (1980).
5. Shimotohno, K., and H. Temin. Formation of infectious progeny virus after insertion of herpes simplex thymidine kinase gene into DNA of an avian retrovirus. Cell 26:67-77 (1981).

DISCUSSION

Q. HATCHER: The LTR flanking sequences of retroviruses have recently been implicated in the induction of leukemias via the same mechanism that led to high expression of the retrovirus genes. What kind of precautions would be necessary in using retrovirus vectors for the introduction of genes to make sure that yet a different type of disease is not created in patients?

A. CLINE: You are referring to some interesting studies using retroviruses which themselves do not contain malignant transforming sequences, but which will cause malignancy in animals over a relatively long period of time rather than a short period of time. It is now known how retroviruses cause malignancy. Probably the retroviruses go through cycles of replication and reinsertion so that they keep inserting at various places in the host genome. And occasionally, fortuitously, one eventually inserts near a so-called "oncogene" of the host cell. All humans and other higher vertebrates have oncogenes in their genome. So the fortuitous insertion of the virus, usually upstream of an oncogene, will turn it on. The gene which is normally silent in adult life will then be activated and induce malignancy. Accordingly, induction of malignancy by retroviruses, as best we know, requires rounds of viral replication, insertion, replication, and insertion. In the model system I suggested earlier, we don't go through those rounds of replication. In fact, the host cell only gets 1 to less than 10 viral units inserting. The chance that a virus will randomly insert near one of the sixteen known vertebrate oncogenes is relatively small. So, statistically, the chance of causing malignancy is very small. But, obviously there has to be caution in the use of this system. Both cell lines and animals will have to be observed for a long period of time. The thinking of people who work in this field is that this mechanism should, in fact, be no more hazardous than DNA mediated gene transfer. Indeed, anytime we introduce a new piece of DNA into the host genome, there is the potential for introducing a promoter which may turn on a host oncogene. I believe we're just going to have to see what happens over the next few years in these experimental model systems.

Q. In thinking along the same lines, have you considered targeting your DNA sequences to specific areas in the chromatin?

A. CLINE: Yes. I have thought, "Wouldn't it be nice to heal a lesion rather than to replace it." If one could get site-specific recombinations, one could bring in, just to the beta-globin gene of sickle cell disease, the corrected sequence and then the recombinational events would change the gene from the mutant to the norm. The evidence that exists suggests that in a genome as complex as that of higher vertebrates, we are unlikely to get site-specific recombination. In much simpler systems, it hasn't worked. Thus, unless somebody comes up with a really new strategy for healing a gene defect, I don't think it's going to work. But, a new strategy might come along that we haven't thought of as yet.

Q. STARLINGER: You mentioned that you estimate that anywhere from 1 and 10 copies were inserted. Do you foresee any problems with gene dosage effects, especially in terms of trying to regulate some enzyme that hypothetically could be in too high amounts; or perhaps a gene expressed inappropriately could cause more harm than good?

A. CLINE: Yes. In some cases there may be problems. For example, the thinking is that in the case of the thymidine kinase system, too many working thymidine kinase genes would be lethal for the cell. It's probably a rare event though. In something like the dihydrofolate reductase system, a cell can clearly function with less than 5% of the normal amount of enzymes, and it can also function with some 300 times the normal amount of enzyme. So, that system will be less sensitive to gene dosage effects. As for beta-globin, there might be an interesting story. We clearly would not want a neuron making a lot of beta-globin. But, if we use a technique which will restrict the beta-globin gene to the bone marrow cells, I don't think that should become a problem. I think the major hurdle now is getting high enough levels of gene expression to achieve what we want. Presently, we are not dealing with the problem of overproduction. It may eventually become important in some cell types.

MONOCLONAL ANTIBODY FOR THE PROTECTION OF NEONATAL PIGS AND CALVES FROM TOXIC DIARRHEA

P.L. Sadowski, S.D. Acres[1], and D.M. Sherman[2]
Molecular Genetics, Inc.
Minnetonka, Minnesota 55343

Monoclonal antibody technology, which allows the unlimited production of an antibody with a very defined specificity, has resulted in a renewed interest in passive immunization as a treatment alternative for disease. However, to date, the widespread implementation of monoclonal antibodies for prophylactic or therapeutic use has not occurred. Because of the acceptance of passive immunization in animal health care as can be demonstrated from the sale of conventional antisera for such use, we were encouraged that monoclonal antibodies could find significant use in veterinary health care.

Our attention has focused on a diarrheal disease of newborn calves caused by enterotoxigenic Escherichia coli (ETEC). This disease is the result of the noninvasive colonization of the small intestine of calves by toxigenic E. coli. The susceptibility to the disease is age-dependent, affecting only newborn animals, and vulnerability decreases markedly after 48 hours of life [17]. This

[1]Veterinary Infectious Disease Organization, University of Saskatchewan, Saskatoon, Saskatchewan; [2]Department of Large Animal Clinical Sciences, College of Veterinary Medicine, University of Minnesota, St. Paul, Minnesota.

sensitivity of neonatal animals correlates with the ability of E. coli to only adhere to intestinal epithelial cells from newborn pigs, calves, and mice [16]. These E. coli adhesins which are known as fimbriae or pili, have been characterized from isolates obtained from pigs, cows, and humans [5]. Pili found on enteropathogenic E. coli of bovine origin are of the K99 type in 76-95% of the isolates [7,12,13]. E. coli K99(+) strains would adhere to intestinal epithelial cells and E. coli which differed only in their lack of pili failed to adhere [10]. Growth of ETEC strains under conditions unfavorable for pilus expression resulted in the failure of the E. coli to bind to calf brush border preparations [3]. Thus, the ability to adhere and resist the purging action of mucus and peristalsis appears to be at least as significant as toxigenicity to the virulence of the E. coli.

A protective immune response has been induced in cows using bacterin vaccines [1,14]. A high degree of correlation was found to exist between anti-K99 colostral titers and the survival of colostrum-fed calves challenged by homologous and heterologous K99(+) ETEC. A similar protective immune response was produced by vaccinating the dam with purified pili [1].

Commercial bacterins which elicit anti-K99 colostral antibody responses in the vaccinate are effective in the protection of neonatal calves from death due to ETEC. These products, though efficacious, have several significant drawbacks. Vaccination of the dams must be done twice within a defined time frame prior to parturition. The disease must be anticipated, as vaccination during calving will not result in protective antibody being stimulated in the dam fast enough to save compromised calves. Additionally, alternate means of therapy are expensive and of limited efficacy. The availability of serum containing anti-K99 antibody which could be fed to newborn calves would overcome several of the shortcomings attributed to the vaccines. Such a passive antibody produced in cows has been demonstrated to be effective in protecting neonatal calves from a challenge by enteropathogenic K99(+) *E. coli* [18].

The object of this research was to produce monoclonal antibodies to the K99 pilus, and then determine the efficacy of orally administered monoclonal antibody in protecting calves from death due to enteropathogenic K99(+) *E. coli*.

Purified K99 pilus protein was used to immunize Balb/c mice [9]. Spleen cells from hyperimmunized mice were fused with a P3-NS-1-Ag 4/1 plasmacytoma [11] by a modification of the method of Gefter *et al*. [6]. Hybridomas producing antibody reacting with the K99 pilus were identified by using an enzyme-linked immunosorbent assay [19]. One of the hybridomas which produced 10-20 mg/ml of immunoglobulin when grown as an ascites tumor in Balb/c mice was chosen for further characterization.

The cross reactivity of the monoclonal antibody with other *E. coli* components or pili was assessed by simple agglutination reactions [15]. As can be seen in Table 1, The monoclonal antibody will agglutinate the K99 prototype strain B44 [12]. The failure to

Table 1

Agglutination of Piliated *E. coli* By a K99-specific Monoclonal Antibody

Strain	Growth Temperature	Agglutination Titer
B44 (Wilson)	37°C	1/8000
	18°C	<1/10
B44 (Acres)	37°C	1/8000
	18°C	<1/10
1751 (Moon)	37°C	<1/10
$K88^+$ (UM)	37°C	<1/10
$987P^+$ (UM)	37°C	<1/10

agglutinate E. coli B44 grown at 18°C under which conditions the pilus is not produced [3] suggested that the agglutination of the K99(+) E. coli was due solely to antibody reacting with the pilus. The K99 monoclonal antibody failed to agglutinate E. coli strains expressing K88, 987P, and the F41 pilus on strain 1751 [2; Harley Moon, personal communication].

To further analyze the specificity of the K99-reactive monoclonal antibody, ^{35}S-methionine labelled extracts of E. coli were immunoprecipitated and the polypeptides analyzed by SDS-PAGE electrophoresis [4,8]. A single polypeptide consistent with the subunit size of 18,500 daltons reported for the K99 pilus [5] was precipitated from the K99(+) E. coli prototype strains B44 and B41 [12] by

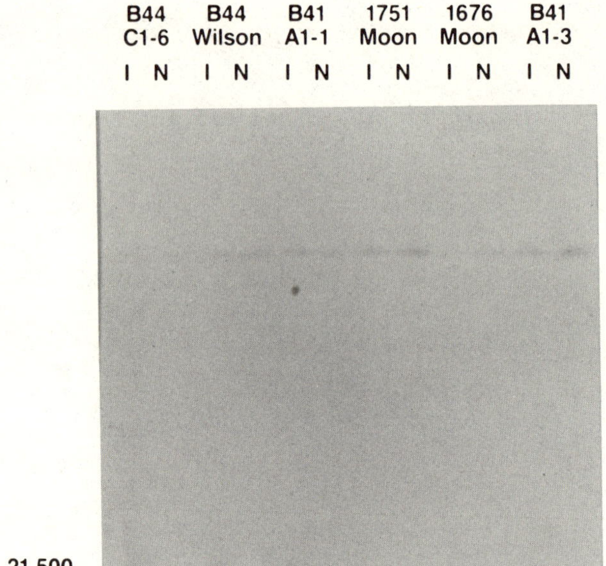

Fig. 1. Proteins in E. coliI immunoprecipitable by a monocolonal antibody reactive with the K99 pilus.

the K99-reactive monoclonal antibody (Lane I). A monoclonal antibody against a heterologous protein failed to precipitate any polypeptides from those lysates (Lane N). The K99 monoclonal failed to immunoprecipitate any polypeptides from lysates of *E. coli* strains 1676 and 1751 which are F41(+).

The ability of this K99-specific monoclonal antibody to protect newborn pigs and calves from death due to enteropathogenic K99(+) *E. coli* was determined. Colostrum deprived, cesarean derived piglets were obtained one day prior to parturition. These piglets were fed 100 mg of monoclonal antibody and challenged with 1×10^{10} viable strain B41 *E. coli* within four hours of birth. As can be seen in Table 2, 11 out of the 14 (79%) piglets receiving the K99-specific monoclonal antibody survived the challenge in contrast to 2 out of 10 survivors in the unprotected group ($0.001 > P > 0.005$, by Chi-squared analysis). Similarly, newborn calves protectd by oral administration of 20 mg of monoclonal antibody within the first 12 hours of birth survived a strain B44 *E. coli* challenge of 2.6×10^{10} viable organisms (Table 3). Six out of seven protected calves (86%)

Table 2

Protection of Newborn Pigs by the Oral Administration of K99-Specific Monoclonal Antibody

Trial Group	Pigs	
	Alive	Dead
Monoclonal antibody	11	3
Placebo	2	8

Table 3

Protection of Newborn Calves by the Oral Administration of a K99-Specific Monoclonal Antibody

Trial Group	Calves	
	Alive	Dead
Monoclonal antibody	6	1
Placebo	2	6

survived as compared with 2 out of 8 survivors in the unprotected group (0.05 > P > 0.01, by Chi-squared analysis).

In summary, a monoclonal antibody reactive with the K99 pilus protein and not crossreactive with any other *E. coli* components has been shown to be efficacious in protecting neonatal animals from death due to enteropathogenic K99(+) *E. coli*. This antibody is effective when administered orally, and establishes the importance of *E. coli* adhesins to pathogenicity in the intestinal tract.

ACKNOWLEDGEMENTS

We wish to thank Dr. R. Isaacson for providing us with the K99-pilus protein. We thank Dr. R. Wilson, and Dr. H. Moon for providing us with bacterial strains.

REFERENCES

1. Acres, A.D., R.E. Isaacson, L.A. Babiuk, and R.A. Kapitany (1979) *Infect. Immun.* 25:121.
2. Awad-Masalmeh, M., H.W. Moon, P.L. Runnels, and R.W. Schneider (1982). *Infect. Immun.* 35:305.

3. Burrows, M.R., R. Sellwood, and R.A. Gibbons (1976). J. Gen. Microbiol. 96:269.

4. Collett, M.S., and R.L. Erikson (1976). Proc. Natl. Acad. Sci. 75:2021.

5. Gaastra, W., and F.K. de Graaf (1982). Microbiol. Rev. 46:129.

6. Gefter, M.L., D.H. Margulies, and M.D. Scharff (1977). Somat. Cell Genet. 3:231.

7. Guinée, P.A.M., W.H. Jansen, and C.M. Agterberg (1976). Infect. Immun. 13:1369.

8. Horwich, A., A.H. Koop, and W. Eckhart (1980). J. Virol. 36:125.

9. Isaacson, R.E. (1977). Infect. Immun. 15:272.

10. Isaacson, R.E., P.C. Fusco, P.C. Brinton, and H.W. Moon (1978). Infect. Immun. 21:392.

11. Kohler, G., and C. Milstein (1976). Europ. J. Immunol. 6:511.

12. Moon, H.W., S.C. Whipp, and S.M. Skartvedt (1976). Am. J. Vet. Res. 37:1025.

13. Myers, L.L., and P.A.M. Guinée (1976). Infect. Immun. 13:1117.

14. Myers, L.L. (1978). Am. J. Vet. Res. 39:761.

15. Nichols, W.S. and R.M. Nakamura (1980). In Manual of Clinical Immunology (N. Rose and H. Friedman, eds.). p 15. Amer. Soc. Microbiol., Washington, D.C.

16. Runnels, P.L., H.W. Moon, and R.A. Schneider (1980). Infect. Immun. 28:298.

17. Smith, H.W., and Halls, S. (1967). J. Pathol. Bacteriol. 93:499.

18. Trainin, Z., J. Brenner, R. Meirom, I. Kornitzer, R. Tamarin, and A. Cohen (1980). "Oral Immunization of Young Calves Against Enteropathogenic E. coli with Immunocol." Presented at, The 11th International Cattle Disease Symposium.

19. Voller, A., D. Bidwell, and A. Bartlett (1980). In Manual of Clinical Immunology (N. Rose and H. Friedman, eds.) p 359. Amer. Soc. Microbiol., Washington, D.C.

MONOCLONAL ANTIBODIES AS PHYSIOLOGIC PROBES

M. Mudgett-Hunter[*2], G.P. Budzik[**3], P.K. Donahoe[**], B.A. Khaw[*], M.N. Margolies, E.C. Ridgeway[+], and E. Haber[*1]

[*]Cardiac Unit, [**]Pediatric Surgical Unit, and [+]Thyroid Unit, Massachusetts General Hospital and Harvard Medical School, Boston, Massachusetts 02114

INTRODUCTION

Clinicians and research scientists alike have for years utilized the immune response to generate antibodies to probe physiologic and biochemical systems. Polyclonal antibody found in the course of the humoral response to an antigen may detect, quantify, and localize small amounts of material in complex mixtures. Were it not for the heterogeneity and unpredictability of the immune reponse, immunologic assays might have had an even greater application. With the introduction of somatic cell fusion most of the

[1]This work was supported by NIH grant HL-19529, NCI grant #CA-17393, USPH grant AM-16791, and the Specialized Center for Research in Ischemic Heart Disease grant #HL-26215. [2] Dr. Mudgett-Hunter is a recipient of Established Investigator Award #79-189 from the American Heart Association. [3] Dr. Budzik is a recipient of the Charles A. King Trust Fellowship, Medical Research Foundation.

problems associated with polyclonal antisera and their application to basic and clinical questions are likely to be overcome.

Antiserum obtained from an immunized animal is a heterogeneous mixture containing many antibodies each with a different affinity for various antigenic determinants. Due to the complexity and dynamic nature of the immune response, each antiserum or bleed differs from the other, even if it is obtained from the same animal.

In 1975 Kohler and Milstein [1] demonstrated that somatic cell fusion could be used to establish continuous cell cultures actively secreting specific antibody. The antibody produced by these cell cultures or hybridomas are fundamentally different from conventional antisera obtained from immunized animals. Each cell line synthesizes and secretes a homogeneous, or monoclonal, antibody which represents only one of the many immunoglobulins produced by the immunized animal. Hybridoma cell lines represent a distinct advantage over antisera in that they may be frozen, later to be thawed and injected into animals, where, like their parental myelomas, they produce ascites. In this manner large amounts of homogeneous antibody can be obtained from the ascites produced. Thus hybridomas provide a potentially unlimited supply of a well-characterized antibody for an indefinite period of time [2].

Prior to their use in various assay systems, traditional antisera often had to be extensively adsorbed with antigens of other specificity in order to prevent unwanted cross reactions. Since a monoclonal antibody is a uniform molecular species, this strategy cannot be applied. Any antigen that reacts will simply result in the removal of all immunoglobulin molecules which are present as a homogeneous population. However, by selection of the appropriate monoclonal antibody the desired range of cross reactivity can be specified. Shared specificities may imply shared structural determinants and cross reactivities may imply functional and evolutionary relationships among macromolecules. Conversely, the capability of selecting a monoclonal antibody for its monospecificity or lack of cross reactivity towards other antigens likewise is a powerful feature of the hybridoma technique. In this case the monoclonal antibody recognizes a unique determinant not found on other macromolecules.

Another distinct advantage of the hybridoma technique is the ability to generate and select for antibody specific for one component of an impure antigen preparation used for immunization. Screening techniques are then designed to select the hybridoma specific for only one of the components. This capability enormously extends the range of antigens for which immunological reagents may be prepared and makes it possible to purify a single antigen from a mixture.

In this paper we review a few applications of monoclonal antibodies and illustrate certain advantages of hybridomas over conventional antisera.

Monoclonal Antibodies Specific for the Drug Digoxin

Digoxin is the drug most often prescribed for patients with congestive heart failure. It is one of a large group of cardiac glycosides each of which are composed of a steroid or aglycone portion and from one to four sugar residues. The pharmacological activity resides in the aglycone portion of the molecule; the attached glycoside residues modify water solubility and potency [3]. One of the important pharmacodynamic properties of cardiac glycosides is to increase the force of myocardial contraction.

Since digoxin intoxication is one of the most prevalent drug reactions encountered in clinical practice [4], high-affinity, anti-digoxin antibodies have been useful in the management of these

Structure 1:

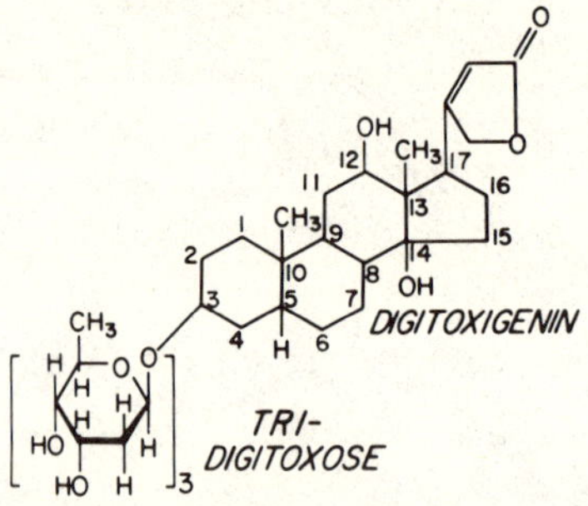

DIGOXIN

patients. Digoxin intoxication frequently occurs because of the narrow margin between therapeutic and toxic doses of digoxin and related cardiac glycosides. Consequently, patients undergoing treatment with digoxin must be closely monitored for levels of circulating digoxin. The production of high-affinity, polyclonal, anti-digoxin antibody has allowed for the detection of digitalis glycosides in serum at subnanogram amounts by radioimmunoassay (RIA) [5]. It would be desirable to obtain an unlimited supply of high-affinity, monoclonal, anti-digoxin antibody with defined specificity.

Using digoxin-protein conjugates as antigen and the somatic cell fusion technique, we have produced several high-affinity, anti-digoxin, monoclonal antibodies (hybridomas). Briefly, spleen cells from A/J mice immunized with digoxin covalently coupled to human serum albumin (Dig-HSA) were fused with either NS-1 (Fusion 25 only) or SP2/0 murine myeloma cell lines (all subsequent fusions) as previously described [6].

Antibody production of subcloned anti-digoxin, monoclonal hybridoma cell lines was augmented in ascites form and anti-digoxin antibody was purified from ascites by affinity chromatography as described previously [6].

Table 1

Monoclonal Anti-digoxin Antibodies

Monoclonal Antibody	H-chain Isotype	Affinity K_0 $(M^{-1})^a$ K_0	S.E.	Specificity
Dig 25-54	γ_1	1.3×10^8	0.4×10^8	digoxigenin/digitoxigenin
Dig 26-10	γ_{2a}	6.9×10^9	0.6×10^9	digoxigenin/digitoxigenin
Dig 35-20	γ_1	1.9×10^9	0.9×10^9	digoxigenin/digitoxigenin
Dig 40-020	γ_1	3.5×10^9	1.4×10^9	digitoxose
Dig 40-040	γ_1	7.5×10^9	0.2×10^9	n.d.[b]
Dig 40-050	γ_{2b}	5.7×10^8	0.9×10^8	n.d.
Dig 40-120	γ_{2a}	4.0×10^9	0.6×10^9	digitoxose

[a]Affinity (K_0) and standard deviations were determined as described previously [6]. [b] n.d.= not done.

The characteristics of seven different monoclonal, anti-digoxin antibodies obtained from such fusions are summarized in Table 1. When assayed for murine H-chain isotypes [6], four monoclonal antibodies had the $\gamma 1$ H-chain isotype, two were the $\gamma 2a$ isotype and one was the $\gamma 2b$ isotype. Average intrinsic association constants (K_0) were determined for each monoclonal, anti-digoxin antibody, using a dextran-coated charcoal binding method for separation of antibody bound from free [^{3}H]digoxin [7]. The data were plotted according to a modified Sips equation [8]. As seen in Table 1, all seven monoclonal anti-digoxin antibodies were found to have relatively high association constants (K_0) (10^8 to 10^9 M^{-1}). Two hybridoma antibodies, Dig 25-54 (K_0 1.3×10^8 M^{-1}) and Dig 40-050 ($K_0 = 5.7 \times 10^8$ M^{-1}), had affinities about an order of magnitude less than the other five. Among these five, the K_0s ranged from 1.9×10^9 to 7.5×10^9 M^{-1}. It is striking that all monoclonal anti-digoxin antibodies characterized to date have high affinities. Since pooled A/J polyclonal, anti-digoxin antibody was also found to have a K_0 of 3×10^9

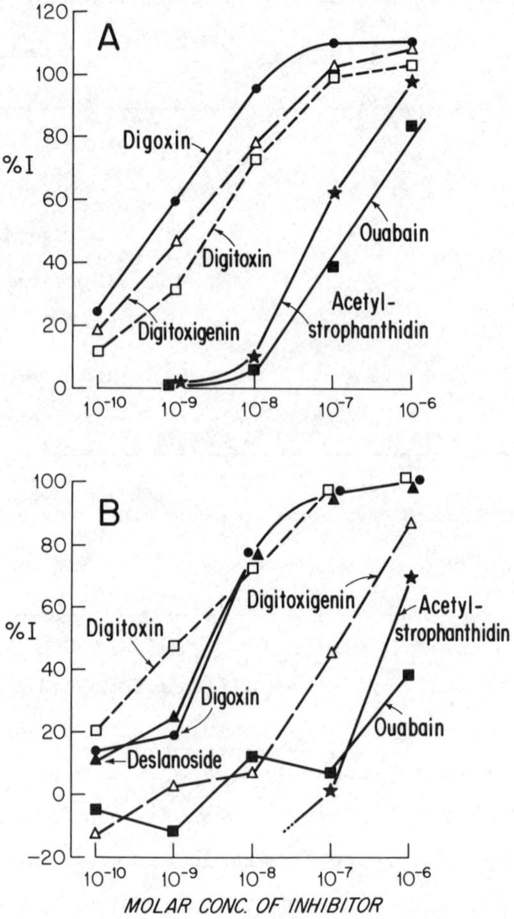

Fig. 1. Inhibition of binding of monoclonal antibody to [^{3}H]-digoxin in the dextran-coated charcoal RIA by various cardic glysosides: digoxin (●), digitoxin (□), digitoxigenin (Δ), deslanoside (▲), acetylstrophanthidin (★), ouabain (■). No inhibition was found for endogenous steroids: cholesterol, testosterone, 17-beta-estradiol, progesterone, cortisol, and 4-androsterone (data not shown). Specificity patterns are shown for two monoclonal anti-digoxin antibodies: Panel A, Dig 35-20, Panel B, Dig 40-120.

M^{-1} [6], it is possible that high-affinity antibodies predominate in the A/J immune response to the digoxin hapten.

A series of monoclonal antibodies reactive toward a well-defined hapten provides a unique model system for probing the fine specificity of an antibody combining site. Digoxin is an ideal hapten because of its rigid steroid backbone structure which is resistant to conformational changes as various functional groups are substituted at various positions on the four-ring structure. Moreover, digoxin and related cardiac glycosides correspond in size to adequately fill the antibody combining site [6]. In an attempt to assess their antigen specificity, each monoclonal antibody was further characterized for its relative affinity for various cardiac glycoside analogs.

Using the dextran-coated charcoal RIA, the binding of monoclonal antibody to [^{3}H]digoxin was inhibited by unlabeled digoxin and related cardiac glycosides such as digitoxigenin, deslanoside, acetylstrophanthidin, and ouabain [6]. Examples of the inhibition profiles obtained are shown in Figure 1, in which the profile for monoclonal antibody Dig 35-20 (panel A) is compared to that obtained for monoclonal antibody Dig 40-120 (panel B). The binding of both antibodies to [^{3}H]digoxin was inhibited equally well by unlabeled digoxin and digitoxin which differ only by a single hydroxyl group present on Carbon 12 of the digoxin steroid-ring structure, but absent in digitoxin (see Structure 1, above). Relative to digoxin, both antibodies are much less reactive to acetylstrophanthidin and ouabain by at least a factor of 100. Ouabain and acetylstrophanthidin differ significantly in the number and nature of the functional groups substituted in rings A and B of the steroid backbone. They also differ in the nature of the attached sugar molecules. In place of the three digitoxose sugars present in digoxin there is one residue of rhamnose in ouabain. In acetylstrophanthidin, the sugar residues are replaced by an acetyl group at C3. Based on this evidence alone, specificity of these two antibodies could be directed to either the digitoxose residues or digoxigenin moieties of digoxin (See Structure 1). The reactivities of these two antibodies, however, differ significantly towards digitoxigenin, the aglycone portion of digitoxin. Since the binding of antibody Dig 35-20 to [^{3}H]digoxin (panel A, Figure 1) is inhibited to the same extent by unlabeled digoxin, digitoxin and digitoxigenin, but to a much lesser extent by acetylstrophanthidin and ouabain, the specificity of this antibody must reside in the aglycone portion of digoxin. On the other hand, Dig 40-120 exhibits a much-reduced affinity to digitoxigenin relative to digoxin and digitoxin (data not shown). Since digitoxigenin, acetylstrophanthidin, and ouabain differ from digoxin and digitoxin either by the absence of sugar (digitoxigenin and acetylstrophanthidin) or presence of a different sugar (rhamnose in ouabain), then digitoxose must be significantly involved in the binding recognition of Dig 40-120. Monoclonal antibodies Dig 25-54 and Dig 26-10 exhibited inhibition profiles similar to Dig 35-20 (see Table 2), and, hence, share a specificity for the aglycone portion of the digoxin. Monoclonal antibody Dig 40-020 was found to have an inhibition profile similar to Dig 40-120 and, hence, is also directed towards the digitoxose moiety of digoxin.

These studies illustrate the utility of monoclonal antibodies in dissecting the fine specificity of a combining site for antigen. Each anti-digoxin antibody thus far analyzed is unique by several criteria including H-chain isotype, isoelectric focusing, affinity determination, partial amino acid sequence of both H and L chains [ref. 9; Margolies, M.N., unpublished data]. Furthermore, since no two antibodies have identical specificity or inhibition patterns (Fig. 1), no two antibodies bind digoxin in exactly the same manner. Although digoxin is a relatively simple antigen, the variation with which an antibody may bind to digoxin is further testimony to the diversity of the immune response. The dissection of this diversity

Table 2

Clinical Assay for Digoxin Using Monoclonal Anti-digoxin Antibody[a]

Anti-digoxin Antibody	Sheep Antisera	Dig 26-10	Dig 35-20
	Digoxin/ml sera		
	ng/ml	ng/ml	ng/ml
Patient Number			
4601	2.8	2.6	n.d.
4615	0.8	0.8	n.d.
5884	1.6	1.6	n.d.
9708	4.8	5.4	6.0
9717	2.3	2.1	1.9
9761	1.5	n.d.	1.6
2020	3.4	3.8	3.5
2045	0.6	0.3	0.8

[a]Monoclonal antibodies Dig 26-10 and Dig 35-20 were compared to the sheep anti-digoxin sera for their ability to quantitate digoxin in patients' sera in a [^{3}H]digoxin-RIA, as previously described [6].

[b]n.d.=not done.

was made possible by the availability of a large set of monoclonal antibodies.

Two monoclonal antibodies possessed sufficient affinity and specificity for digoxin to be useful in a clinical RIA for determining serum digoxin levels. The results of the RIA [5] which utilized either sheep anti-digoxin sera or hybridomas Dig 26-10 and Dig 35-20 as anti-digoxin antibody to detect digoxin levels in sera from eight patients is shown in Table 2. Both monoclonal anti-digoxin antibodies detected levels of digoxin in human serum samples comparable to that detected by a polyclonal sheep antiserum. Thus, monoclonal anti-digoxin antibodies are useful reagents in a clinical RIA used to monitor patients undergoing digitalis treatment, particularly as they promise to be available in unlimited supply with unaltered specificity.

Although frequent determination of digoxin serum levels has reduced the incidence of digoxin intoxication, management of patients with acute digoxin intoxication remains a major clinical problem. Since one of the mechanisms of action of cardiac glycosides is the inhibition of the membrane sodium-potassium ATPase system [10], it was thought that antibodies directed to digoxin could compete with the digoxin receptor for digoxin and reverse its biological effect. In fact, reversal of cardiac glycoside effects by specific antibody has been demonstrated in several systems including: *in vitro* erythrocyte cation transport, isolated Purkinje fibers, atrioventricular-node preparations, isolated papillary muscles and atrial strips [10]. Established digoxin-induced ventricular tachycardia in intact dogs was reversed upon the administration of polyclonal sheep anti-digoxin antibody and Fab derived from it. Recently, Fab prepared from affinity-purified sheep antidigoxin antibodies have been successfully used to rescue several patients from severe digoxin intoxication resulting from an overdose of digoxin [11,12]. For example, sheep anti-digoxin Fab successfully reversed intoxication in an otherwise lethal overdose in a 39-year-old male who took 90 0.25-mg digoxin tablets with suicidal intent [11]. Monoclonal anti-digoxin antibodies with K_0s of 10^9 or greater should be useful as therapeutic reagents for the reversal of digoxin intoxication. One monoclonal anti-digoxin antibody, Dig 26-10, is currently undergoing tests for its ability to reverse established digoxin intoxication in animal models. Digoxin intoxication was experimentally induced in cats by intravenous administration of 0.15-0.20 mg digoxin per kg. Following an IV injection of one-fold stoichiometric excess of monoclonal anti-digoxin antibody Dig 26-10, digoxin-induced sustained ventricular tachycardia was rapidly reversed in 2 out of 3 cats. Equivalent amounts of normal mouse IgG, however, did not reverse digoxin intoxication in this model system [13]. The ability of Fab prepared from Dig 26-10 to reverse digoxin intoxication in a guinea pig model system is also being tested (Smith, T., unpublished results). The ability of Fab to neutralize the deleterious effects of an exogenous drug provides impetus for the production of monoclonal antibodies specific for other drugs and toxins for which there is no known antidote. Since the production of large quantities of ascites is relatively simple and preparation of Fab straightforward, the commercial development and production of monoclonal Fab as therapeutic or detoxifying drugs is particularly attractive.

In summary, the anti-digoxin hybridoma system illustrates three important applications of monoclonal antibodies. First, a series of different monoclonal antibodies to a simple hapten can serve as a model system for studying the fine specificity of the antigen-antibody combining site. Second, high-affinity monoclonal antibody can serve as a reliable reagent in a clinical assay for the determination of drug levels such as digoxin in patients' sera. Finally, Fab prepared from monoclonal anti-digoxin antibody may serve as a therapeutic drug for the reversal of digoxin intoxication.

Monoclonal Antibody in Search of the Fetal Regressor, Mullerian Inhibiting Substance (MIS)

Mullerian inhibiting substance (MIS) is an embryonic regulator which is secreted by the embryonic testis and is essential to male differentiation. MIS causes the regression of the Mullerian duct [14-16] which, in the female, develops into the fallopian tubes, uterus, and vagina. Cancers derived from these organs histologigically resemble tissue obtained from the Mullerian duct. When fractions containing biologically active MIS were incubated with human ovarian cancer cells, a significant cytotoxicity index was obtained [17-19]. This effect was not observed when these MIS-containing fractions were tested against human glioblastoma or fibroblast lines [17]. Monoclonal antibodies to MIS might thus serve as a probe in the study of the cytotoxic effect MIS has on ovarian and other cancerous tumors.

Efforts to purify MIS have been extremely difficult. In spite of a 30,000-fold purification following affinity chromatography on Matrex-gel-Green A (Amicon) [20], fractions containing biologically active MIS remain a complex mixture of proteins when analyzed by SDS gel electrophoresis (Budzik, G.P, unpublished observations). Antibody specific for MIS would be useful in the purification and study of this embryonic hormone. However, the impurity of the MIS-containing preparation prohibits the production of traditional polyclonal antisera. Antibody with the requisite specificity might be obtained, however, by technique of somatic cell fusion in spite of the impurity of the immunizing antigen. The successful production of monoclonal anti-MIS antibodies by the hybridoma technique has recently been reported [21].

Hybridoma IVA6 was the product of a fusion between spleen cells from BALB/c mice immunized with a crude MIS preparation (approximately 1% MIS) and the NS-1 myeloma cells as previously described [21]. On subcloning, IVA6, monoclonal hybridoma IIIB3, which secreted antibody directed against crude MIS, was identified and expanded in the ascites form.

Specificity of antibody IIIB3 for MIS was assessed by both an RIA [21] and by an organ culture assay [22]. In a solid-phase RIA, several proteins were tested for their ability to inhibit the binding of IIIB3 to an MIS preparation. Bound IIIB3 was detected by ^{125}I-goat antimouse IgG_1 as previously described [21]. As seen in Table 3, MIS preparation Green 2, which contained biologically

Table 3

Cross-reactivity of Monoclonal anti-MIS Antibody IIIB3[a]

Inhibitor	Protein Concentration mg/ml	Maximum % Inhibition
MIS (Green 1)	0.98	21
MIS (Green 2)	0.11	65
Myoglobin	1.0	10
Insulin	1.0	3
Hemocyanin-Digoxin	1.0	25
Horse serum	1%	0

[a]Cross reactivity of monoclonal anti-MIS antibody was determined by inhibition of binding of antibody IIIB3 to MIS preparation (Green 2). Bound IIIB3 was detected with ^{125}I-goat-antimouse IgG, as previously described [21].

active MIS, resulted in 65% inhibition of binding of IIIB3. Solutions of myoglobin and insulin, at ten times the total protein concentration, did not significantly inhibit the binding of monoclonal antibody IIIB3 to MIS. Although MIS preparation Green 1 did not contain biologically active MIS, 21% inhibition of the binding of antibody IIIB3 was found when the total protein concentration of this fraction was ten times that of Green 2. At a 1:10 dilution, Green 1 gave less than 10% inhibition [21]. It is possible that this fraction eluted from the same matrex gel-Green A column contains forms of MIS which, although biologically inactive, remain immunologically reactive. The cross reactivity of antibody IIIB3 with hemocyanin coupled to digoxin at a concentration of 1 mg/ml (25% inhibition) is unexplained. It is conceivable that MIS and hemocyanin share a common antigenic determinant. Within the limited scope of proteins tested, it appears that monoclonal antibody IIIB3 is relatively specific for MIS.

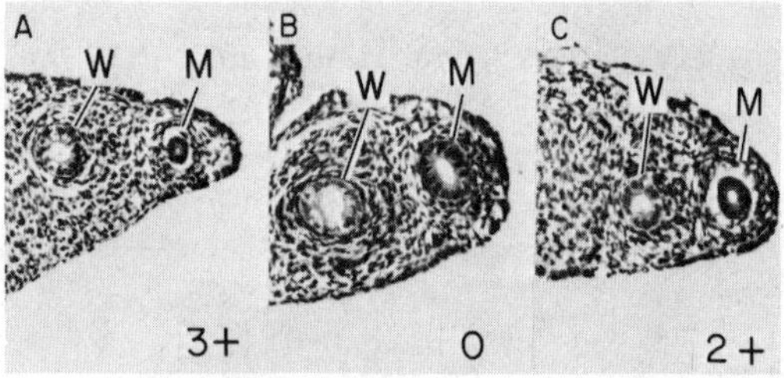

Fig. 2. Organ culture assay of 14-day urogenital ridge using samples of 500-fold purified MIS before and after affinity chromatography on a column prepared from the DEAE fraction isolated from ascites produced by the monoclonal anti-MIS-IIIB3 hybridoma. Panel A: MIS preparation prior to affinity chromatography. Mullerian duct (M) shows 3+ regression. Panel B: MIS preparation following affinity chromatography on antiMIS-IIIB3 Sepharose column (PBS-eluted fraction). Mullerian duct shows no regression in the organ culture assay due to the absence of biologically active MIS. Panel C: MIS preparation following affinity chromatography on the control column. The PBS-eluted fraction gave a 2+ regression of the Mullerian duct in the organ culture assay.

The specificity of IIIB3 for MIS was confirmed by this antibody's ability to absorb biologically active MIS by affinity chromatography. IgG monoclonal IIIB3 antibody was purified from ascites by DEAE chromatography and coupled to a solid support to produce an anti-MIS immunoadsorbant column [21]. A 500-fold purified fraction of MIS was tested for biological activity in the organ culture assay [22] before and after passage through the anti-MIS-IIIB3 affinity column. As seen in Fig. 2, the unabsorbed MIS preparation demonstrated a degree of activity scored as 3^+ (maximum score is 5^+) while the PBS-eluted fraction from the anti-MIS-IIIB3 affinity column demonstrated no biological activity (Panel B). As a control, the same MIS preparation was absorbed by an affinity column prepared from a monoclonal anti-digoxin antibody. In this case, the PBS-eluted fraction demonstrated an activity scored as 2^+ (Panel C). This apparently diminished activity eluted from the control column is expected and is probably due to dilution or denaturation by the affinity chromatography manipulations. Although repeated attempts to elute MIS from the anti-MIS-IIIB3 affinity column failed to yield biologically active MIS, biologically active MIS was successfully eluted with 3 M NH_4SCN from an affinity column prepared from another monoclonal anti-MIS antibody, IB2 [21]. The production of a monoclonal antibody with the requisite specificity for MIS is an example of the power of the hybridoma technique since less than 1% of the immunizing MIS preparation was MIS protein.

In order to test monoclonal anti-MIS antibody IIIB3 for its ability to inhibit biological activity, anti-MIS-IIB3 was first mixed with an MIS preparation and then added to the media surrounding the tissues in the organ culture assay. Although antibody IIIB3 did adsorb biologically active MIS, repeated attempts to demonstrate that this antibody will directly block biological activity have failed [21]. These results suggest that anti-MIS antibody IIIB3 binds MIS at determinants distant from the biologically active site in a manner that does not interfere with MIS activity.

Recently, the capability of antibody IIIB3 to bind a single component of an MIS preparation was demonstrated. An MIS preparation which represented a 30,000-fold purification (Green 2) was radiolabeled with ^{14}C by reductive methylation procedures (^{14}C-MIS) [23]. Antibody IIIB3 was first incubated with the ^{14}C-MIS fraction and then precipitated with excess goat-antimouse IgG reagent. The pellet was solubilized and then subjected to SDS electrophoresis. Results of autoradiography of the gel patterns showed a single component of the original Green 2 preparation to be precipitated by antibody IIIB3 (Budzik, G.P., personal communication).

The ability of monoclonal anti-MIS antibody to probe the

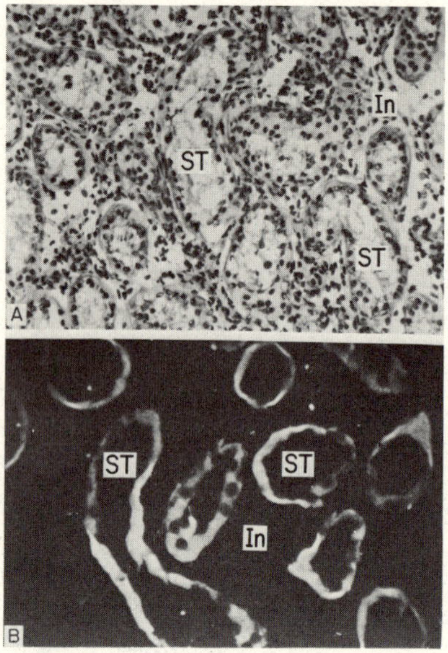

Fig. 3. Immunofluorescent localization of the anti-MIS-IIIB3 monoclonal antibody in the newborn calf testis. Panel A. The normal morphology of the newborn calf testis with seminiferous tubules and interstitial cells. Panel B. Specific localization of anti-MIS antibody IIIB3 to the seminiferous tubules. There was no labeling with normal mouse serum or with antibody raised against digoxin (data not shown).

morphology of embryonic tissues was also investigated. A fresh frozen section of newborn calf testis was first incubated with monoclonal antibody IIIB3 and washed. Any bound antibody IIIB3 was detected with a fluorescein-labeled second antibody, FITC-goat-antimouse immunoglobulin. As seen in panel B, Fig. 3, fluorescence staining was specifically localized to the seminiferous tubules. Fluorescent labeling by antibody IIIB3 was not detected in chicken, human, rat or mouse testis when similarly prepared. Since seminiferous tubules secrete MIS [24,25] and anti-MIS-IIIB3 was raised against calf MIS, the species specificity shown by antibody IIIB3 is striking (Shima, H., personal communication).

In summary, these studies are but a few examples of how monoclonal antibodies to MIS may serve as physiologic probes in many ways. Monoclonal anit-MIS antibody will facilitate the purification of MIS by affinity chromatography. Monoclonal anti-MIS antibodies can aid in the detection of both the site of cellular production of MIS and the receptors for MIS. Monoclonal anti-MIS antibody will also allow the development of a clinically useful RIA for the detection of MIS in tissue extracts, serum, and urine. Perhaps, most importantly, anti-MIS monoclonal antibodies will serve as physiologic probes in the study of the potential role of MIS as a chemotherapeutic reagent.

Probing the Physiologic Role of TSH

The glycoprotein hormones, thyrotropin stimulating hormone (TSH), luteinizing hormone (LH), follicle stimulating hormone (FSH), and chorionic gonadotropin (CG), consist of immunologically and biologically unique beta subunits noncovalently associated with identical alpha subunits. Although antisera to these hormones have been characterized as having great sensitivity and high specificity, these polyclonal antisera all have varying degrees of affinity for the common alpha subunit. Consequently, cross reactivity of antisera against TSH, for example, with the other glycoprotein hormones (LH, CG, and FSH) is inevitable [26]. Polyclonal antisera are thus limited in precisely determining the small amounts of one hormone in the presence of the other hormones. The hybridoma technique has the potential of resolving these problems by means of selecting monoclonal antibodies specific for the beta subunit of interest. In fact we recently reported the production of a high-affinity monoclonal antibody specific for human TSH (hTSH) [27].

Monoclonal antibody anti-hTSH 1/1 was the product of a fusion between spleen cells from a Balb/c mouse immunized with hTSH and the NS-1 myeloma cell line [27]. The original mixed hybridoma was cloned by limiting dilution. Antibody production from the selected clone, anti-hTSH 1/1, was augmented in the ascites form. Following purification from ascites by DEAE chromatography, anti-hTSH 1/1 was further characterized for affinity and specificity.

Scatchard analysis of homologous displacement curves resulted in a linear plot from which the average affinity constant K_D was determined to be 4.0×10^{-9} M/L. Interestingly, monoclonal antibody anti-hTSH 1/1 ($gamma_1$, kappa) was found to have a slightly reduced affinity ($K_D = 2.6 \times 10^{-8}$ M/L) for the beta subunit of hTSH [27]. The specificity of anti-hTSH 1/1 was assessed by the inhibition of binding of ^{125}I-hTSH to anti-hTSH 1/1, by both human and nonhuman glycoprotein hormones and their alpha and beta subunits. The resulting specificity profile shown in Fig. 4, is remarkable in its unique specificity for the beta subunit of human TSH (hTSH) and the lack of cross reactivity to the corresponding TSH alpha subunit (hTSH-alpha), other human glycoprotein hormones and their subunits (i.e., hCG, hCG, hLH, and hFSH) and nonhuman glycoprotein hormones including bovine (b) and rat (r) TSH beta subunits. Although hTSH-alpha, hFSH, and hLH/FSH LER 907 did not inhibit monoclonal antibody binding in amounts up to 10^3 ng/tube, they did displace ^{125}I-hTSH at 10^4 ng/tube which corresponds to a calculated cross reactivity of 1-2%. It is likely that the cross reactivity in these samples is due to known hTSH contamination in these preparations.

The production of monoclonal anti-hTSH 1/1 is a prime example of a monoclonal antibody with unique monospecificity. Apparently the determinant this antibody recognizes is specific for the beta subunit of hTSH. Since anti-hTSH 1/1 does not cross react with TSH-beta from other species, this structural determinant was not conserved in the evolution of hTSH-beta. It should be noted that in general monoclonality of an antibody does not necessarily result in monospecificity; however, desired specificity may be selected by appropriate screening of fusion products.

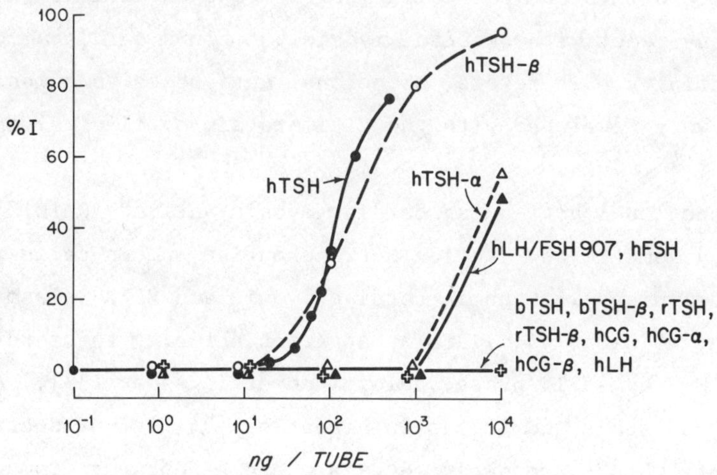

Fig. 4. Inhibition of binding of ^{125}I-labeled hTSH from anti-hTSH 1/1 antibody by unlabeled hTSH and various other human and nonhuman glycoprotein hormones as indicated in the figure and text.

The high degree of specificity for hTSH-beta should allow for studies on structure/function relationships, detection, and analysis of hTSH or hTSH-beta in the presence of other human glycoprotein hormones. The reduced affinity of anti-hTSH-beta 1/1 together with its specificity should permit the purification of hTSH or hTSH-beta by affinity chromatography. Another application is the use of the antibody as an immunofluorescent probe for hTSH-producing cells in the anterior pituitary.

Diagnosis of Myocardial Infarction Using Monoclonal Anti-myosin Antibody

The utilization of polyclonal anti-cardiac myosin antibodies for localization and visualization of experimental myocardial infarction has been reported [28-32]. Although affinity-purified, anti-cardiac myosin antisera are available, the quantity is limited and the specificity of the antisera is not consistent with respect to cross reactivity with skeletal myosin. The somatic cell fusion technique offers the possibility of finding an antibody which did not cross react with skeletal myosin but bound cardiac myosin with high affinity. Therefore, monoclonal antibodies to human cardiac myosin were developed with the ultimate aim of clinical application.

Monoclonal anti-human cardiac myosin antibody R11D10 was developed by somatic cell fusion between murine spleen cells from a mouse immunized with human cardiac myosin and SP2/0 plasmacytomas. Antibody R11D10 (IgG_{2a}) has an apparent affinity for cardiac myosin of 10^9 M^{-1} by solid-phase radioimmunometric assay [33]. Antibody R11D10 was subjected to papain digestion [34] for production of Fab fragments which were purified by protein A-Sepharose immunoadsorption [33,35]. Prior to labeling with technetium-99m (^{99m}Tc), R11D10-Fab was derivatized with diethylene triamine pentaacetic acid (DTPA) [32,36], a bifunctional chelating agent. Then DTPA-R11D10-Fab was labeled with ^{99m}Tc pertechnetate by the dithionite reduction method using ^{99m}Tc pertechnetate [32]. Anti-human cardiac myosin antibody R11D10 was observed to have 100% cross reactivity with canine cardiac myosin. Therefore, R11D10 was first tested in canine experimental myocardial infarct visualization studies.

Experimental myocardial infarction was induced in dogs under pentobarbitol anesthesia by ligation of the left anterior descending coronary artery for 3 hr after which the occlusive ligature was removed and the thoracotomy closed [28]. One hr later, 6-10 mCi of ^{99m}Tc-DTPA-R11D10-Fab was administered intravenously and gamma images in the left lateral position were obtained every minute for the first 10 min, and then at 1, 2, and 18 hr post injection. At 2 and 18 hr, anteroposterior images were also obtained for comparison. Figure 5 illustrates the results of one such study. The top panel represents 1-min images obtained at 0, 5, and 10 min post injection. Right (RV) and left ventricular (LV) activities can be observed in these early images. However, by 2 hr post injection, the left lateral (LL) image shows redistribution of radioactivity in the

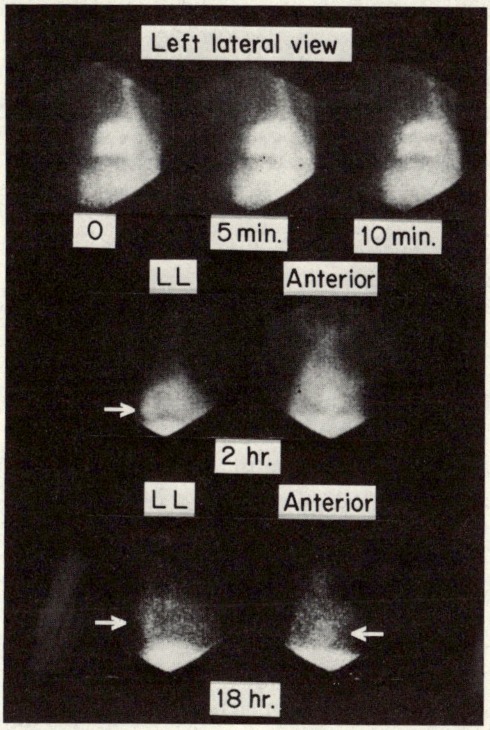

Fig. 5. Gamma images of canine experimental myocardial infarction using ^{99m}Tc-DTPA-R11D10 Fab. Arrows denote region of monoclonal anti-myosin localization at various times.

region of the heart. An area of increased radioactivity can be observed at the anteroapical region of the heart (arrow) which was the site of the experimental myocardial infarction. The corresponding anterior view at 2 hr is less distinct due to persistent blood activity. However, by 18 hr post injection, the radioactivity associated with anti-myosin localization can be observed distinctly in the left lateral (arrow) as well as in the anterior views (arrow). The lower central radioactivity is that of the liver due to blood pool activity as well as the possible presence of some denatured ^{99m}Tc-labeled DTPA-R11D10-Fab in the injected dose.

Thus, somatic cell fusion has permitted the selection of an anti-cardiac myosin antibody which does not cross react with skeletal myosin. Moreover, these studies have shown that this anti-cardiac myosin hybridoma can distinguish infarct from normal myocardium. Regions of infarction can be first visualized as early as 2 hr post injection in this canine experimental myocardial infarct model. The application of the method of labeling monoclonal anti-myosin with ^{99m}Tc is being applied to labeling other monoclonal antibodies for tumor detection and visualization.

CONCLUSION

It has been estimated that there are more than one hundred million different antibody combining sites. The power of this incredible array of selectivity and specificity has been only minimally utilized in biological research over the last century in that the only reagent available was the polyclonal antiserum. Now, antibodies need no longer be considered mixtures of varying properties but may be obtained as defined molecular entities. The small amount of serum from a particular animal is replaced by an indefinite quantity of a homogeneous protein. Selection from the many clones that can be examined in a series of cell fusion experiments allows for identification of precisely the antibody that has the properties of interest. Of the many potential applications of these methods, four have been described here: 1) the dissection of the molecular structure of a single organic compound through the employment of monoclonal antibodies that recognize small segments of the molecule: 2) the isolation of a protein from a mixture by selecting antibody-secreting cells on the basis of their antibody's biologic specificity rather than by fractionating protein molecules; 3) identification of a protein on the basis of unique epitopes that differentiate it from other proteins that have many common epitopes; 4) application of specificity for recognition of new antigenic structures exposed *in vivo*. The reader will have little difficulty in envisioning many additional applications of this most powerful tool.

REFERENCES

1. Kohler, G., and C. Milstein. 1975. Continuous cultures of fused cells secreting antibody of pre-defined specificity. Nature 256:495-497.
2. Yelton, D.E., and M.D. Scharff. 1981. Monoclonal antibodies: A powerful new tool in biology and medicine. Ann. Rev. Biochem. 50:657-680.
3. Hoffman, B.F., and J.T. Bigger, Jr. 1980. Digitalis and allied cardiac glycosides. In The Pharmacological Basis of Therapeutics. 6th edition. (A.G. Gilman, Y.S. Goodman, and A. Gilman, Eds.) MacMillan, New York. pp729-760.
4. Smith, T.W., and E. Haber. 1973. Digitalis. New Engl. J. Med. 289:945, 1010, 1063, 1125.
5. Smith, T.W., V.P. Butler, Jr., and E. Haber. 1969. Determination of therapeutic and toxic serum digoxin concentrations by radioimmunoassay. New Engl. J. Med. 281:1212-1216.
6. Mudgett-Hunter, M., M.N. Margolies, A.Ju, and E. Haber. 1982. High affinity monoclonal antibodies to the cardiac glycoside digoxin. J. Immunol., (in press).
7. Smith, T.W. 1972. Ouabain-specific antibodies: Immunochemical properties and reversal of NA+, K+-activated adenosine triphosphatase inhibition. J. Clin. Invest. 51:1583-1593.
8. Nisonoff, A., and D. Pressman. 1958. Heterogeneity and average combining constants of antibodies from individual rabbits. J. Immunol. 80:417-428.
9. Novotny, J., M. Mudgett-Hunter, E. Haber, and M.N. Margolies. 1981. Primary structure of a mouse antidigoxin hybridoma antibody. Fed. Proc. 40:1098.
10. Schwartz, A., G.E. Lindenmayer, and J.C. Allen. 1975. The sodium-potassium adenosine triphosphatase: Pharmacological, physiological and biochemical aspects. Pharmacol. Rev. 27:3-134.
11. Smith, T.W., E. Haber, L. Yeatman, and V.P. Butler, Jr. 1976.

Reversal of advanced digoxin intoxication with Fab fragments of digoxinspecific antibodies. New Eng. J. Med. 294:797-800.

12. Burchiel, S.W., B.A. Khaw, B.G. Rhodes, T.W. Smith, and E. Haber. 1981. Immunopharmacokinetics and radiolabeled antibodies and their fragments. In Tumor Imaging: Radioimmunochemical Detection of Cancer. Edited by S.W. Burchiel, B.A. Rhodes, and B. Friedman. Masson, New York.

13. Margolies, M.N., M. Mudgett-Hunter, J. Novotny, and E. Haber. 1981. Monoclonal antibodies directed against the cardiac glycoside digoxin. In Monoclonal Antibodies and T Cell Hybridomas. (G. Hammerling, U. Hammerling, and J.F. Kearney, Eds.) Elsevier, New York.

14. Jost, A. 1946. Sur la differenciation sexuelle de l'embryon de lapin experiences de paraboise. CR Soc. Biol. 140:463-464.

15. Jost, A. 1946. Sur la differenciation sexuelle de l'embryon de lapin remarques au sujet de certaines operations chirurgical. CR Soc. Biol. 140:460-462.

16. Jost, A. 1947. Sur les derives mulleriens d'embryons de lapin des deus sexes castres a 21 jours. CR Soc. Biol. 141:135-136.

17. Donahoe, P.K., D.A. Swann, A. Hayashi, and M.D. Sullivan. 1979. Mullerian duct regression in the embryo correlated with cytotoxic activity against a human ovarian cancer. Science 205:913-915.

18. Donahoe, P.K., A.F. Fuller, Jr., R.E. Scully, S.R. Guy, and G.P. Budzik. 1981. Mullerian inhibiting substance inhibits growth of a human ovarian cancer in nude mice. Ann. Surg. 194:472-480.

19. Fuller, A.F. Jr., S.R. Guy, G.P. Budzik, P.K. Donahoe. 1982. Mullerian inhibiting substance inhibits colony growth of a human ovarian cancer cell line. J. Clin. Endo. Metab. 54:1051-1055.

20. Donahoe, P.K., G.P. Budzik, R.L. Trelstad, M. Mudgett-Hunter, A.F. Fuller, Jr., J.M. Hutson, H. Ikawa, A. Hayashi, and D.T. MacLaughlin. 1982. Mullerian inhibiting substance: An

update. In Recent Progress in Hormone Research, Vo. 38. (R.O. Greep, Ed.), New York: Academic Press, pp 279-330.

21. Mudgett-Hunter, M., G.P. Budzik, M. Sullivan, and P.K. Donahoe. 1982. Monoclonal antibody to mullerian inhibiting substance. J. Immunol. 128:1327-1333.
22. Donahoe, P.K., Y. Ito, S. Marfatia, and W. H. Hendren. 1977. A graded organ culture assay for the detection of Mullerian inhibiting substance. J. Surg. Res. 23:141-148.
23. Finger, J.M., and K.H. Choo. 1981. Double-label reductive methylation of tissue proteins for precision two-dimensional polyacrylamide-gel electrophoretic analysis. Biochem. J. 193:371-374.
24. Blanchard, M., and N. Josso. 1974. Sources of the anti-Mullerian hormone synthesized by the fetal testis: Mullerian inhibiting activity of fetal bovine Sertoli cells in tissue culture. Ped. Res. 8:968-971.
25. Price, J.M. 1979. The secretion of Mullerian inhibiting substance by culture isolated Sertoli cells of the neonatal calf. Am. J. Anat. 156:147-157.
26. Pierce, J.G., and T.F. Parsons. 1981. Glycoprotein hormones: Structure and function. Ann. Rev. Biochem. 50:465-495.
27. Ridgeway, E.C., L.J. Ardisson, M.J. Meskell, and M. Mudgett-Hunter. 1982. Monoclonal antibody to human thyrotropin. J. Clin. Endo. Metab. 55:44-48.
28. Khaw, B.A., G.A. Beller, E. Haber, and T.W. Smith. 1976. Localization of cardiac myosin-specific antibody in myocardial infarction. J. Clin. Invest. 58:439-446.
29. Khaw, B.A., G.A. Beller, and E. Haber. 1978. Experimental myocardial infarct imaging following intravenous administration of Iodine-131 labeled antibody (Fab')2 fragments specific for cardiac myosin. Circulation. 57:743-750.
30. Khaw, B.A., J.T. Fallon, H.W. Strauss, and E. Haber. 1980. Myocardial infarct imaging with Indium-111-diethylene triamine pentaacetic acid-anticanine cardiac myosin antibodies. Science.

209:295-297.

31. Khaw, B.A., J.T. Fallon, H. Katus, D. Elmaleh, H.W. Strauss, E. Locke, G.M. Pohost, and E. Haber. 1979. Positron imaging of experimental myocardial infarction with 68Ga-DTPA-antimyosin antibody. Circulation. 59 and 60 (Suppl II): 139.

32. Khaw, B.A., H.W. Strauss, A. Carvalho, E. Locke, H.K. Gold, and E. Haber. Labeling anti-cardiac myosin Fab and human fibrinogen with Technetium-99m. J. Nucl. Med. (submitted for publication).

33. Wands, J.R., and V.R. Zurawski. 1981. High affinity monoclonal antibodies to hepatitis B surface antigen produced by somatic cell hybrids. Gastroent. 80:225-232.

34. Porter, R.R. 1959. The hydrolysis of rabbit gamma-globulin and antibodies with crystalline papain. Biochem. J. 73:119-126.

35. Ey, P.L., S.J. Prowse, and C.R. Jenkin. 1978. Isolation of pure IgG1, IgG2a and IgG2b immunoglobulins from mouse serum using protein A Sepharose. Immunochem. 15:429-436.

36. Krejcarek, G.E., and Tucker, K.L. 1977. Covalent attachment of chelating groups to macromolecules. Biochem. Biophys. Res. Comm. 77:582-585.

DISCUSSION

Q. Did I hear you correctly that for the production of monoclonal anti-digoxin antibodies you used A/J mice? Was that a conscious choice?

A. HUNTER: Yes. It was a conscious choice. Initially we used a variety of strains to examine the neonatal response to digoxin. The A/J mouse seemed to respond best when compared to the other strains. Although the Balb/c mice did make antibody to digoxin the antidigoxin response in terms of titer were best in A/J mice. The other reason is purely personal -- Balb/c mice fight a lot, and A/J mice are very docile.

Q. T. SEALE: I was wondering, what would be the efficacy of

removing the digoxin in cases of overdose. Perhaps two monoclonal antibodies of two different isotypes could be used instead of one. Do you expect a complimentation or some type of competition in a situation such as that?

A. HUNTER: I'm not sure I understand your question. Do you mean something to do with another digitalis?

Q. T. SEALE: I mean if you show/use two monoclonal antibodies at the same time, instead of one.

A. HUNTER: In that case, I don't think you would want to see two because of the possibility of forming small aggregates, which would be more difficult for the body to eliminate. The studies by Tom Smith with baboons indicate that the Fab fragment is cleared very quickly, bound to digoxin. So you wouldn't want to set up a situation where you could form aggregates. You would want to use only a single monoclonal Fab fragment at a time.

Q. T. SEALE: Would that be more help for purification? In the purufication of your hormone of interest, would it be helpful in purification to use two different monoclonal antibodies?

A. HUNTER: Sure. If you want to achieve an effective higher affinity, you wouldn't use Fab, but you'd use intact antibodies. There are theoretical approaches where you can get around the problem of lower affinity by covalently coupling more than one antibody. This rational is based on the avidity shown by IgM. In this approach you would use two antibodies that recognize different determinants on the same molecule. That is certainly feasible.

Q. P. GUIRE: Can you easily avoid the need for purified antigen in selecting the proper clone?

A. HUNTER: You need purified antigen to select for the proper clone or a bio-assay.

Q. P. GUIRE: Okay. When you made the point of one advantage of monoclonal antibodies being they do not require purified immunogen, you still will need it for selection of a clone.

A. HUNTER: Yes, if you use an RIA for selection. In the case of the MIS, we used the bioassay in order to demonstrate specificity.

Q. J. MARTINIS: I had two questions about digoxin. One is, do you have any ideas on why you got such nice affinity antibodies? The second is, you said that the digoxin fills the binding site. Were you able to simultaneously bind two of your antibodies to digoxin?

A. HUNTER: In answer to your second question, we haven't tried that. Now that we have two that recognize different determinates, I certainly will try it. I'm not sure why I get high affinity, I've looked at the polyclonal responses of the A/J mouse and found it to have an average affinity of 10^9. It could simply be that this particular strain responds with a high affinity variable region gene for this antigen.

Q. Is there any problem growing the hybridoma as ascites tumor, since it's from an A/J mouse?

A. HUNTER: You wouldn't choose the Balb/c mouse. Instead you grow them in CAF mice which are the F_1 generation of a cross between A/J and Balb/c mice.

NOVEL APPLICATIONS OF MONOCLONAL ANTIBODIES

Joanne Martinis, Gary S. David, Richard M. Bartholomew, and Robert Wang
Hybritech Incorporated
11085 Torreyane Road
San Diego, California 92121-1197

INTRODUCTION

The rationale for hybridoma technology is the inherent properties of the mammalian immune system: the antibody response to a foreign antigen is clonal, committed, and heterogeneous. Although a given antibody producing cell will secrete an antibody of one, and only one, specificity regardless of subsequent exposure to another antigen, any given antigen will stimulate many independent antibody producing cells, resulting in the heterogeneous, polyclonal antibody response observed in immune serum (Fig. 1). If an individual antibody producing cell could be immortalized, it would then make homogeneous monoclonal antibody indefinitely. This is essentially the hybridoma process (Fig. 2). As shown by Kohler and Milstein in 1975 [1], when a lymphocyte secreting a specific antibody is fused with a myeloma cell the resulting hybrid shows dominant expression of two critical parental traits, specific antibody production (from the lymphocyte) and immortal growth (from the myeloma). The ability to

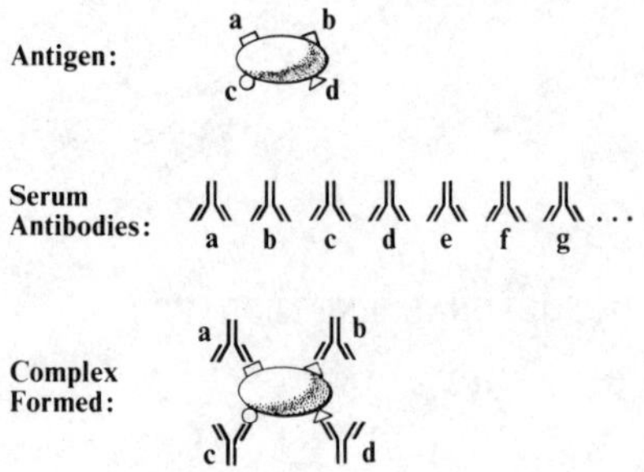

Fig. 1. Polyclonal antibody response in immune serum. Antigen containing determinants a, b, c, and d is used to immunize a rabbit. Serum antibodies made in response to this immunization contain specificity for determinants a-d as well as other specificities (e-g, ...). In addition, there are many antibodies with varying affinities made to each determinant.

immortalize specific antibody producing cells allows the dissection of the immune response and the production of antibodies with precisely defined characteristics. In turn, the ability to select such antibodies opens the door to novel applications in diagnostics, therapeutics, and separation technology.

In Vitro Diagnostics

The ability to select site specific antibodies of varying affinities to the different epitopes of a multi-determinant antigen has several implications for *in vitro* diagnostic assays. First, two antibodies reactive with an antigen can be selected such that neither interferes with the binding of the other to the antigen, allowing the development of a simultaneous immunometric assay. Second, because the affinity of a monoclonal antibody is precisely defined, an assay can be engineered with a desired range of sensitivity by judicious selection of the antibodies involved. Third,

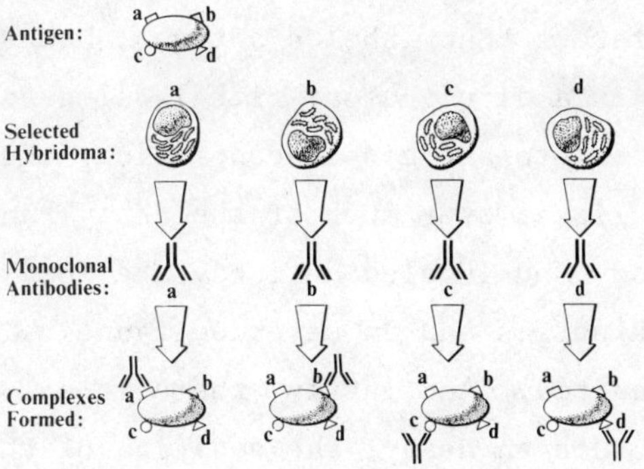

Fig. 2. Monoclonal antibody made by hybridomas. Antigen containing determinants a, b, c, and d is used to immunize a mouse. Hybridoma derived monoclonal antibodies made in response to this immunization contain specificity for only one determinant (a or b or c or d).

the consistent and predictable binding of a monoclonal antibody to its antigen allows the engineering of homogeneous assays.

The most commonly used clinical radioassay is the competitive binding radioimmunoassay (RIA). In this assay the patient's sample is mixed with radiolabeled antigen and specific antiserum. The antigen in the patient sample is quantitated by its ability to inhibit binding of the labeled antigen. However, this assay has several technical limitations. First, because it is an indirect assay, the dose response curve is nonlinear. Second, the labeled antigen and specific antibody must be critically balanced to allow the required specificity; thus, the reaction cannot be driven by excess reagents and the range is limited. Furthermore, this critical balance means that these assays are subject to multiple pipetting errors in the clinical setting. Third, purified antigen is necessary and must be able to be radiolabeled without loss of specific immunoreactivity and stability.

In contrast, an immunoradiometric assay (IRMA), utilizing labeled antibody rather than labeled antigen, has several advantages. First, it is a direct assay with labeled antibody binding directly proportional to antigen concentration; thus the dose-response curve is linear over much of the assay range. Second, solid phase antibody and labeled antibody are in excess giving such assays favorable kinetics and an extended range. Third, labeled antigen is not required. And lastly, there is only one critical pipetting step in such an assay, the addition of the patient's sample.

Although the advantages of immunometric assays are formidable, they have not found widespread usefulness in clinical diagnostics because of two major drawbacks: the large quantities of antibodies required and the necessity for affinity chromatography. Affinity purification, with its resulting loss of high affinity antibody and potential for denaturation, and the inability, even with laborious immunization and/or antibody purification and adsorption protocols to remove all steric interference of the solid phase and labeled antibody have limited immunometric assays using polyclonal antisera. However, such assays take full advantage of monoclonal antibodies because of their unlimited availability and simplicity of purification and the ability to select a pair of high affinity antibodies directed at distinct sites such that neither antibody interferes with the binding of the other (Fig. 3). This allows the assay to be performed in many instances as a simultaneous assay, rather than as the sequential two-step assay generally required with polyclonal antisera (Fig. 4 and 5).

The ability to select for antibodies at sterically distinct sites on a multi-determinant antigen is illustrated in Fig. 6 which shows the effect of solution-phase antibodies on the binding ^{125}I-labeled IgE to solid-phase monoclonal antibody C. The control

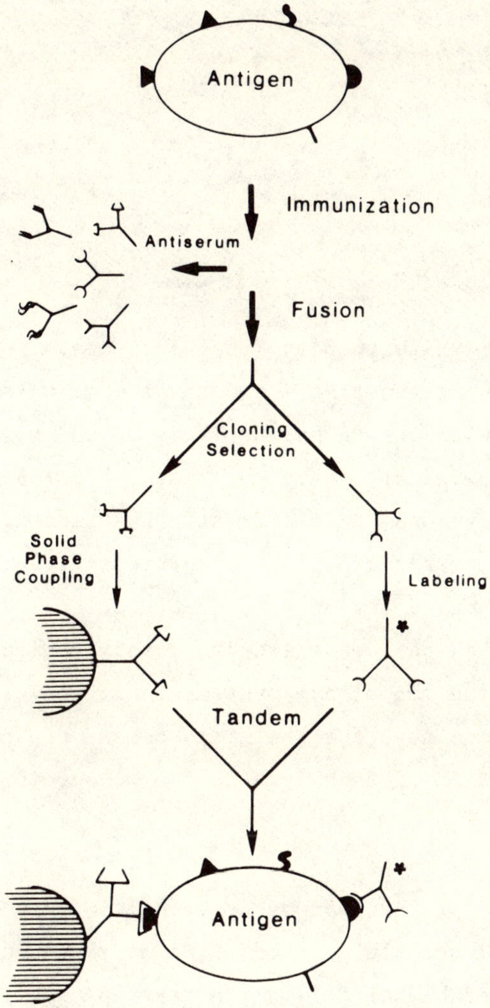

Fig. 3. Schematic representation of the selection of an antibody pair for use in a simultaneous immunometric assay. After immunization and fusion, two hybridoma lines are selected that secrete antibodies specific for sterically distinct determinants on the antigen molecule. The antibody product of one of these cell lines is coupled to a solid phase, while the antibody product of the other cell line is labeled (e.g., with a radioisotope).

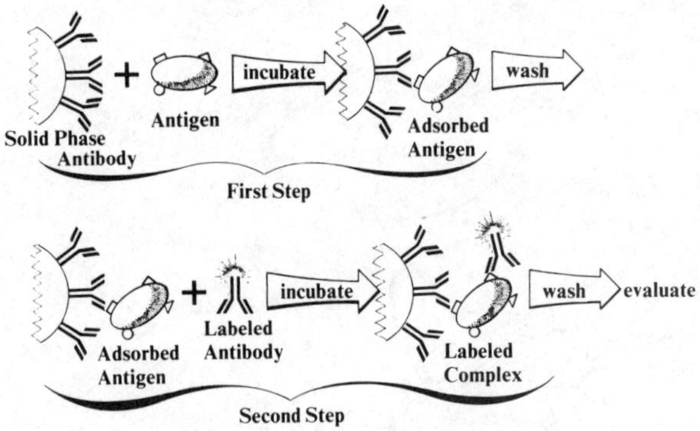

Fig. 4. Two step IRMA with polyclonal antisera. Solid-phase antibody and antigen react to form an insoluble complex (first step). With monoclonal antibody on the solid-phase, all antigens will attach by the same determinant, while solid-phase polyclonal antiserum attaches randomly. In the second step, the solid-phase adsorbed antigen reacts with excess labeled antibody to form the labeled complex. No competition between solid-phase and labeled antibodies is seen in the monoclonal system, while polyclonal antiserum reagents compete for the sites unless separate affinity-purification of each reagent can be accomplished.

antibody (specific for PAP) had no detectable effect on the binding of the IgE to the insoluble antibody. Similarly, monoclonal antibody D had no detectable effect, demonstrating that it was specfic for a determinant on IgE sterically distinct from that recognized by the solid phase antibody. Monoclonal antibody E partially inhibited antigen binding, which suggested that it was recognizing a different, but spatially close, determinant such that its presence on the antigen caused some steric inhibition of the binding of the antigen to the insoluble antibody C. Monoclonal antibody C (that antibody present on the solid phase) drastically inhibited antigen binding, as predicted. Figure 7 shows data from simultaneous and sequential IRMAs for human IgE, using antibodies C and D. As would be expected if the two antibodies bind completely independently to the antigen,

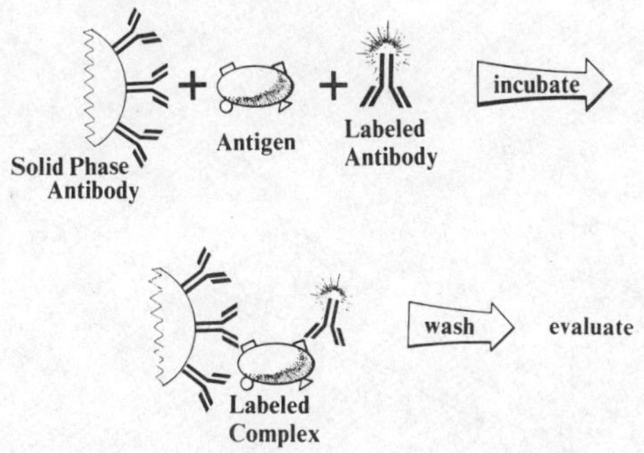

Fig. 5. Simultaneous IRMA with monoclonal antibodies. In a single step, all reagents and the sample are combined. Polyclonal reagents compete for the various antigenic sites while monoclonal antibodies bind separate independent sites. Thus, only a single incubation and wash step is necessary since there will be no interference with appropriately chosen monoclonal antibodies.

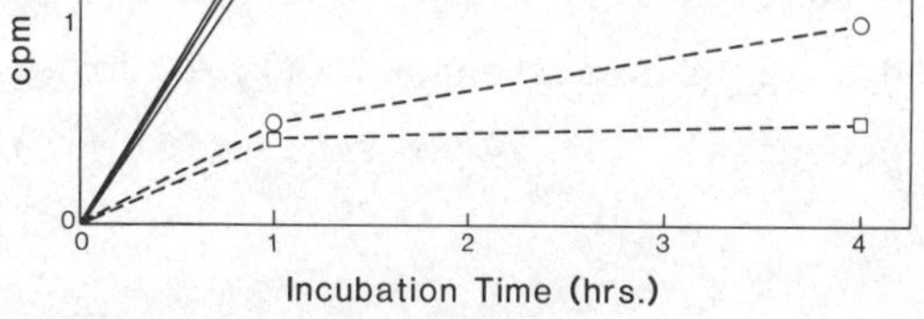

Fig. 6. Steric effects of solution-phase monoclonal antibodies on the binding of ^{125}I-labeled IgE to solid-phase monoclonal antibody C. No antibody (buffer control) (Δ); PAP-specific antibody (■) IgE-specific antibody D (●); IgE-specific antibody C (□); IgE-specific antibody E (O).

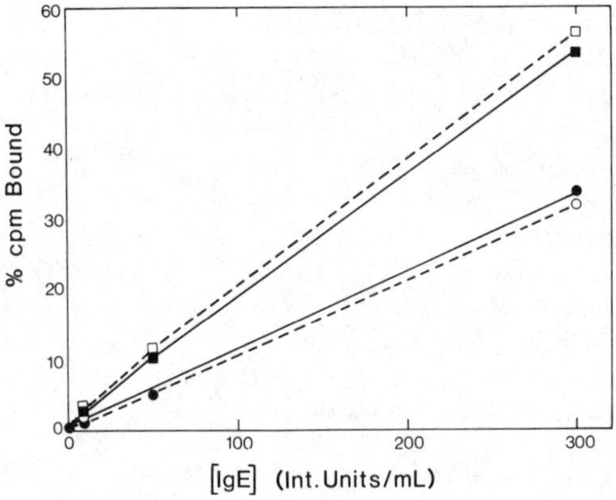

Fig. 7. Comparison of sequential and simultaneous IRMAs with monoclonal antibodies. Solid-phase antibody was obtained from hybridoma clone C, and antibodies produced by clone D were radiolabeled with ^{131}I. Approximately 10 ng of the iodinated antibody were used per data point. In the simultaneous incubation experiments, all reagents were mixed and incubated at 37°C for either 5 or 24 hr. The samples were then washed and counted for ^{131}I-labeled antibody. In the sequential incubation experiments the solid-phase antibody was first incubated with IgE calibrator for either 5 or 24 hr at 37°C. Each solid-phase antibody ball was washed then incubated in an identical manner in the presence of ^{131}I-labeled antibody. After the second incubation period, the samples were washed and counted for ^{131}I-labeled antibody. 5 hr simultaneous (●); 24 hr simultaneous (■); 5 hr sequential (O); 24 hr sequential (□).

the results of the simultaneous assays at both 5 and 24 hr time points are virtually identical to those of the sequential assays.

The range and sensitivity of such an assay can be engineered by the appropriate choice of the antibody pair involved. Immunoradiometric assays involving different combinations of three monoclonal antibodies are illustrated in Fig. 8. When radiolabeled clone A

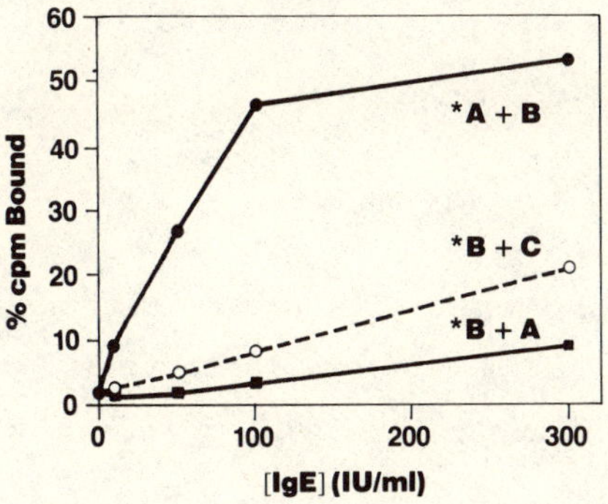

Fig. 8. Effect of monoclonal antibody pairs on sensitivity and quantitation range of an IRMA. *A and *B refer to radiolabeled antibody derived from clones A and B, respectively. A,B, and C refer to solid-phase antibodies derived from clones A, B, and C.

antibody is used in conjunction with solid-phase clone B antibody, a highly sensitive but short-range assay is obtained. On the other hand, when these antibodies are reversed and radiolabeled clone B antibody is used with solid-phase clone A antibody, the results are strikingly different: an assay with very low sensitivity but broad range. When radiolabeled clone B antibody is paired with solid-phase clone C antibody, results are intermediate. Thus by choosing appropriate pairs of antibodies for use in an immunometric assay, one can engineer an assay with finely tuned sensitivity.

An additional advantage of this system is shown by the development of an IRMA for HCG that quantitates only the intact molecule. RIAs for HCG are hampered by the difficulty of preparing HCG specific antiserum because antiserum raised to HCG will cross-react with the pituitary hormones FSH, LH, and TSH because these hormones share a common alpha subunit and differ only in a portion of their beta subunits. One solution to this problem has been to use purified β subunit as a immunogen to raise antisera to that portion of the β subunit that is unique to HCG [2]. Generally with the aid of

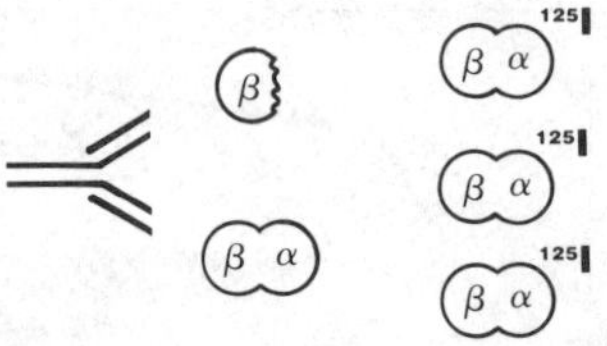

Fig. 9. HCG ASSAY: Competitive Radio-Immunoassay. β-specific RIA for HCG. In this assay, both free β subunit and intact HCG will compete for labeled intact HCG.

adsorption procedures, antisera have been produced that have minimal cross reactivity to these structurally similar pituitary hormones. However, such antisera will react with both the free β subunit and the intact HCG molecule in a competitive binding RIA (Fig. 9). There can be considerable discrepency between an HCG value as determined by a β-specific RIA and that determined by a bioassay. This discrepency is due to the presence of free β subunits in the sample. The WHO International Standard (IS) and the WHO International Reference Preparation (IRP) currently in use give identical values when measured in a bioassay but the IRP measures 105 IU while the IS measures 200 IU in a β-specific RIA.

One way to circumvent interference from free β subunit in an RIA would be to use an antiserum that recognizes only intact HCG and not free α or β subunits. Such assays have been reported [3,4] but are not generally available, most likely due to technical difficulties in producing such an antiserum that is also adequately sensitive. We developed an alternative approach, utilizing an immunoradiometric assay specific for native HCG based on two monoclonal antibodies, one directed at a binding site unique to the β region of the HCG molecule (and not cross reactive with lutropin, thyrotropin, and follitropin), and the other directed at a binding site unique to the α region (Fig. 10). The requirement for two binding sites inherent in the IRMA, coupled with the specificity of the monoclonal antibodies, has resulted in an assay that is specific for only

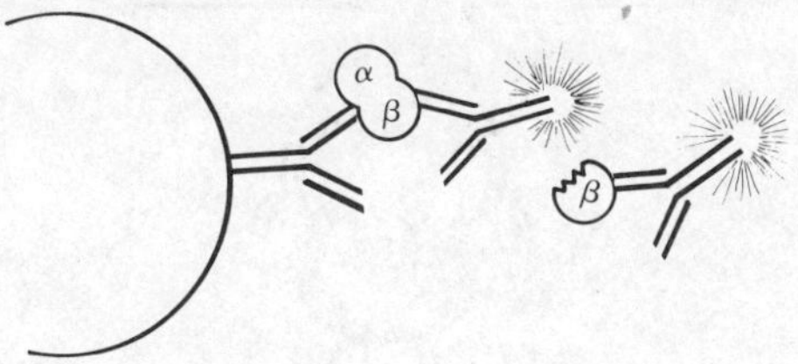

Fig. 10. HCG ASSAY: Solid Phasae 2-Site Immunometric Assay. Intact HCG specific IRMA. In this assay, only intact HCG is quantitated because of the necessity for simultaneous binding of both the α and β specific antibodies.

intact HCG. Free α or β subunits, lutropin, follitropin, and thyrotropin do not interfere with the assay. In this assay the WHO IS and IRP give identical calibration curves from 5 to 100,000 IU, because only HCG and not β subunit is measured by this IRMA. Hence the HCG concentration determined for a sample should be the same regardless of which reference preparation is used to calibrate the IRMA.

Similarly, we have developed an assay that is specific only for the free β subunit, by utilizing a different pair of monoclonal antibodies. One of these is specific for a cryptic binding site on the β subunit that is only exposed on free β subunits; the other is specific for a determinant which is exposed on both free and intact β subunits.

Homogeneous Assay

Homogeneous assays are those in which no separation step is required because the bound and the free form of the label are differentially quantitatable [5]. These are operationally the simplest clinical test and the easiest to automate. For example, if an

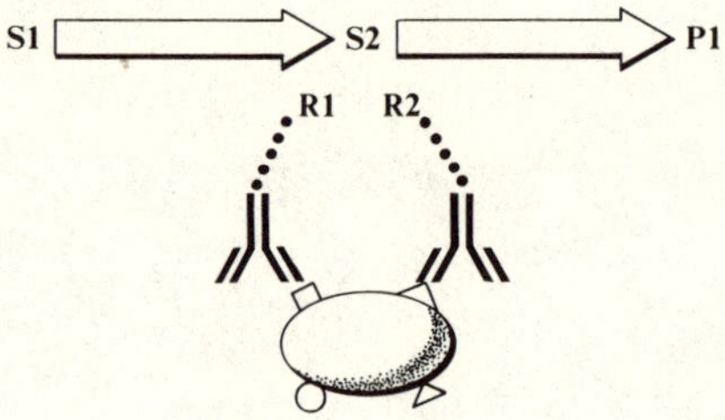

System	R1	R2	S1	S2	P1
Fluorescence quenching	Fluorescein	Rhodamine	340 nm	460 nm	520 nm
Proximal enzyme linking	Hexokinase	Glucose-6P-de hydrogenase	ATP + glucose	Glucose-6P + NAD^+	Gluconolac- tone-6P + NADH
Proximal enzyme linking	Glucose oxidase	Peroxidase	Glucose	Peroxide + DAB	Oxidized DAB
Bioluminescence	NAD oxidore- ductase	Luciferase	NADH + FMN	$FMNH_2$	$h\nu$
Allosteric activation	Phosphofructo- kinase	Phosphoenol- pyruvate carboxylase	Fructose-6- phosphate	Phosphoenol- pyruvate NADH (MDH)	NAD^+
Allosteric inhibition	Aspartate aminotrans- fersae	Phosphoenol- pyruvate carboxylase	Oxalacetate + glutamate	Phosphoenol- pyruvate + NADH	Oxalacetate + NAD^+
Enzyme/substrate	Peroxidase	Luminol	Peroxide	(Luminol)	$h\nu$

Fig. 11. Proximal linkage immunometric assays. Monoclonal antibodies that are conjugated to specific compounds and bind proximal antigenic sites can be used to produce homogeneous immunometric assays. R1 and R2 are fluorophores, enzymes, or enzyme/substrates, while S1 can be light or substrates. S2 is a product of R1 and a substrate for R2. S2 can also be transferred or emitted light. P1 is the measurable substance: light ($h\upsilon$), NAD^+, NADH, chromophores, etc. See graph above for specific examples.

enzyme can be attached covalently to a specific region of an antigen, an antibody directed against an adjacent determinant may cause a consistent and predictable inhibition or enhancement of enzymic activity; free antigen (in a patient's serum, for example) would inhibit the effect of the antibody. Moreover, all antibodies in the monoclonal population recognize the same precise determinant; only a small fraction of antibodies present in polyclonal antiserum would be expected to be specific for that determinant.

The IRMA technology can also be translated into homogeneous assays such as those based on fluorescence quenching and proximal enzyme linking. These assays rely on reactions that only occur maximally when the indicator molecules are correctly positioned (Fig. 11). By conjugating the indicator molecules to a pair of monoclonal antibodies that bind adjacent determinants on the antigen allowing the proper spacing for interaction, the concentration of antigen could be measured by the signal generated by the indicator pair.

Bifunctional Antibodies

The potential advantages of monoclonal antibodies in *in vivo* immunodiagnostics and immunotherapeutics have been recognized since hybridomas were first described [1]. Many of these proposed advantages have now been realized. For instance, tumor localization studies using radiolabeled monoclonal antibodies show improved levels of specific localization into the tumor [6]. These improvements over the results found with polyclonal antiserum are in part attributable to the absence of the large amounts of non-specific immunoglobulin found in polyclonal antisera. Although such antisera can be affinity purified, the desorption procedures normally result in some antibody denaturation, increasing non-specific tissue localization and rapid serum clearance. However, even with monoclonal antibodies, non-specific tissue localization continues to be a significant problem, and is likely due to normal metabolic events, some of which are the result of slight structural changes that occur with radiolabeling or conjugation of the antibody molecule.

One approach to help alleviate these problems in tumor immunotherapy is to generate hybrid antibodies containing two different antigen binding sites, one specific for the tumor, the other for the toxin, drug, or radioactive reagent. Such antibodies have two immediate advantages. First, no chemical modifications or potential denaturating conditions occur when antibody-therapeutic agent complexes are made by this procedure. Second, antibody and therapeutic agent administration can be separated temporally, allowing antibody to localize to tumor and clear from other tissue, followed by subsequent low dose injection of the toxin, drug, or radioactive reagent, which will then concentrate to therapeutically significant doses in the tumor.

Although hybrid antibodies can be made by chemical means, involving production of half molecules and subsequent renaturation to whole antibody [7], the conditions necessary are fairly drastic and result in a significant amount of irreversible denaturation. Furthermore, with monoclonal antibodies the yields are often low and vary according to the nature of the antibodies involved. An alternative to this method is to trick plasma cells into making such antibodies biologically, under completely non-denaturing conditions, using hybridoma technology. Such a procedure will produce hybrid monoclonal antibody molecules which possess, in addition to their dual specificity, the many advantageous characteristics of monoclonal antibodies.

The development of one such hybridoma producing hybrid antibody was as follows. Initially, spleen cells obtained from Balb/c mice hyperimmunized with human prostatic acid phosphatase (PAP) were fused with P3.653 myeloma cells [8]. Fused cells were seeded into 96 well microtiter plates in hypoxanthine-aminopterin-thymidine (HAT) selective medium [9] at concentrations estimated to yield less than 33% hybridoma positive wells. The resulting hybridomas were screened for their ability to bind ^{125}I-labeled PAP by a solid phase second antibody radioimmunoassay [10]. One clone, PAC 017, was selected and subcloned.

Subclone PAC 017.1 originally isolated in HAT selective medium was back-selected to HAT sensitivity. First, it was transferred to HT medium for 1 week, then to nonselective medium. After several weeks of growth under non-selective conditions cells were placed in medium containing 10^{-4}M 8-azaguanine. Cells which survive in this medium have usually segregated the hypoxanthine-guaninine phosphoribosyl transferase (HPRT) gene and become HAT sensitive. Clones that grew out were tested for HAT sensitivity and antibody production. One clone, PAC 017.1 BS, was shown to retain production of antibody specific for PAP, but exhibited HAT sensitivity with a reversion frequency of less than $4x10^{-8}$. This clone was subcloned, and the subclones behaved like the parent. One subclone, PAC 017.1 #50, was chosen for fusions and is designated BSP.

Finally BSP cells were fused with spleen cells obtained from Balb/c mice hyperimmunized with hepatitis B surface antigen (HBsAg) as described above. All hybridomas were screened for their ability to bind ^{125}I-labeled HBsAg and ^{125}I-labeled PAP. Two of 220 hybridomas tested exhibited specificity for both PAP and HBsAg. Five of the 220 hybridomas tested were unable to bind PAP, indicating some instability of antibody production in the back-selected parental cell line. Although the frequency of wells positive for hybridoma growth in the fusion was only 25%, the possibility still existed that those wells showing binding activity for both PAP and HBsAg contained two independent clones. On subcloning by limiting dilution, however, both hybridomas yielded subclones which still bound both antigens. When ascites derived from these subclones were analyzed by Orstein Davis polyacrylamide gel electrophoresis (PAGE) [11,12], they yielded the multiple banding patterns that were characteristic of the parent clones.

That the antibody products from these two clones retained

Table 1

Simultaneous Binding of Two Different Antigens Demonstrating the Presence of Hybrid Antibody

ascites	specificity	*HBsAg	*PAP	*PAP + PAP-017
IEU 025	IgE (control)	15,340	2,145	2,930
PAC 017	PAP	16,280	2,956	5,128
HBI 456	HBsAg	73,020	2,973	2,870
BSH 016	test for dual	78,900	82,533	2,936

* ^{125}I-labeled

200 μl of each of the above ascites were incubated overnight with 12 polystyrene balls containing immobilized HBsAg (Abbott Laboratories). Following extensive washing, triplicate samples were incubated with 100,000 cpm of each of the indicated trace labels for 4 hours. The resulting cpm bound in each case are reported. Data indicate that the BSH 016 ascites contains antibody molecules with dual specificity for hepatitis and PAP antigens, the PAP reactivity being against the same epitope as the back selected parental line used in the fusion.

binding specificity for PAP and HBsAg during cell dilution, subcloning, and ascites production is evidence that a single hybridoma was responsible for the two antigen specificities. A dual specificity such as this could result from a single cell synthesizing: a) two distinct antibody molecules, one with only PAP specificity and one with only HBsAg specificity, b) hybrid molecules that actually contain one binding site specific for hepatitis and the other binding site specific for PAP, or c) a combination of hybrid molecules and the two separate antibodies.

To determine if hybrid antibody molecules are produced in these clones, the ability of one of these clones (BSH 016) to bind both antigens simultaneously was tested by employing solid phase HBsAg and various radiolabeled antigens, including radiolabeled PAP (Table 1). Results showed that solid phase HBsAg incubated with BSH 016 ascites could efficiently bind ^{125}I-labeled PAP. The specific nature of this binding and the retention of the same recognition

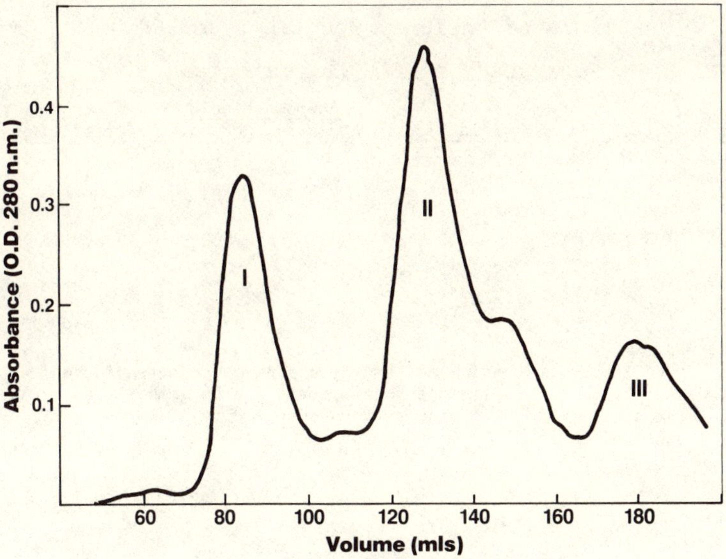

Fig. 12. Protein profile by OD_{280} of DEAE purified BSH 016 antibody moieties.

site expressed by the back-selected hybridoma used in the fusion was confirmed by the fact that prior incubation of the PAP label with PAC 017 (the monoclonal antibody secreted by the parental line) prevented the label from binding to the HBsAg hybrid antibody matrix. In contrast, neither PAC 017 ascites (only PAP specificity) nor HBI 456 ascites (only HBsAg specificity) when incubated with solid phase HBsAg yielded significant amounts of PAP antigen binding. These results verified the presence of hybrid molecules, but yielded no information concerning the proportion of the total antibody in the hybrid form. The observation that incubation of BSH 016 with the solid phase HBsAg also leads to HBsAg label binding is strong evidence that the cell is also producing antibody molecules with only HBsAg specificity.

Because of the differences in mobilities noted on PAGE, we next attempted to separate the BSH 016 antibody moieties on a preparative

Table 2

Analysis of Antibody Species from BSH 016

Separated on DEAE Chromatography

Pool	Fractions	Yield (μg)	Antigen Binding† *PAP(%)	*HBsAg(%)	Specificity
I	81-90	2,020	10	91	HBsAg
IIa	116-131	2,000	100	100	Hybrid
IIb	132-152	4,170	---	---	
IIc	153-164	945	82	98	Hybrid
III	171-197	1,942	93	4	PAP

† 100 ng of the corresponding antibody pools were incubated for 4 hours with ^{125}I-PAP or ^{125}I-HBsAg then overnight with immobilized horse anti-mouse antibody to determine antigen specificity.
* ^{125}I-labeled

scale by DEAE ion exchange chromotography. Figure 12 shows the resulting 3 well separated peaks, the middle one evidently composed of at least two species. When these peaks were analyzed on PAGE, each yielded a single band corresponding to one of the bands present in the starting material.

Each of the DEAE peaks was subsequently tested for antigen binding using radiolabeled HBsAg and PAP. The first peak could bind HBsAg, but not PAP, the second peak (and the peak shoulder) could bind both PAP and HBsAg, while the third peak could bind PAP and not HBsAg (Table 2). These results demonstrate that well over 50% of the antibody is "hybrid" in nature, and roughly approximates the 1:2:1 ratios expected if all heavy chains are synthesized in equal amounts and randomly associate with each other, regardless of origin.

The antibody hybrid (peak II) was radiolabeled and 85% of the radioactivity from peak II could bind PAP and 88% could bind to HBsAg, indicating that the vast majority of immunoreactive antibody in this peak is hybrid. The affinity of the hybrid for the PAP antigen was found to be slightly lower than that of the parental PAC 017 antibody. This slightly lower affinity of the hybrid in comparison to its parental PAC 017 antibody is probably due to the univalence of the antibody for PAP and it is about the same difference as we have seen to occur between an antibody and its Fab fragment. The hybrid molecule appears to be stable, with no observable changes in its electrophoretic gel characteristics or in its dual specificity even after prolonged storage.

When these experiments were begun, it was not immediately obvious that such large amounts of hybrid antibody would be made. In fact, we were not even certain that any hybrid molecules would be formed. If the assumptions are made that all heavy and light chains are synthesized in equal amounts and their association with one another is totally random, and if correct heavy and light chain pairing is necessary for antigen binding, then only 1/8 of the synthesized immunoglobulin should be hybrid molecules capable of efficiently binding both antigens. The observation that well over half of the antibody is comprised of functional hybrid molecules implies that either association is not totally random, or that correct heavy and light chain pairing is not necessary for antigen binding, or both. It is likely that heavy chain pairing is essentially random between molecules of the same IgG subclass, since such pairing occurs before light chain addition and involves only constant region interactions. However, the association of light with heavy chain probably favors homologous combination, since it appears to involve specific interactions between both constant and variable regions [13] and follows two step kinetics [14]. In addition, incorrect light chain pairing could lower the affinity of binding without completely eliminating it, and the resulting antibody would still appear antigen specific in our test systems. In this regard, the shoulder of the hybrid peak from DEAE appeared to have a slightly lower K_a for PAP antigen than did the major peak. In any case, the large percentage of hybrid molecules formed and the ease with which they can be produced and separated on a preparative scale is encouraging.

Currently, several hybridoma lines that secrete antibodies against tumor associated antigens are being back-selected. These will be fused with spleen cells from mice immunized with antigens such as toxins or therapeutic drugs, and the resulting hybrid monoclonal antibodies tested in vivo in tumor localization and therapeutic programs. The use of these hybrid antibodies may eliminate much of the non-specific localization previously observed in such systems.

Another potential use of such bifunctional antibodies is their application to homogeneous assays as described above. If the antibodies used were bifunctional and bound the antigen and the indicator molecules in the correct orientation, the problems associated with stably coupling the indicators to the antibodies without inactivating them would be lessened.

Immunoaffinity Chromatography

Immunoaffinity chromatography provides an ideal tool for the exceedingly specific isolation of minor antigenic species from a heterogeneous mixture of biological materials. In the past, immunoaffinity chromatography has suffered from one dilemma: highly efficient adsorption from dilute solution necessitates using high affinity antibodies, while efficient desorption of a biologically active antigen from the antibody requires low affinity antibodies. Even antibodies of moderate affinity often require rather drastic elution conditions, such as low pH or high concentrations of chaotropes, often resulting in some denaturation of the antigen and a reduced lifetime of the immunoadsorbent.

It has been reported that single amino acid substitution (ser→leu) in type A influenza virus caused a change in affinity of a monoclonal antibody of about 5 orders of magnitude [15]. This data implies that a very minor change in the primary sequence of either an antigen or an antibody can enormously affect the interaction of a specific antigen-antibody pair. Relatively minor changes in pH conditions, which would be expected to titrate certain amino acids such as his or lys, can similarly effect major changes in antigen-antibody interactions. Such "switches" would not be noted in a population of polyclonal antibodies, due to the hetereogeneity of the population; but, because of the homogeneity of monoclonal antibodies, these simple alterations in the charges of specific amino acids can permit the "switch" of a high affinity antigenantibody interactin to one of extremely low affinity. This capability permits the use of high affinity antibodies for immunopurification purposes, and provides a means for efficient desorption of antigen under relatively mild conditions.

Figure 13 shows the sensitivity of one monoclonal antibody (072) specific for hGH to mildly acidic conditions. The control antibody, 352, retained its high affinity for the antigen under these conditions. Figure 13b illustrates the desorption of ^{125}I-hGH from a monoclonal antibody (101) which is sensitive to moderately basic conditions. The control antibody in this experiment, 033, retained its high affinity for the antigen even at pH 10.5, under which conditions the antigen had almost completely eluted from the 101 antibody ball adsorbent. K_a's for all four antibodies were $\geq 10^{10}$ M^{-1} at pH 7. Table 3 illustrates the rate of desorption of a PAP specific antibody. At the shortest experimentally feasible incubation period, 1.3 minutes, essentially all of the ^{125}I-PAY-276 (K_a, pH 7 $\approx 5 \times 10^{10}$ M^{-1}) had desorbed from the insolubilized PAP. Because of the short time involved, the balls were not washed prior to counting, leading to the increased counts present at the 30 ng/ml PAP concentration.

It is apparent from this data that the alterations in pH affect

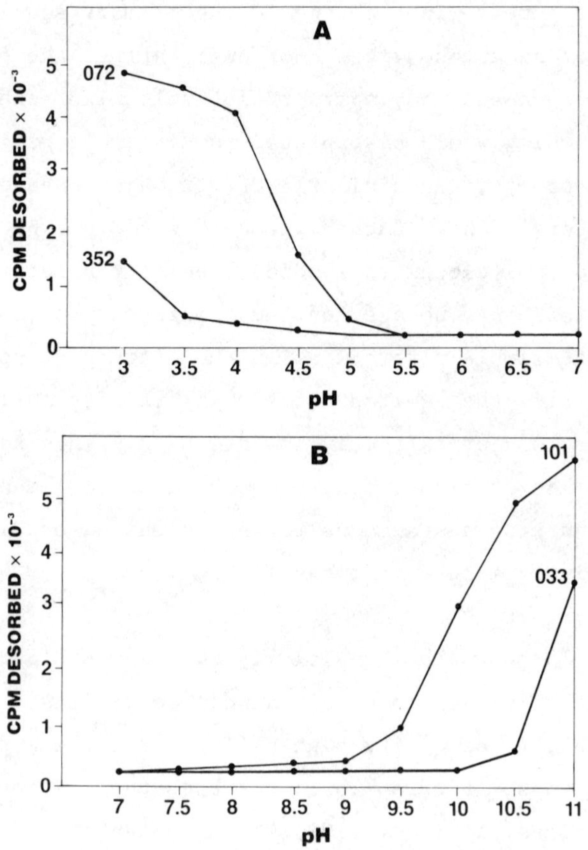

Fig. 13. Desorption of ^{125}I-hGH from insoluble monoclonal antibodies. Monoclonal antibodies to human growth hormone (hGH) bound to polysyrene balls were incubated with ^{125}I-hGH, (Cambridge Nuclear, 50 μCi/μg) then washed to remove unbound antigen. Each ball was allowed to adsorb approximately 0.1 to 0.2 ng of antigen, representing a condition of gross antibody excess. Triplicate balls were incubated with 1.0 ml of buffer at various pH conditions for 4 hr at room temperature, then 800 μl of each supernatant fraction was counted for ^{125}I-hGH.

specific antigen-antibody interactions dramatically and almost instantaneously. The ability to rapidly "switch" from high to low

Table 3

Desorption of ^{125}I-PAY-276 from Insoluble PAP

PAP conc. (ng/ml)	cpm untreated	cpm treated *		
		1.3 min	10 min	
		pH 4.0	pH 4.0	pH 6.5
0	1,711	1,260	1,328	1,502
1	4,128	1,594	1,456	3,494
5	13,261	2,136	1,766	11,858
10	22,423	1,970	2,036	19,282
20	39,121	2,728	2,476	35,338
30	53,061	2,734	3,154	49,780

^{125}I-antibody desorption. A series of calibration curves for prostatic acid phosphatase (PAP) were set up in the range of 0 to 30 ng/ml. Calibrators were incubated with ^{125}I-anti-PAP monoclonal antibody (10-15 μCi/μg) in the presence of a polystyrene ball to which a second monoclonal antibody had been bound. The ^{125}I-labeled antibody had previously been demonstrated to desorb at pH 4.0 to 4.5, while the solid phase antibody (against a distinct epitope on PAP) had been shown to retain its high affinity under these conditions. After 4 hours at room temperature, each ball was washed 2 times with saline containing 0.1% Tween-20, then duplicate balls were treated for either 1.3 minutes or 10 minutes at pH 4.0 or for 10 minutes at pH 6.5. Unbound radiolabeled antibodies were removed by aspiration, and the balls were counted for residual ^{125}I-antibody without washing.

affinity will provide an ideal tool for immunoaffinity chromatographic procedures.

The concept of affecting the strength of an antigen-antibody reaction is not necessarily limited to the titration of charged amino acids, but would also apply to other kinds of interactions. For example, low concentrations of urea or chaotropes could be used which would result in highly specific inhibition reactions, rather than general alterations in antigen and antibody properties. Another example would include aromatic nonionic detergents such as Triton X-100 for the dissociation of antigen-antibody complexes where binding reactions require aromatic pi-bonding. Borate would inhibit the binding of certain carbohydrate specific antibodies or interactions where one of the ligands displays a very specific tertiary structure as in serine proteinases [11].

The specific amino acids affected by a given elution condition, such as pH titration of histidine or lysine, may be present on either the antigen or the antibody. In addition, the specific amino acid(s) affected need not reside on either the antigen epitope or within the antibody combining site. For example, Rudikoff et al. [17] reported a glu→ala substitution which destroyed the affinity of a myeloma protein for phosphocholine by destabilizing H-L chain interactions.

Only through the homogeneity of monoclonal antibodies can the "switch" phenomenon be efficiently utilized. Proper selection procedures could yield a population of polyclonal antibodies which behaved similarly, but the selection procedure would require much antigen, would probably be tedious, and would result in a mixture of intrinsically low affinity antibodies and high affinity "switch" antibodies. The opportunity to select for "switch" antibodies sensitive to specific conditions, such as mildly acidic or basic pH conditions, provides flexibility in tailoring an affinity matrix to deal with antigens which are stable only under certain conditions. For example, PAP is quite sensitive to even mildly basic conditions, but is extremely stable under mildly acidic conditions. Thus, an immunoaffinity purification system designed for the isolation of PAP would incorporate an antibody which "switches" in mild acid. In fact, we have carried out semi-preparative purification of PAP from diluted seminal fluid using PAY-276 bound to Sepharose with excellent results. On the other hand, human growth hormone appears to be stable to both acidic and basic conditions, and an immunopurification system could readily use either hGH specific antibody 072 or 101 for efficient purification.

The usefulness of immunoaffinity chromatography is likely to experience a major advance due to the onset of monoclonal antibody technology, and to the ability to select for "switch" antibodies.

SUMMARY

The ability to "engineer" antibodies, using the techniques of somatic cell genetics and cell fusion, has opened a new era in immunochemistry. No longer are immunologists limited by the vagaries of polyclonal antibody production. Using hybridoma technology, consistent preparations of precisely defined monoclonal antibodies are now available. Immunochemists are free to pick and choose those precisely defined characteristics of a homogeneous species of antibody that are best suited for a given application. To date, monoclonal antibodies have been used primarily as research chemicals. However, the implications of this new technology for diagnostic, therapeutic, and separation systems are rapidly becoming apparent.

ACKNOWLEDGEMENT

The authors would like to thank Karyl LaPinska for preparing the manuscript, and our co-workers at Hybritech for discussions and advice.

REFERENCES

1. Kphler, G., and C. Milstein. Continuous cultures of fused cells secreting antibody of pre-defined specificity. Nature 256:485-497 (1975).
2. Vaitukaitis, J.L., G.D., Braunstein, and G.T. Ross. A radioimmunoassay which specifically measures human chorionic gonadotropin in the presence of human luteinizing hormone. Am. J. Obstet. Gynecol. 113:751-757 (1972).
3. Storring, P.L, R.E. Gaines-Das, and D.R. Bangham. International reference preparation of human chorionic gonadotropin for immunoassay: Potency estimates in various bioassay and protein binding assays; and international reference preparations of the α and β subunits of human chorionic gonadotropin for immunoassay. J. Endocrinol. 84:295-310 (1980).
4. Reuter, A.M., J. Schoonbrood, and P. Franchimont. Specific radioimmunoassay of HCG and its α and β subunits: Methods and

results. In Cancer Related Antigens, P. Franchimont, Ed., Elsevier-North Holland Biomedical Press, Amsterdam and New York, pp. 237-250 (1976).

5. Rubenstein, K.E., R.S. Schneider, and E.F. Ullman. "Homogeneous" enzyme immunoassay. A new immunochemical technique. Biochem. Biophys. Res. Commun. 47:846-851 (1972).
6. Ballou, B., G. Levine, T.R. Hakala, and D. Solter. Tumor location detected with radioactively labeled monoclonal antibody and external scintigraphy. Science 206:844-847 (1979).
7. Palmer, J.L., and A. Nisonoff. Science 143:376 (1973).
8. J. F. Kearney, A. Radbrach, B. Liesegang, and K. Rajenaky. A new mouse myeloma cell line that has lost immunoglobulin expression but permits the construction of antibody-secreting hybrid cell lines. J. Immunol. 123:1548-1550 (1979).
9. Littlefield, J.W. Selection of hybrids from matings of fibroblasts in vitro and their presumed recombinants. Science 145: 709-710 (1964).
10. Wang, R., E.D. Sevier, R.A., Reisfeld, and G.S. David. Semi-automatic solid-phase radioimmunoassay for carcinoembryonic antigens. J. Immunol. Methods 18:157-164 (1977).
11. Ornstein, L. Disc electrophoresis-I. Background and theory. Ann. N.Y. Acad. Sci. 121:321-349 (1964).
12. Davis, B.J. Disc electrophoresis-II. Method and application to human serum proteins. Ann. N.Y. Acad. Sci. 121:404-427 (1964).
13. Alexander, I., D.I.C. Kells, K.J. Dorrington, and M. Klein. Mol. Immunol. 17:1351 (1980).
14. Watt, R.M., and E.W. Voss, Jr. J. Biol. Chem. 254:7150 (1979).
15. Laver, W.G., W.G. Gerhard, R.G. Webster, M.E. Frankel, and G.M. Air. Proc. Natl. Acad. Sci. USA, 76:1425-1429 (1979).
16. Akparov, V.KH., and V.M. Stepanov, J. Chromatograph, 155:329-336. (1978).
17. Rudikoff, S., A.M. Giusti, W.D. Cook, M.D. Sharff, Proc. Natl. Acad. Sci. USA 79:1979-1983 (1982).

BIOTECHNOLOGY FOR AGRICULTURE
OVERVIEW BY CONVENER

Roger Kleese
Molecular Genetics, Inc.
Minnetonka, Minnesota 55343

There are four points which I think are important as an overview if we are to think ahead to the applications we might make with biotechnology.

Point 1: The magnitude of the effort to develop these new technologies with crop species has, as I'm sure you know, been very minimal to date. Certainly, in contrast to recombinant DNA work with *E. coli* or microorganisms in general, our efforts are not extensive. We're going to see considerable activity in the future and I am very positive about the prospects for this area of research. But we do need to understand a great deal more about gene structure and function, how genes are put together and how they are regulated in plants. If we were to select a particular plant gene to transfer, today there would not be very many choices. I'm thinking of the genes that would have economic importance. Many of those genes are not easily isolated.

Genes for disease resistance are often mentioned as important candidates for gene transfer. However, there are very few genes for disease resistance or any other single-gene trait which could even be isolated with current laboratory techniques. Working with the complex traits that are important to plant breeders, is a much more difficult task. Let me give you an example of what I'm thinking about. "Standability" in cereal species is, as the name suggests, the ability of the plant to stand up through the entire growing season. This greatly facilitates harvest and can result in increased productivity. It can be a serious problem in many crop species. Standability not only involves good stems or stalks, but also good roots. It may involve resistance to insects or diseases which are probably unrelated genetically to desirable morphological or anatomical features of the stalks or the roots. Even if we were working in a disease- or insect-free environment, we do not have a clear understanding of the genetic control of good stalk strength or good root development. When we begin to look at some of the important economic traits in which plant breeders are interested we quickly find they are physiologically and genetically very complex. Manipulating these genes will not be easy.

Point 2: Species specificity seems to be playing a very major role in what we can or cannot do, especially with plant tissue culture. If we are to use biotechnology on a broad scale with crop species, we have to be able to manipulate a dozen or fifteen major crop species, plus a few minor crop species. Within these crop species we have many important genotypes. In corn alone, a species with which I'm more familiar, it would be nice if we could work with at least the most important inbred lines. But, if we were really efficient with our technologies, it would be desirable to work with two to three dozen different inbreds. This is much different than working with a limited number of microorganisms.

Point 3: Many of the applications of gene transfer will be done with genes which need to be appropriately regulated in development. In our place of business, we are interested in making subunit animal vaccines so one of the things we must do is raise the level of expression of the gene for the antigenic protein in the host bacterium. We want to maximize the production of that protein.

This is very different than altering traits which lead to improvements in crop species. Consider yield as an example. Yield is physiologically and genetically extremely complex so we have tried to work instead with the components of yield. We can think of these components as either morphological or physiological. Morphological components of yield are seed size, seed number, and perhaps the number of inflorescence per plant, i.e., the number of spikes, ears, etc. Examples of physiological components are rate of photosynthate production and rate of translocation of that photosynthate from the leaf to the grain. As we've worked with these components we have looked for variability which gives us, for example, maximum seed number or maximum photosynthetic rate. This approach has not been very profitable. I believe we do not want to maximize the components but rather only the end point of these components; that is, yield.

Because the components interact with each other we would like to optimize their rate or number with respect to each other so that maximum yield is generated. Genes with regulatory functions will be instrumental in controlling these variables. But how does one determine these optimal rates or numbers bearing in mind there may be many combinations which result in superior yield? We simply don't have an answer for this question. Understanding and controlling the regulation of these components will be important if we are to successfully alter such complex traits.

Point 4: It is absolutely essential to know and understand the marketplace and the plant breeders'current practices and needs. The plant breeder is in a position to be knowledgeable about the market. If he is going to be producing varieties or hybrids for ten or fifteen years hence he must have an understanding of the market needs for that time. It is through his eyes, his knowledge of germplasm and his knowledge of the agricultural scene that one can obtain valuable feedback for the laboratory. This can give focus and direction to the kinds of research we want to do.

The chapters that follow will deal with some aspects of gene transfer, but there are a number of plant breeders who are not greatly interested in gene transfer. They would rather have help in the selection and evaluation of their material. They would like to make their selections more efficiently and to evaluate them more rapidly and precisely. Are there ways that our new technology can help them in these and other areas where they express a need?

I would summarize this fourth point by urging the interaction among molecular biologists, those working with tissue cultures, and plant breeders. It is important that each of us begins to know and understand each other's needs and capabilities.

BIOCHEMICAL STUDIES ON THE SUCROSE SYNTHASE GENE IN *ZEA MAYS* L. AND ON CONTROLLING ELEMENT *Ds* INSERTED AT THIS LOCUS

U. Courage-Tebbe, H-P. Döring, M. Geiser,
P. Starlinger, E. Tillmann, E. Weck, and W. Werr

Institut fur Genetik, Universitat Köln
Federal Republic of Germany

The molecular biology of plants has not yet been studied as extensively as in animals. Techniques to introduce isolated genes at will into cells or even into whole animals via the germ line have only beginnings of counterparts in plants. As it would be very desirable to develop such techniques, it will be useful to examine the existing genetic knowledge for possible approaches. Such approaches will be especially welcome in monocotyledonous plants which include some of the most important crop plants.

One of the phenomena worth studying in this context are "controlling elements" in *Zea mays L*. They were discovered by B. McClintock in studies of unstable mutations. In a long series of very detailed investigations, McClintock and a few other corn geneticists established that the unstable mutations are due to the insertion of transposable genetic elements at the gene loci. At the site of insertion, they can exert various effects on adjacent genes. These effects extend from complete or partial inactivation of genes to enhancement of gene action and may be subject to controlling influences exerted by other genetic elements which in many cases have proved to be transposable themselves [17,21,23].

While the genetic and physiological properties of controlling elements in corn were established by genetic means in the 1940s and 1950s, transposable elements were studied by biochemical means in the 1960s and 1970s, first in bacteria [1,13,14,24] and later in a variety of eucaryotic organisms, most thoroughly in yeast and in *Drosophila melanogaster*. It was established that transposable elements consist of DNA. Many of them were sequenced and by sequence analysis and physiological studies certain features of their behavior were elucidated [5,16,25,]. The comparison of their properties with those of controlling elements in *Zea mays L*. showed a similarity to the elements in corn. Studies at the DNA level, however, were lacking [22,25]. It would be desirable to study the maize controlling elements for their inherent interest. In addition, maize elements may also bear a vast potential for application. One of these lies in the fact that spontaneous mutations in corn can be caused by the insertion of these elements at a gene locus rather than by other means. Thus, the additional creation of genetic variability may be aided by a detailed understanding of these elements and possibly by ways to use them in mutagenesis.

In addition, it would be desirable to introduce DNA into single plant cells and regenerate whole plants. This is certainly difficult in itself, but once achieved, it will be useful only if this DNA is incorporated into plant chromosomes. It is not yet clear, whether this will happen spontaneously. If transposable elements are present in the newly introduced DNA, and if it will become possible to produce *in vitro* manipulated controlling elements with recognizable inserted genes, this might eventually aid in genetic manipulation of plants.

For all these reasons, we have looked for means to study corn controlling elements at the molecular level. The starting point for the biochemical study of transposable elements in corn must be the isolation and identification of a DNA sequence. At present there is no direct way to do this. An indirect way, however, is conceivable [9]. Methods are available to isolate genes with an identifiable gene product. If mutants are known, in which a specific gene is inactivated by the insertion of a controlling element, the DNA of this gene and surrounding sequences could be isolated both from the wild type and the mutant. DNA present at the gene locus in the latter, but not in the former, might then belong to the controlling element. This might be proven using the cloned DNA as a starting material.

For our studies, we chose the gene Sh which encodes endosperm sucrose synthase [7,8]. McClintock had isolated mutants of this gene which are caused by the insertion of controlling element Ds in their vicinity [18,19]. She could show this because Ds causes chromosome breaks and the consequent loss of genes located on the part of the chromosome distal to the break. These breaks, however, occur only if another controlling element, Ac, is present in the same cell. Ac activates Ds in position trans.

From the genetic point of view, these mutations are not ideal for our studies. They have arisen in a complicated series of events to be described below. In addition, the pattern of forward and backward mutation of these unstable mutants cannot be followed as easily as in those cases where a gene responsible for color formation of the kernels is involved. We reasoned, however, that these disadvantages would be more than compensated by the fact that sucrose synthase is a major endosperm protein and that this would facilitate the preliminary steps of gene isolation.

As a first step, we showed that developing endosperm contains the mRNA for sucrose synthase using cell-free translation in reticulocyte lystates and immunoprecipitation of the product [28]. In the next step, we prepared cDNA from the mixture of endosperm mRNAs and cloned it in pBR322, using GC tailing. From a collection of approximately 250 clones obtained by transformation of *E. coli*, we isolated one clone that contained an insert transcribed from the sucrose synthase gene. This was shown by its ability to specifically bind the sucrose synthase mRNA which, after subsequent elution, gave the correct product upon translation and immunoprecipitation [11].

The cDNA clone was nick-translated and used as a probe in Southern hybridization experiments with genomic DNA obtained from the wild type and several mutants caused by the insertion of *Ds* at the sucrose synthase gene. One major band, and in a few cases some minor bands, were observed. While these latter bands stayed constant, the major band was altered in the mutants, indicating: (i) that this band probably contains the sucrose synthase gene and (ii) that the mutations investigated are indeed caused by a DNA rearrangement rather than by a point mutation. This latter statement had to await confirmation, because restriction polymorphisms are observed in maize DNA and a restriction pattern deviation is not solid proof for a DNA rearrangement. We could, however, establish a limited restriction map around the hybridizing region by single and double digestion with several restriction endonucleases. These restriction maps show regions of homology between all three mutants and differences in another segment of the restriction map, thus lending support to the hypothesis of a DNA rearrangement [10]. Similar results have been reported by Burr and Burr [3] and by Chaleff *et al*. [6].

Starting from these observations, we size-fractionized genomic DNA after digestion with the appropriate restriction endonuclease and tried to clone the DNA in *λ1059*, a BamHI replacement vector which allowed the selection of those phages in which the internal fragment of the phage DNA has been replaced [15]. Plaque-hybridization of the *in vitro* packaged phage thus allowed us to isolate *λ* phages carrying DNA hybridizing to our cDNA clone from the wild type and the two mutants, sh-m5933 and sh-m6233. The first two DNA inserts have, up to now, been characterized more extensively and will be described below (M. Geiser, E. Weck, H.-P. Döring, U. Courage-Tebbe, E. Tillmann, P. Starlinger, manuscript in preparation).

Restriction maps have been constructed of the DNA inserts. These coincide with those deduced from Southern blotting of genomic DNA with regard to the order of cleavage sites, though size determinations could be made more accurately by summing up small fragments rather than measuring large ones. The wild type phage carries a 16kb BamHI fragment. This has been subcloned in pBR322 for further studies. The clone obtained from mutant sh-m5933 carries a 21kb BclI fragment. From it, several subfragments have been subcloned in pBR322. The following results have been obtained:

1. Restriction analysis and DNA-DNA hybridization experiments have shown that the DNA segment of 6kb located at the right of the map of sh-m5933 is homologous to corresponding segments of the wild type DNA extending to the BciI site.

2. The region hybridizing to the cDNA clone is located about 4kb to the left of the BclI site. The BglII site separating a 6kb BglII fragment and a 3,3kb BglII fragment is present on the cDNA clone.

3. A HindIII site located just to the right of the BglII site is not found in the cDNA clone. It may belong to an intron not represented in the cDNA.

4. Several fragments from the DNA region presumably containing the sucrose synthase gene were isolated and subjected to exonuclease

VII and endonuclease S1 mapping [2,27]. Though these experiments are not yet complete, the presence of at least one intron and an extension of the gene of 800bp to the right of the *Bgl*II site separating the 3.3 and the 6.0kb fragments have been established. The number of introns and extension of the gene to the left of the *Bgl*II site have not been determined yet with certainty (W. Werr, unpublished).

5. Approximately 2kb to the left of the *Bgl*II site mentioned above, the homology between mutant and wild type DNA terminates. Mutant DNA located to the left of this junction does not show homology to the DNA of the wild type clone. This DNA has a length of approximately 15kb. It may either be DNA of transposable element *Ds*, or else it may be DNA of the maize chromosome rearranged under the influence of the controlling element which in the wild type is located at another position.

6. The availability of a cloned 16kb fragment containing the sucrose synthase gene enabled us to extend our study of genomic DNA by means of Southern blotting analysis. We found that several restriction fragments of this DNA contain repetitive sequences. In addition, a few DNA segments used as probes gave unique patterns of DNA.

Using the evidence presently available, we arrive at the following conclusions: No part of the DNA detectable in the wild type is missing in the DNA of mutants *sh-m5933* and *sh-m6233* as far as the resolution of the blotting analysis allows us to detect. These mutants differ from mutant *shbz-m4*, the DNA of which does not hybridize to the DNA of the wild type clone, and thus carries a deletion of at least 16kb length. No such deletion is present, however, in the other two mutants, contrary to our hypothesis deducted from limited data obtained by Southern blotting with the cDNA clone. From these data, we had hypothesized that all mutants at the sucrose synthase gene had originated by adjacent deletions to the right of Ds located at some distance from the sucrose synthase gene [10]. This hypothesis is no longer tenable, and we must assume that in addition to deletions other rearrangements can be caused by Ds.

7. The 15kb segment of DNA that is present in the cloned DNA of mutant sh-m5933 but not in the cloned DNA of wild type and may be Ds DNA has been characterized to a limited extent. Restriction mapping and hybridization experiments have shown that at least two inverted repeats of several hundred base pairs each are present of this DNA segment. The rightmost member of the first pair is located around a BamHI site, located no more than 300 base pairs to the left of the junction point between wild type and non-wild type DNA. The first 100bp of these 300bp segments are part of the inverted repeat. This could be shown by DNA sequencing. It is possible, but not yet proven, that this member of the inverted repeat extends up to the junction point. This is presently being investigated by further DNA sequencing.

The other pair of inverted repeats is located to the left and to the right, respectively, of the left member of the first pair of inverted repeats.

8. The availability of a DNA fragment that possibly (but by no means certainly) belongs to Ds has enabled us to study the question of whether this DNA is represented in genomic DNA only once or in several copies. We have done hybridization experiments with genomic DNA of several maize lines using subcloned fragments of the "non-wild type" DNA of the cloned segment of mutant sh-m5933 as a probe.

Our probes hybridize to a limited number of DNA fragments. With several probes and maize lines, we count between 10 and 25 bands.

The actual number may be larger due to overlapping bands. If a 2.25kb *Bam*HI-*Hind*III fragment carrying the junction is used as a probe, all bands are of similar, low intensity. If a 4.4kb *Eco*RI-*Bam*HI fragment or a 2.7kb *Bam*HI fragment internal to the putative *Ds* DNA are used, the intensity of the bands varies from weak to strong. This may reflect different lengths of homologous DNA in various fragments, while the 2.25kb junction fragment does not contain more than approximately 300bp of *Ds* DNA and thus cannot hybridize to extended regions in the genomic DNA. Other explanations including different degrees of homology, or the presence of several DNA fragments of identical size are not excluded, however.

The observation that a limited number of DNA fragments hybridizes to our probes is interesting. The DNA cannot be unique DNA from the vicinity of the shrunken gene that is placed next to this gene by DNA rearrangement in the mutants. Neither does this DNA hybridize to the many bands usually observed with repetitive DNA. The presence of a limited number of copies of *Ds* would explain our data.

There are difficulties with this interpretation, however. If all copies of *Ds* were identical, the use as probes of internal fragments should lead to the appearance of only one strong band. This band should represent the internal DNA fragment cleaved from all copies of *Ds* DNA. The hybridization pattern will be complicated if internal fragments crosshybridize. Only the 2.25kb fragment carrying the junction between the sucrose synthase gene and *Ds* DNA should reveal as many bands as there are copies of *Ds* (or twice this number if the termini of *Ds* should be identical).

The presence of many bands hybridizing to internal fragments might indicate a structural heterogeneity of several copies of *Ds*. Functional heterogeneity of different *Ds* was described by McClintock as "states" of the element [17,21]. At the DNA level, the cloning of these sequences will be necessary to support the above assumptions. One additional clone available was obtained from sh-m6233 (E. Weck, unpublished). In addition to the wild type clone, it also hybridizes to subcloned mutant DNA of sh-m5933. The restriction maps of the two mutant DNAs are, however, different.

The present studies have laid the foundation for further investigations which will lead to a better understanding of the DNA structure of transposable element Ds in Zea mays L.

ACKNOWLEDGEMENT

These investigations were supported by the Landesamt für Forschung des Landes Nordrhein-Westfalen and the Kommission der Europäischen Gemeinschaft.

REFERENCES

1. Adhya, S.L., J.A. Shapiro, (1969) The galactose operon of E. coli K12, I. Structural and pleiotropic mutations of the operon, Genetics 62:231-247.
2. Berk, A.J., P.A. Sharp, (1978) Spliced mDNAs of Simian virus 40, Proc. Natl. Acad. Sci. USA, 75:1274-1278.
3. Burr, B., F. Burr, (1981) Detection of maize controlling element events at the shrunken locus, Genetics 98:143-156.
4. Calos, M.P., L. Johnsrud, J.H. Miller, (1978) DNA sequences at the integration sites of the insertion element IS1, Cell 13:411.
5. Calos, M., J.H. Miller, (1980) Transposable Elements, Cell 20:579-595.
6. Chaleff, D., J. Mauvais, S. McCormick, M. Shure, S. Wessler, N. Fedoroff (1981) Controlling elements in maize, Carnegie Inst. Wash. Yearbook 80:158-174.

7. Chourey, P., O. Nelson, (1976) The enzymatic deficiency conditioned by the shrunken-1 mutation in maize. Biochem. Genetics 14:1041-1055.

8. Chourey, P., D. Schwartz, (1971) Ethyl methane sulfonate-induced mutation of the Sh protein in maize. Mutat. Res. 12:151-157.

9. Döring, H.P, R. Ehring, M. Geiser, P. Starlinger, J. Wostemeyer (1979) The gene encoding endosperm sucrose synthetase in Zea mays as a tool to study controlling elements. In The Plant Genome, p. 72 (Eds. D.R. Davies and D.A. Hopwood).

10. Döring, H.P., M. Geiser, P. Starlinger, (1981) Transposable element Ds at the shrunken locus in Zea mays, Mol. Gen. Genet. 184:377-380.

11. Geiser, M., H.P. Döring, J. Wostemeyer, U. Behrens, E. Tillmann, P. Starlinger, (1980) A cDNA clone from Zea mays endosperm sucrose-synthase mRNA, Nucl. Acids. Res. 8:6175-6188.

12. Grindley, N.D.F. (1978) IS1 Insertion generates duplication of nine base sequence at its target site, Cell 13:419.

13. Jordan, E., H. Saedler, and P. Starlinger, (1967) Strong-polar Mutations in the transferase gene of the galactose operon in Escherichia coli, Mol. Gen. Genet. 100:296-306.

14. Jordan, E., H. Saedler, P. Starlinger (1968) 0°- and strong-polar mutations in the gal operon are insertions, Mol. Gen. Genet. 102:353-363.

15. Karn, J., S. Brenner, L. Barnett, G. Cesarini, (1980) Novel bacteriophage λ cloning vector. Proc. Natl. Acad. Sci., USA 77:5172-5176.

16. Kleckner, N (1981) Transposable elements in prokaryotes, Ann. Review of Genetics 15:341-404.

17. McClintock, B. (1951) Chromosome organization and genetic expression, Cold. Spring Harbor Symp. Quant. Biol. 16:13-47.

18. McClintock, B. (1952) Mutable loci in maize, Carnegie Inst. Wash. Yearbook 51:212-219.

19. McClintock, B. (1953) Mutation in maize, Carnegie Inst. Wash. Yearbook 52:227-237.

20. McClintock, B. (1955) Controlled mutation in maize, Carnegie Inst. Wash. Yearbook 54:245-255.

21. McClintock, B. (1965) The control of gene action in maize, Brookhaven Symp. Biol. 18:162-184.

22. Nevers, P.,and H. Saedler (1977) Transposable genetic elements as agents of gene instability and chromosomal rearrangements, Nature 268:109-115.

23. Peterson, P.A. (1953) A mutable pale green locus in maize, Genetics 38:682.

24. Shapiro, J.A. (1969) Mutations caused by the insertion of genetic material into the galactose operon of *Escherichia coli*, J. Mol. Biol. 40:93-205.

25. P. Starlinger, (1980) A re-examination of McClintock's "Controlling Elements" in maize in view of recent advances in molecular biology. *In* Genome organization and expression in plants (Ed. C.J. Leaver) pp 537-551, Plenum Press.

26. Starlinger, P., (1980) IS-elements and transposons, Plasmid 3:241-259.

27. Weaver, R.F., C. Weissmann, (1979) Mapping of RNA by a modification of the Berk-Sharp procedure: The 5'termini of 15 S β-globin mRNA premature and mature 10 S β-globin mRNA have identical map coordinates, Nucl. Acids Res. 7:1175-1193.

28. Wöstemeyer, J., U. Behrens, A. Merckelbach, M. Müller, P. Starlinger, (1980) Translation of *Zea mays* endosperm sucrose synthase mRNA *in vitro*, Eur. J. Biochem. 114:39-44.

DISCUSSION

Q. P. CLEARY: Is the *Ac* locus similar to the G-loop locus in μ? I mean, do you think of it that way, as a sort of transposase gene?

A. P. STARLINGER: The G-loop does nothing for transpostion. Another gene doesn't transpose the G-loop. I would not draw too much of an analogy to maize in this particular case.

Q. H. GINSBURG: Do you think that there is any relationship between the Ds element and things like enhancers that have been discovered in SV40 that possibly exist in retroviruses in other organisms?

A. STARLINGER: There is a transposable element in maize which is called "enhancer" which has been discovered by Peter Peterson in Ames, Iowa. It is identical to an element which McClintock has studied, called Spm, is this what you are referring to?

Q. GINSBURG: I'm talking about SV40, the 72 base pair repeated element that will effect or enhance the expression of genes.

A. STARLINGER: Well, again, I think we would need to know much more in order to draw some analogies. Ac certainly is an element that contains a whole gene with a trans-acting function. For Ds, to the best of our knowledge, there is not any strong evidence that it can act as a promoter for any gene. In that case, it would at this point become meaningful to ask "How is this gene controlled and does it have this 72-base pair enhancing sequence?" At the moment, it is mainly an element that can be inserted, removed, maybe internally rearranged, and in these functions, to the best of my knowledge at the moment, the sequence doesn't have a part. But it is simply too early to say whether this will come out in the future.

Q. J. WOODMAN: If you have two mutable loci in the same background, do they both respond to Ac at the same time, or are mutable loci autonomous?

A. STARLINGER: That is an experiment that has been done by McClintock, and the answer was yes. Two different Ds loci in the same cell respond at the same time, so probably the rare event, this stochastic event, is happening at Ac and not at the Ds. Let's not forget, in all this transposition business, that we are dealing with something that certainly needs a function, but the function is rarely exerted - in only every thousandth or fewer cells. Yet how do you keep the function down; just by a repressor? How can it be done when such a function is expressed so very rarely?

Q. GINSBURG: Are there any mutants of the Ac locus that have altered the frequency of its expression? You say it's a rare event, and when it happens, all the Ds's in the cell pop out. Can you alter that frequency mutationally at the Ac locus?

A. STARLINGER: Well, again, this is really old work by McClintock and the answer is yes. The situation is complicated. You can vary the dosage of Ac within the cell. The dosage effects a reverse effect. If you have two copies of it, the events are later and rarer than if you have only one copy. There are mutants or changes of Ac state in which a singular seed behaves as two usually do.

Q. S. LEE: Right now, it seems to be the case in bacterial systems that DNA bracketed by insertion sequences has the ability to transpose. Do you think that the element TE may be something like that?

A. STARLINGER: Yes, I think the element TE is somehow similar. But the additional complication that is also present in bacteria is that certain pieces, which have nothing to do with the transposition function - maybe because of evolution - have been fixed to the part of insertion elements. They have a tendency to stick to it for a long time. You find that in transposons.

Q. G. WALKER (MIT): Have you used your Ds probe to get DNA from a variety of different strains that you think might contain insertions?

A. STARLINGER: Up to now, no; we have only looked at a variety of maize lines and the patterns are largely similar, but there are differences. We, of course, want to look at teosinte as well as other species, but this has not yet been done.

THE USE OF TI-PLASMIDS FOR THE GENETIC ENGINEERING OF PLANTS

Joachim Schröder[1], Henri De Greve[2], Jean-Pierre Hernalsteens[2], Jan Leemans[2], Marc Van Montagu[2,3], Léon Otten[1], Gudrun Schröder[1], Lothar Willmitzer[1], and Jozef Schell[1,3]

INTRODUCTION

Crown gall is a neoplastic disease of many dicotyledonous plants and is caused by the soil bacterium *Agrobacterium tumefaciens*. A large extrachromosomal plasmid in these bacteria was found to be responsible for its tumor-inducing capacity and was, therefore, called Ti-plasmid [36]. Bacteria-free crown gall cells can be cultured in the absence of phytohormones like auxines and cytokinines, and this hormone-independent growth defines tumorous growth in plants [1]. Sterile tumor tissues have been shown to contain a DNA segment (called T-DNA) which is homologous and colinear with a defined fragment of the Ti-plasmid, and it is covalently linked to plant DNA [4,23,29,33,34,44,46]. The T-DNA has been localized in the nucleus [5,37] and is directly responsible for

1. Max-Planck-Institut für Züchtungsforschung, D-5000 Köln 30, Federal Republic of Germany;
2. Laboratorium Genetisch Virologie, Vrije Universiteit, Brussels, Belgium;
3. Laboratorium voor Genetika, Rijksuniversiteit, Gent, Belgium

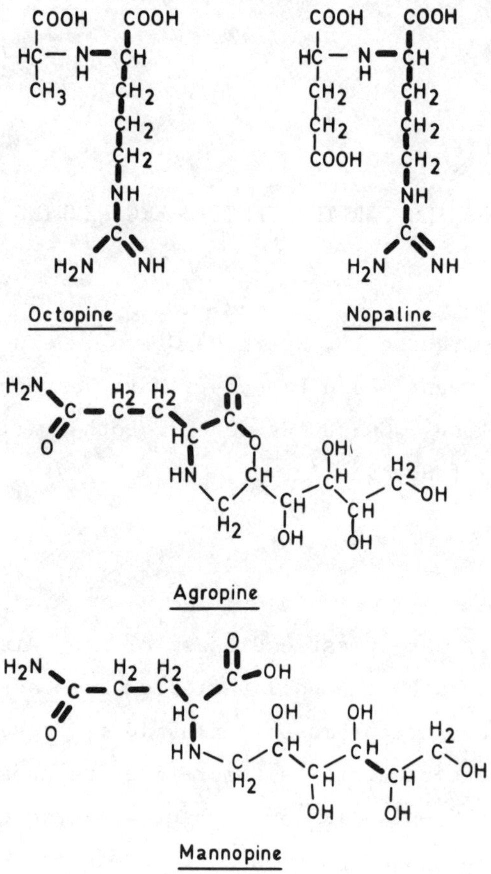

Fig. 1. Chemical structures of some opines found in crown gall tumors.

the hormone-independent growth of the cells. It is also responsible for the synthesis of a number of low molecular weight compounds, called opines, which are not found in normal plant tissues. The opine produced defines crown galls as octopine, nopaline, or agropine type tumors [15](Fig. 1). Opines can be utilized by Agrobacterium tumefaciens selectively as sources for carbon, nitrogen, and energy; thus, the interaction between these bacteria and plants can be seen as a special parasitic relationship which benefits the bacteria [29]. Figure 2 summarizes some of the salient

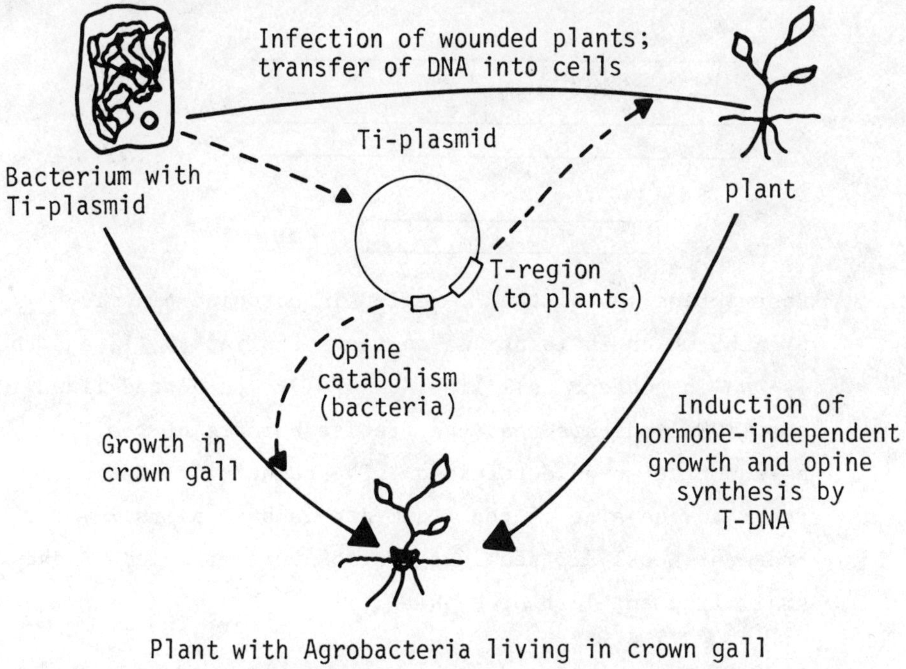

Fig. 2. Genetic colonization of plants by *Agrobacterium tumefaciens*.

features of the biological system.

We describe some recent advances in understanding this system: The functions of the T-DNA in plant tumor cells and the use of Ti-plasmids as vectors for the controlled genetic engineering of plants.

FUNCTIONS OF THE T-DNA

Previous work has shown that the T-DNA is transcribed in transformed plant cells [10,13,14,38], but in most cases the number, sizes, and locations of the coding regions were not known. Recently, these questions were investigated in some cell suspension cultures from tobacco which harbor the T-DNA from pTiA6, a Ti-plasmid inducing octopine synthesis. The cells contain only the TL-fragment of

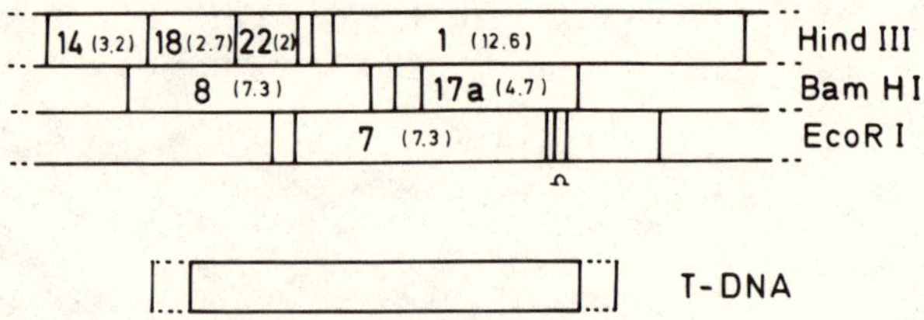

Fig. 3. Restriction map of the T_L-region in octopine plasmid pTiAch5 which is identical to that of pTiA6 [9,11] and the T_L-DNA in tobacco cell line A6-S1[6]. The dotted lines in the T-DNA indicate that the precise borders of the T-DNA have not yet been determined. The numbers in brackets refer to the size of the fragments in base pairs x 10^{-3}. Fragment EcoRI 32 (see last part of this article) is the small fragment left of EcoRI 7.

the T-region [6,33] (Fig. 3). Tumor-specific RNAs were detected and mapped by hybridization of ^{32}P-labelled Ti-plasmid fragments to polyadenylated RNA which had been separated on agarose gels and then transferred to DBM paper. The results [39], summarized in Fig. 4, show that the cells contained a total of seven distinct transcripts which differ markedly in their relative abundance and in their sizes. They all bind to oligo(dT)-cellulose, indicating that they are polyadenylated, and thus, that the T-DNA which was transferred from a prokaryotic organism must provide specific poly(A)-addition sites. The direction of transcription was determined for six of the seven transcripts, and the locations of the approximate 5'- and 3'-ends were mapped on the T_L-DNA.

All seven RNAs mapped within the T-DNA sequence. This and the observation that transcription is inhibited by low concentrations of α-amanitin [40] seems to suggest that each transcript is determined by a specific promoter site on the T_L-DNA recognized by plant RNA

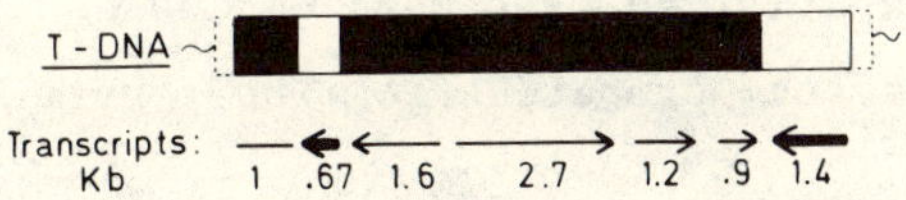

Fig. 4. Transcripts in octopine tumor line A6-S1. The numbers refer to the size of the RNAs in bases X 10^{-3}. The thickness of the lines indicates the relative abundance of the RNAs, and the arrows describe the direction of transcription of the six transcripts where this has been determined.

polymerase II. The data presented here do not rule out that some T-DNA promoters serve for transcription of more than one RNA. Considering the groupwise orientation of several transcripts (Fig. 4), the simplest model would assume one promoter site per group of transcripts. If so, one would expect that inactivation of a 5'-proximal gene of a group would also lead to disappearance of the transcripts from the 5'-distal genes. However, analysis of some cell lines containing the T-DNA of Ti-plasmid mutants indicates that groupwise inactivation of genes did not occur [22]. The results available so far are consistent with the assumption that each gene of the T_L-DNA has its own signals for transcription in the eukaryotic plant cells.

To understand the mechanisms of T-DNA it is important to know whether these RNAs are translated into proteins and to analyze their functions. The hybridization studies and a previous report on T-DNA derived translatable RNAs [24] indicated that the concentrations of these RNAs are very low in transformed plant cells. It was, therefore, necessary to develop a hybridization selection procedure sufficiently sensitive and specific to detect mRNAs which represent about 0.0001% of the total mRNA activity in the plant cells. This procedure was used to enrich for T-DNA derived mRNAs by hybridization to Ti-plasmid fragments covalently bound to microcrystalline cellulose; the hybridized RNAs were eluted and translated *in vitro* in a cell-free system prepared from wheat germ.

The results obtained with this approach are summarized in Fig. 5 [32]. The octopine tumor cells contained at least three T-DNA derived mRNAs which are translated *in vitro* into distinct proteins, and the coding regions correlate with those of three transcripts. The protein encoded at the right end of the T_L-DNA (M_r 39,000] was of specific interest since previous genetic analysis indicated that this part is responsible for octopine synthesis [7,12,20] and since the size of the *in vitro* synthesized protein is identical with that of the octopine-synthesizing enzyme in octopine tumors. Immunological studies showed that this protein was recognized by antiserum against the tumor-specific enzyme [31]. These results were confirmed recently [25] and demonstrate that the structural gene for the octopine-synthesizing enzyme is on the Ti-plasmid. So far, this is the only protein product of the T-DNA with known enzymatic properties; the possible functions of the two smaller T-DNA derived proteins are not known. The region coding for the octopine-synthesizing enzyme has recently been sequenced (De Greve *et al*., manuscript in preparation). According to these data, the sequences for initiation and termination of transcription reveal signals of eukaryotic rather than prokaryotic types, suggesting that this gene is designed for expression in eukaryotic cells.

However, this is not necessarily true for all genes of the T-region, since transcripts were also detected in *Agrobacteria* [13]. It was therefore of interest whether the T-DNA derived mRNAs isolated from plant cells shared properties with typical prokaryotic or eukaryotic mRNAs. The fact that translation of all three mRNAs was inhibited by the cap analogue pm^7G [32] suggests but does not prove that they contain a cap structure at the 5'-end. This would be typical for eukaryotic mRNA, since caps have not been described in prokaryotic RNA. All three mRNAs were found in polyadenylated as well as in nonpolyadenylated RNA fractions; this cannot be used for such a tentative classification, since both types of RNA have been described in eukaryotic as well as in prokaryotic cells.

The mRNAs for the three proteins each represent about 0.0001% of the total mRNA activity in polyribosomal RNA, and this appears to be the detection limit at present for translatable RNA. The other four transcripts detected by hybridization experiments are present at even lower concentrations, and, assuming that they possess mRNA activity, this is likely to be the reason why, so far, the corresponding proteins could not be identified by *in vitro* translation.

A different approach was therefore developed to search for coding regions on the T-DNA and their protein products. Fragments from the T-region were cloned into *E. coli* plasmids and analyzed for gene expression in *E. coli* minicells [30]. Some of the results are also summarized in Fig. 5. There are at least four different coding regions within the T_L-DNA which can be expressed in minicells into distinct proteins from promoters which are active in the prokaryotic cells. The four regions expressed in *E. coli* correlate with four regions transcribed in plant cells into RNA. The plant transcripts are larger than the proteins in *E. coli*, and the regions expressed in minicells appear to lie within the regions transcribed in plant cells. Although other explanations are not ruled out, one may speculate that plant cells and *E. coli* express at least partly the same coding regions.

A fifth coding region was obtained as fusion between part of a bacterial gene from the vector plasmid and part of the structural gene for the octopine-synthesizing enzyme [30]. The gene product of this hybrid in minicells is a fusion protein of the amino-terminal part of the bacterial protein and the carboxy-terminal part of the

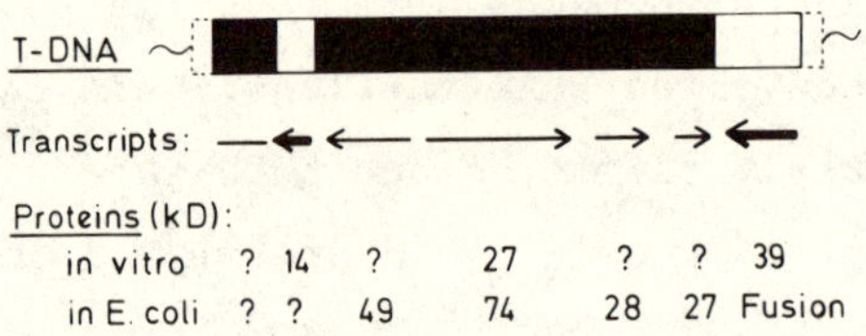

Fig. 5. Correlation of transcripts with proteins encoded on T_L-DNA. Proteins were identified either by translation of hybrid-selected mRNA from tobacco cell line A6-S1 (*in vitro*) or by expression of coding regions in *E. coli* minicells (*E. coli*). The numbers refer to the size of the proteins in Daltons x 10^{-3}. Question marks indicate that it has not been possible so far to demonstrate proteins correlating with the transcripts. The protein with M_r 39,000 represents the octopine-synthesizing enzyme.

plant tumor-specific protein, as shown by specific immunoprecipitations with antisera against both the plant and the bacterial protein. This demonstrates by independent evidence that the structural gene for this protein is on the Ti-plasmid.

In summary, these results clearly show that *Agrobacterium tumefaciens* performs a true genetic manipulation of plants by transfering genes which are actively expressed in plant cells.

As discussed above, the exact functions of most T-DNA gene products are not known. However, the action of the genes leading to hormone-independent growth may be formally compared with the effects of a balanced addition of cytokinins plus auxins to the growth medium of normal cells, since this leads to undifferentiated growth with non-transformed plant cells. If this comparison is meaningful, it should be possible to identify the DNA sequences responsible for the "hormone-like" effects by analyzing tumors induced with mutant

Ti-plasmids with a T-region modified by deletion or insertion of DNA in defined locations. This general approach to identify functions of the T-DNA has been worked out in several laboratories [8, 16,17,18,26,27] and had led to a rough localization of the regions responsible for octopine and nopaline synthesis [7,12,19,20] in the plant cells.

Now the transcripts of the T-DNA have been identified and mapped (Fig. 4), and thus it is possible to assign the mutational inactivation of functions to specific genes [21,22,39]. With respect to the "hormone-like" effects of the T-DNA it is of considerable interest that inactivation of two specific genes led to tumors producing shoots, and this resembles the effect of supplying normal cells with excess cytokinins but no auxins. Thus the inactivated genes appear to produce in undifferentiated tumors with a complete T-DNA an "auxin-like" effect by suppressing shoot formation. Correspondingly, inactivation of a third gene led to tumors producing roots, and this resembles the effect of supplying normal cells with excess auxins but very little cytokinins. Apparently this gene codes for a product suppressing root formation, a "cytokinin-like" effect. Thus it is possible to assign "auxin-like" and "cytokinin-like" effects to specific genes of the T-DNA [22].

The general approach to define functions of the T-DNA which is briefly described here has been extended to other genes as well, and the results will not only assist in the eventual analysis of the exact function of the gene products, but they are also important for the development of new Ti-plasmid derived gene vectors which allow subsequent regeneration of plants from single cells.

GENETIC ENGINEERING OF PLANTS WITH TI-PLASMIDS

There is considerable interest in using Ti-plasmids as vectors for the introduction of desired genes into plants, and it has been shown that foreign DNA can be inserted into the T-region of the plasmid and thus be cotransferred to the plant nucleus [17,21]. Since one of the goals of such experiments is the production of normal plants with interesting new properties, it is important to establish whether cells transformed with T-DNA can be regenerated into plants and whether the additional genetic information is maintained during sexual reproduction. These requirements are difficult to meet when using Ti-plasmids containing the genes for tumorous growth, probably because the activities of these genes cannot be entirely repressed [2,3,35,41-43,45]. Since DNA transfer and tumorous growth are separate functions [22], an alternative approach is to alter Ti-plasmids genetically so as to inactivate the tumor genes in the T-region without interfering with the transfer of the T-DNA to the plant cells.

Such a pTi-mutant has been obtained by Tn7 mutagenesis [7]; it contains the large transposon Tn7 inserted into the fragment EcoRI 32 of pTiB6S3 (see Fig. 3), an octopine type plasmid. Tumors induced on tobacco with this plasmid are morphogenetically very active and produce numerous shoots.

The vast majority of these shoots can, upon separation from the tumor, develop roots and grow into normal plants. These shoots do not contain any measurable T-DNA linked activity or function and are, therefore, presumably derived from either untransformed cells present in the initial, uncloned tumor tissue or from cells which have lost the T-DNA by deletion. By extensive screening of several hundred of these shoots, some were found to contain and express the gene for octopine synthase. These plants have been called rGV1-5 (De Greve _et al._, manuscript in preparation) and one of them, rGV-1, has been studied in great detail. It was found to regenerate into a morphologically normal tobacco plant which contained the additional enzyme activity in all cells of all the organs tested [28].

Table 1

Transmission of the Gene for Octopine Synthesis in Tobacco Plant rGV-1. The Plant is Fertile and the Gene is Transmitted to Progeny as a Dominant Mendelian Gene which is Present Once per Haploid Genome.

Crosses	No. of progeny tested	Octopine synthesis +		-
rGV-1 ♂ x rGV-1 ♀	145	110 (76%)		35 (24%)
rGV-1 ♂ x Wildtype ♀	248	124 (50%)		124 (50%)
rGV-1 ♀ x Wildtype ♂	187	81 (43%)		106 (57%)
Haploid plantlets from anther cultures	102	47 (46%)		55 (54%)
rGV-1 ♂ x rGV-1 ♀	200	++* 42 (21%)	+* 95 (48%)	- 63 (31%)

* Estimated from a semi-quantitative assay of enzyme activity.

Analysis of the T-DNA showed that it has an internal deletion which eliminated the Tn7 insertion and adjacent DNA sequences, but the octopine gene is present and also its transcripts, as would be expected from the presence of the enzyme activity (De Greve *et al.*, manuscript in preparation). The experiments proved that the stable incorporation of a well defined additional gene into higher plant cells is possible without affecting the morphogenetic potential of the cells.

The plant flowered and set seeds quite normally, and it was investigated whether the progeny also contained the additional gene activity. The results, summarized in Table 1, show that the gene was transmitted as a stable, dominant Mendelian gene which is present once per haploid genome. Such experiments have been continued for several generations with the same result, indicating that the foreign gene in fact has become a stable part of the plant genome.

The results summarized here clearly indicate that a stable introduction of foreign genes via Ti-plasmids into plant cells is possible without affecting the morphogenetic potential of the cells These are important prerequisites for successful genetic engineering of plants. Construction of Ti-plasmid derivatives in which the genes for tumorous growth are replaced by other selectable markers for genetically altered plant cells is underway.

REFERENCES

1. Braun, A.C. 1956. The activation of two growth substance systems accompanying the conversion of normal to tumor cells in crown gall. Cancer Res. 16:53-56
2. Braun, A.C. 1959. A demonstration of the recovery of the crown gall tumor cell with the use of complex tumors of single cell origin. Proc. Natl. Acad. Sci. USA 45:932-938.
3. Braun, A.C., and H.N. Wood. 1976. Suppression of the neoplastic state with the acquisition of specialized functions in cells, tissues and organs of crown gall teratomas of tobacco. Proc. Natl. Acad. Sci. USA 73:496-500.
4. Chilton, M.-D., H.J. Drummond, D.J. Merlo, D. Sciaky, A.L. Montoya, M.P. Gordon, and E.W. Nester, 1977. Stable incorporation of plasmid DNA into higher plant cells: the molecular basis of crown gall tumorigenesis. Cell 11:263-271.
5. Chilton, M.-D., R.K. Saiki, N. Yadav, M.P. Gordon, and F. Quetier. 1980. T-DNA from Agrobacterium Ti-plasmid is in the nuclear DNA fraction of crown gall tumor cells. Proc. Natl. Acad. Sci. USA 77:4060-4064.

6. De Beuckeleer, M., M. Lemmers, G. De Vos, L. Willmitzer, M. Van Montagu, and J. Schell. 1981. Further insight on the transferred-DNA of octopine crown gall. Mol. Gen. Genet. 193:283-288.

7. De Greve, H., H. Decraemer, J. Seurinck, M. Van Montagu, and J. Schell. 1981. The functional organization of the octopine _Agrobacterium tumefaciens_ plasmid pTiB6S3. Plasmid 6:235-248.

8. Dhaese, P., H. De Greve, H. Decraemer, J. Schell, and M. Van Montagu. 1979. Rapid mapping of transposon insertion and deletion mutations in the large Ti-plasmids of _Agrobacterium tumefaciens_ Nucleic Acids Res. 7:1837-1849.

9. De Vos, G., M. De Beuckeleer, M. Van Montagu, and J. Schell. 1981. Restriction endonuclease mapping of the octopine tumor-inducing plasmid pTiAch5 of _Agrobacterium tumefaciens_. Plasmid 6:249-253.

10. Drummond, M.H., M.P. Gordon, E.W. Nester, and M.-D. Chilton. 1977. Foreign DNA of bacterial plasmid origin is transcribed in crown gall tumors. Nature 269:535-536.

11. Engler, G., M. Van Montagu, I. Zaenen, and J. Schell. 1977. Homology between Ti-plasmids of _Agrobacterium tumefaciens_: hybridization studies using electron microscopy. Biochem. Soc. Trans. 5:930-931.

12. Garfinkel, D.J., R.B. Simpson, L.W. Ream, F.F. White, M.P. Gordon, and E.W. Nester. 1981. Genetic analysis of crown gall: fine structure map of the T-DNA by site-directed mutagenesis. Cell 27:143-153.

13. Gelvin, S.B., M.P. Gordon, E.W. Nester, and A.I. Aronson. 1981. Transcription of the _Agrobacterium_ Ti-plasmid in the bacterium and in crown gall tumors. Plasmid 6:17-29.

14. Gurley, W.B., J.D. Kemp. M.J. Alber, D.W. Sutton, and J. Gallis. 1979. Transcription of Ti-plasmid derived sequences in three octopine-type crown gall tumor lines. Proc. Natl. Acad. Sci. USA 76:2828-2832.

15. Guyon, P., M.-D. Chilton, A. Petit, and J. Tempé. 1980. Agropine in "null-type" crown gall tumors: evidence for the generality of the opine concept. Proc. Natl. Acad. Sci. USA 77:2693-2697.

16. Hernalsteens, J.P., H. De Greve, M. Van Montagu, and J. Schell. 1978. Mutagenesis by insertion of the drug resistance transposon Tn7 applied to the Ti plasmid of Agrobacterium tumefaciens. Plasmid 1:218-225.

17. Hernalsteens, J.P., F. Van Vliet, M. De Beuckeleer, A. Depicker, G. Engler, M. Holsters, M. Van Montagu, and J. Schell. 1980. The Agrobacterium tumefaciens Ti-plasmid as a host vector system for introducing foreign DNA in plant cells. Nature 287:654-656.

18. Hille, J., and R. Schilperoort. 1981. The use of transposons to introduce well-defined deletions in plasmids: possibilities for in vivo cloning. Plasmid 6:151-154.

19. Holsters, M., B. Silva, F., Van Vliet, D. Genetello, M. De Block, P. Dhaese, A. Depicker, D. Inzé, G. Engler, R. Villarroel, M. Van Montagu, and J. Schell. 1980. The functional organization of the nopaline Agrobacterium tumefaciens plasmid pTiC58. Plasmid 3:212-230.

20. Koekman, B.P., G. Ooms, P.M. Klapwijk, and R.A. Schilperoort. 1979. Genetic map of an octopine Ti-plasmid. Plasmid 2:347-357.

21. Leemans, J., Ch. Shaw, R. Deblaere, H. De Greve, J.P. Hernalsteens, M. Maes, M. Van Montagu, and J. Schell. 1981. Site-specific mutagenesis of Agrobacterium Ti-plasmids and transfer of genes to plant cells. J. Mol. Appl. Genet. 1:149-164.

22. Leemans, J., R. Deblaere, L. Willmitzer, H. De Greve, J.P. Hernalsteens, M. Van Montagu, and J. Schell. 1982. Genetic identification of functions of T_L-DNA transcripts in octopine crown galls. EMBO J. 1:147-152.

23. Lemmers, M., M. De Beuckeleer, M. Holsters, P. Zambryski, A. Depicker, J.P. Hernalsteens, M. Van Montagu, and J. Schell.

1980. Internal organization, boundaries and integration of Ti-plasmid DNA in nopaline crown gall tumors. J. Mol. Biol. 144:355-376.

24. McPherson, J.C., E.W. Nester, and M.P. Gordon. 1980. Proteins encoded by Agrobacterium tumefaciens Ti-plasmid DNA (T-DNA) in crown gall tumors. Proc. Natl. Acad. Sci. USA 77:2666-2670.

25. Murai, N., and J.D. Kemp. 1982. Octopine synthase mRNA isolated from sunflower crown gall callus is homologous to the Ti-plasmid of Agrobacterium tumefaciens. Proc. Natl. Acad. Sci. USA 79:86-90.

26. Ooms, G., P.M. Klapwijk, J.A. Poulis, and R.A. Schilperoort. 1980. Characterization of Tn904 insertions in octopine Ti plasmid mutants of Agrobacterium tumefaciens. J. Bact. 144:82-91.

27. Ooms, G., P.J.J. Hooykaas, G. Moolenaar, and R.A. Schilperoort. 1981. Crown gall plant tumors of abnormal morphology, induced by Agrobacterium tumefaciens carrying mutated octopine Ti plasmids; analysis of T-DNA functions. Gene 14:33-50.

28. Otten, L., H. De Greve, J.P. Hernalsteens, M. Van Montagu, O. Schieder, J. Straub, and J. Schell. 1981. Mendelian transmission of genes introduced into plants by the Ti-plasmids of Agrobacterium tumefaciens. Mol. Gen. Genet. 183:209-213.

29. Schell, J., M. Van Montagu, M. De Beuckeleer, M. De Block, A. Depicker, M. De Wilde, G. Engler, C. Genetello, J.P. Hernalsteens, M. Holsters, J. Seurinck, B. Silve, F. Van Vliet, and R. Villarroel. 1979. Interactions and DNA transfer between Agrobacterium tumefaciens, the Ti-plasmid and the plant host. Proc. Roy. Soc. Lond. B 204:251-266.

30. Schröder, J., A. Hillebrand, W. Klipp, and A. Pühler. 1981. Expression of plant tumor-specific proteins in minicells of Escherichia coli: a fusion protein of lysopine dehydrogenase with chloramphenicol acetyltransferase. Nucleic Acids Res. 9:5187-5202.

31. Schröder, J., G. Schröder, H. Huisman, R.A. Schilperoort, and J. Schell. 1981. The mRNA for lysopine dehydrogenase in plant tumor cells is complementary to a Ti-plasmid fragment. FEBS Letters 129:166-168.

32. Schröder, G., and J. Schröder. 1982. Hybridization selection and translation of T-DNA encoded mRNAs from octopine tumors. Mol. Gen. Genet. 185:51-55. 33. Thomashow, M.F., R. Nutter, A.L. Montoya, M.P. Gordon, and E.W. Nester. 1980a. Integration and organization of Ti-plasmid sequences in crown gall tumors. Cell 19:729-739.

34. Thomashow, M.F., R. Nutter, K. Postle, M.-D. Chilton, F.R. Blattner, A. Powell, M.P. Gordon, and E.W. Nester. 1980b. Recombination between higher plant DNA and the Ti-plasmid of *Agrobacterium tumefaciens*. Proc. Natl. Acad. Sci. USA 77:6448-6452.

35. Turgeon, R., H.N. Wood, and A.C. Braun. 1976. Studies on the recovery of crown gall tumor cells. Proc. Natl. Acad. Sci. USA 73:3562-3564.

36. Van Larebeke, N., G. Engler, M. Holsters, S. Van den Elsacker, I. Zaenen, R.A. Schilperoort, and J. Schell. 1974. Large plasmid in *Agrobacterium tumefaciens* essential for crown gall-inducing ability. Nature 252:169-170.

37. Willmitzer, L., M. De Beuckeleer, M. Lemmers, M. Van Montagu, and J. Schell. 1980. The Ti-plasmid derived T-DNA is present in the nucleus and absent from plastids of plant crown gall cells. Nature 287:359-361.

38. Willmitzer, L., L. Otten, G. Simons, W. Schmalenbach, J. Schröder, G. Schröder, M. Van Montagu, G. De Vos, and J. Schell. 1981. Nuclear and polysomal transcripts of T-DNA in octopine crown gall suspension and callus cultures. Mol. Gen. 182:255-262.

39. Willmitzer, L., G. Simons, and J. Schell. 1982. The T_L-DNA in octopine crown gall tumors codes for seven well-defined polyadenylated transcripts. EMBO J. 1:139-146.

40. Willmitzer, L., W. Schmalenbach, and J. Schell. 1981. Transcription of T-DNA in octopine and nopaline crown gall tumors is inhibited by low concentrations of α-amanitin. Nucleic Acids Res. 9:4801-4812.

41. Wood, H.N., A.N. Binns, and A.C. Braun. 1978. Differential expression of oncogenicity and nopaline synthesis in intact leaves derived from crown gall teratomas of tobacco. Differentiation 11:175-180.

42. Wullems, G.J., L. Molendijk, G. Ooms, and R.A. Schilperoort. 1981. Differential expression of crown gall tumor markers in transformants obtained after *in vitro* *Agrobacterium tumefaciens*-induced transformation of cell wall regenerating protoplasts derived from *Nicotiana tabacum*. Proc. Natl. Acad. Sci. USA 78:4344-4348.

43. Wullems, G.J., L. Molendijk, G. Ooms, and R.A. Schilperoort. 1981. Retention of tumor markers in F1 progeny plants from *in vitro* induced octopine and nopaline tumor tissues. Cell 24:719-727.

44. Yadav, N.S., K. Postle, R.K. Saiki, M.F. Thomashow, and M.-D. Chilton.1980. T-DNA of crown gall teratoma is covalently joined to host plant DNA. Nature 287:458-461.

45. Yang, F., A.L. Montoya, D.J. Merlo, M.H. Drummond, M.-D. Chilton, E.W. Nester, and M.P. Gordon, 1980. Foreign DNA sequences in crown gall teratomas and their fate during loss of the tumorous traits. Mol. Gen. Genet. 177:707-714.

46. Zambryski, P., M. Holsters, K. Kruger, A. Depicker, J. Schell, M. Van Montagu, and H.M. Goodman. 1980. Tumor DNA structure in plant cells transformed by *Agrobacterium tumefaciens*. Science 209:1385-1391.

DISCUSSION

Q: STARLINGER: Could you comment on the amount of opines in plants since you said that the concentration of the mRNA was rather low. My question is: How much of the opines is made and why is it of advantage to the bacteria to live on that rather than on other metabolites present in larger amounts in the cell like glucose or its derivatives?

A: SCHRÖDER: The amounts of opines in the plant cells vary, depending on the type of opine. Agrophine or mannopine can represent up to 5 to 7% of the dry weight of the cells, and nopaline is usually about 1%. Octopine is often present in lower concentrations, and thus its synthesis does not represent a significant load on metabolism. This may well be one reason why the "octopine plant" shows the same vigor as a normal plant. Of course the Agrobacteria can also utilize other substances, but the capacity to metabolize opines is of advantage since these substances are excreted by the tumor cells and thus are readily available to bacteria living in the tumors.

Q: Do you mean to say that the auxin and the cytokinin requirement is replaced by some product of the genes, some proteins?

A: SCHRÖDER: In principle, yes, but at present we can be only very vague about the mechanism. The simplest explanation for the hormone independence of the tumor cells would be that some of the gene products of the T-DNA are hormone-synthesizing enzymes, but we have no direct evidence for that. It could well be that those proteins act indirectly, for example, by activating the plant genes responsible for hormone biosynthesis. Other models are also possible. It will not be very simple to analyze this since we know very little about hormone action in plants on the molecular level. It appears that the genes on the T-DNA represent a good system to investigate these questions, since they obviously affect growth and differentiation.

Q: MURPHY: All these studies were done on tobacco, but are the bacteria species-specific at all?

A: SCHRÖDER: You are referring to the host range of Agrobacteria. It is very broad: Agrobacteria can infect probably all dicots and most gymnosperms, but no monocots. This is, of course, very unfortunate, since many important crop plants are monocots. The reason for this limitation is now known.

Q: WALKER: You talked about this tumor line that differentiated into a plant which formed octopine. I didn't quite follow the role of the Tn7-insertion; could you clarify this point?

A: SCHRÖDER: That was an experiment which was started for quite a different reason. The ti-plasmid used here contained Tn7 inserted in the tumor genes, and since this transposon codes for methotrexate resistance, it was hoped that the transformed plant cells would be resistant to this drug. Surprisingly, some of the cells showed the capacity to differentiate into plants which synthesized octopine. This was very unusual, and therefore the T-DNA was analyzed: the only gene which could be identified was that for octopine synthesis. The transposon, Tn7, was absent as were the tumor genes. We do not really know how all of thse genes were eliminated; but we know that this result is reproducible. It seems possible that the presence of the large transposon made the DNA unstable in the plant cells. Thus, an experiment originally designed to confer drug resistance to plant cells led to the possibility of gene transfer without transfer of the genes coding for tumorous growth.

Q: I was wondering about your expression experiments in E. coli: was that done by producing fusion proteins or with flanking sequences recognized by E. coli promoters?

A: SCHRÖDER: We started out with analyzing whether proteins could be expressed with fragments from T-region which were available. We found right away a fusion protein with the octopine-synthesizing enzyme and also expression of other coding regions seemingly transcribed with promoters which were recognized in E. coli.

Q: Which selective markers did you have in mind to replace the tumor genes in the T-DNA?

A: SCHRÖDER: Several transposons, among others Tn5 and Tn7, have been transferred via Ti-plasmid into plant cells, and we are testing whether the resistance genes encodedon them are expressed in the eukaryotic cells.

Q: HATCHER: Did you notice any changes in the octopine plant with respect to susceptibility to infection by Agrobacteria?

A: SCHRÖDER: The octopine plant could be infected by Agrobacteria and form tumors. This is perhaps not too surprising since all of the genes responsible for tumorous growth were either deleted or inactive, and these genes are likely to be responsible for the fact that "real" tumor cells cannot be superinfected with other Ti-plasmids.

Q: WILLIAMS: Is anything known about the insertion sites of the T-DNA within the plant genome?

A: SCHRÖDER: T-DNAs have been detected in unique, middle repetitive DNA-sequences; thus there seems to be no preference in this point. There is some evidence that there are short DNA sequences somewhat outside the T-region which may play a role in recognition of short sequences in the plant DNA, and this type of specificity may be necessary for recombinational integration of the T-DNA.

Q: BRUCE: Can the octopine plant that you described be regenerated on the synthetic medium without any of the growth hormones?

A: SCHRÖDER: Yes. The shoot cultures were sometime maintained on a medium with cytokinin solely to suppress rapid growth. Roots were induced by transferring these shoots to medium without any hormones.

Q: BURCELL: Do you have comparable results with nopaline strains or with *Agrobacterium rhizogenes*?

A: SCHRÖDER: There are a number of experiments with nopaline plasmids and with plasmids from *A. rhizogenes*, but these systems have not been analyzed in great detail yet.

Q: What is the evidence that the proteins expressed in *E. coli* are not artifacts which are not expressed in plant cells?

A: SCHRÖDER: We have no direct evidence for that yet. However, there are three points consistent with the assumption that plant cells and *E. coli* express the same coding regions: (i) the sizes of the transcripts in plants correlate well with the sizes of the proteins expressed in *E. coli*, (ii) in some cases we know that the region expressed in *E. coli* is within the region transcribed in plants, and (iii) in some cases we know that the coding strand is the same in plants and in *E. coli*.

NEW DEVELOPMENTS IN PLANT TISSUE CULTURE AND PLANT REGENERATION

C.E. Green
Department of Agronomy and Plant Genetics
University of Minnesota
St. Paul, Minnesota 55108

Increased interest and progress have been widespread in the field of plant tissue culture in recent years. Although much of this effort preceded recent excitement about "genetic engineering," this field has been significantly stimulated by the broad interest in new biotechnology. This presentation could be devoted to anyone of at least five areas of tissue culture and plant regeneration. It could, for example be devoted to plants which produce secondary products. These are of interest because they are the source of valuable chemicals, often important in medicine. It might also be a discussion focused on recent studies in model systems like tobacco, carrot, petunia, and a few other plant species in which much fundamental information has been generated over the years in plant tissue culture. Thirdly, it could be focused on crop plants. Increased efforts to develop cell and tissue culture systems to manipulate valuable agricultural crops have coincided with the increased interest in new biotechnology in general. A fourth area could focus on plants which have relatively well developed genetic systems. Some obvious candidates include: corn, tomato, barley, wheat and a few others. Lastly, a fifth possibility could be the horticulture/floriculture industry where tissue culture and plant regeneration have become commercially valuable tools for plant propagation, disease control, and germplasm preservation. Rather than attempt to cover all of these areas, I will convey some general observations about the field as well as describe a few specific examples from our experience at the University of Minnesota.

Biotechnology as it applies to plants includes many areas of science. We have already heard that the power of new biotechnology is dependent on the integration of appropriate disciplines and people. Molecular biology and recombinant DNA technology applied to plants and specific plant genes are extremely important areas of research as is the development of appropriate vectors through which to move genes into plants. Unless we have extremely powerful methods to affect the direct transfer of genes into plants, we will need a well-developed tissue culture technology as another part of the biotechnology equation in plants.

The rationale behind developing the technology to propagate plant cells *in vitro* is relatively straightforward, especially from a microbiological viewpoint. Simple stated, it provides a means to continuously propagate large populations of cells in a defined environment and with a short generation time. One of the ultimate goals of plant cell and tissue culture systems is to provide the means to manipulate these eukaryotic organisms at the cellular level. One of the continuing challenges in this field is to extend cell culture methods frequently worked out in model systems to plants with well-developed genetics or which are agriculturally important.

General Aspects of Tissue Culture

A general outline of the field of plant tissue culture is presented in Figure 1. Irrespective of the plant of interest there are

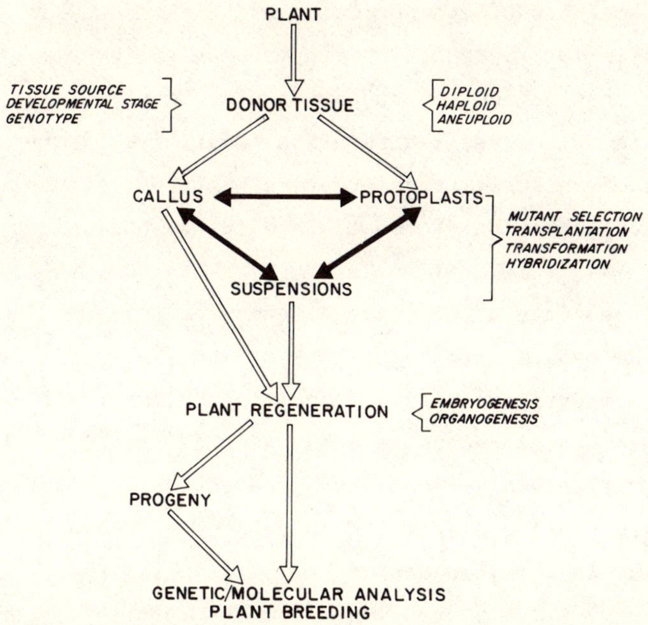

Fig. 1. Diagram of the tissue culture process from the donor plant through to the analysis of regenerated plants and their progeny.

a number of general methods and goals that apply to most tissue culture programs. The success of any program is dependent on the choice of donor tissue from which cultures are initiated. At least three factors influence the potential of particular donor tissues including the genotype, source, and developmental stage of the tissue.

The genetic constitution of cells grown in culture is also determined by the origin of the donor tissue. The initiation of haploid, diploid, or aneuploid cultures such as monosomics or trisomics is possible by the appropriate choice of donor tissues.

The basic manipulations of a tissue culture system include callus, protoplast, and suspension culture (Figure 1). These refer to different methods of growing cells each of which will be discussed later in more detail. The importance of these manipulations is that they provide new opportunities with which to study and manipulate plants. These manipulations might include the selection and analysis of mutants, transformation with DNA, transplantation of organelles, or formation of somatic hybrids by protoplast fusion.

One of the features of plant as compared to mammalian tissue culture is the capacity to regenerate a sexually viable organism. Thus, under appropriate cultural conditions plant cells can express all the developmental events associated with forming a complete plant. After plants are regeneratd, one of their important uses, at least for seed bearing plants, is to produce progeny which can then be analyzed by genetic, molecular, or plant breeding methods. The capacity to regenerate plants and to produce progeny is obviously vital to the application of biotechnology to agriculture.

Tissue Cultures of Corn

In corn, the development of tissue cultures capable of plant regeneration was possible only after the identification of appropriate donor tissues. The first and perhaps most successful donor tissue was the immature embryo isolated from developing ears [5,8]. Immature embryos, 1 mm in length, at the time of isolation are shown in Figure 2a. The tissue cultures in Figure 2b developed from scutellum tissue of similar embryos after three weeks of growth. The resulting cultures are developmentally heterogenous and contain a variety of different tissue types. When the hormone 2,4-dichloroacetic acid (2,4-D) is removed from the growth medium, large numbers of plants are regenerated from these cultures which can be grown to maturity.

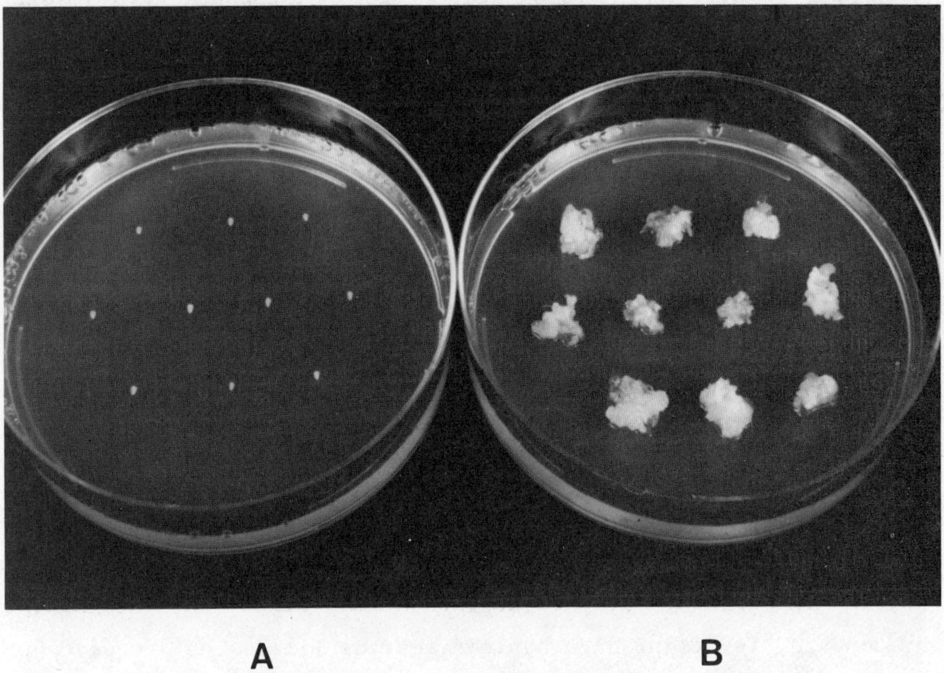

Fig. 2. Tissue cultures initiated from immature embryos of the corn inbred A188.

Another donor tissue from which regenerable tissue cultures of corn have been initiated are immature tassels [12]. This tissue is the male flower and as it matures it is responsible for pollen production. Immature embryos, inflorescences, and other tissues in cereals that have been used to initiate regenerating cultures all have the common characteristic of being developmentally young and meristematically active. Therefore, if we concentrate on young, actively growing tissues the probability of success in tissue culture is increased. This may also account for the many failed attempts to grow cereal protoplasts isolated from leaves. These cells are highly differentiated and not normally growing. Regenerated plants obtained from tissue cultures can be grown to maturity in a glasshouse, growth chamber, or field. The progeny seed produced in crosses with regenerated plants permits the evaluation of subsequent generations. This basic tissue culture approach developed for corn has been extended to many other cereal species and has provided a basis for continuing progress in this field [2,3,13,17].

The basic tissue culture method described above has also been used in other in vitro studies in corn. This includes using genetic methods to produce haploid immature embryos for the initiation of haploid cultures [12]. This is one of two approaches used to obtain haploid cultures. The other more commonly used approach involves the isolation and culture of anthers which contain haploid microspores at appropriate stages of development.

These microspores will multiply under appropriate cultural conditions to produce haploid cultures and plants. The alternative approach in corn is to use stocks containing the gene indeterminant gametophyte, ig, to produce haploid embryos [11]. The frequency of haploids among the progeny in crosses is greatly increased by ig. When ig is combined with genetic markers like the Rsc allele at the R locus and alcohol dehydrogenase, $Adh1^F$, it is possible to systematically identify haploid from diploid embryos in crosses with male parents carrying the r-g and $Adh1^S$ alleles. Selection of haploids is based on anthocyanin pigmentation and Adh1 isoenzyme patterns. The primary purpose of having haploid cells in culture is that they facilitate the direct isolation of recessive mutations.

Friable Callus and Somatic Embryo Genesis

An interesting development in recent years in cereal tissue culture has been the occurence of somatic embryogenesis [3,16]. Although relatively new in cultures of cereal and grasses, this phenomenon was initially described in carrot cultures more than twenty years ago [14,15]. Somatic embryogenesis is the process where cells from callus, suspension, or protoplast cultures develop into complete embryos which are developmentally very similar to zygotic embryos produced in seeds. Tissue culture capabilities have improved in corn so that now it is possible to initiate cultures which have two important characterics [6]. One is that the callus cultures are friable, meaning that they are soft and lose in texture (Figure 3a). This property is important because it can be an indicator of the degree of differentiation in the cells and it facilitates the initiation of suspension cultures. The other valuable attribute of these cultures is that they form very large numbers of somatic embryos. Careful examination of these cultures with a low power microscope permits the recognition of small, organized structures on the surface of the callus. Further examination reveals that this organization of somatic embryos at a range of developmental stages from early globular to those with clearly differentiated suspensors, scutellum, and embryonic axes (Figure 3b). These friable cultures have retained their embryogenic potential for as long as two years and have shown the capacity to produce extremely large numbers of somatic embryos.

A variety of cell types and organizational patterns can be seen when this friable callus is examined by scanning electron microscopy. Many regions on the surface of the callus contain only small cells. The cultures also contain a variety of large elongated cells which do not appear to grow actively nor are they directly associated with embryo development. Embryo formation appears to be exclusively associated with regions containing only small cells.

The embryos do not mature beyond the early stages of development shown in Figure 3b when left on the MS medium containing 2,4-D which is normally used for propagation of the cultures. They undergo, however, further development when transferred to N6 medium without hormones which contain a higher osmotic environment of 5 to 6 percent sucrose. After approximately two weeks of growth on this medium, many embryos have become quite mature (Figure 3c). At this

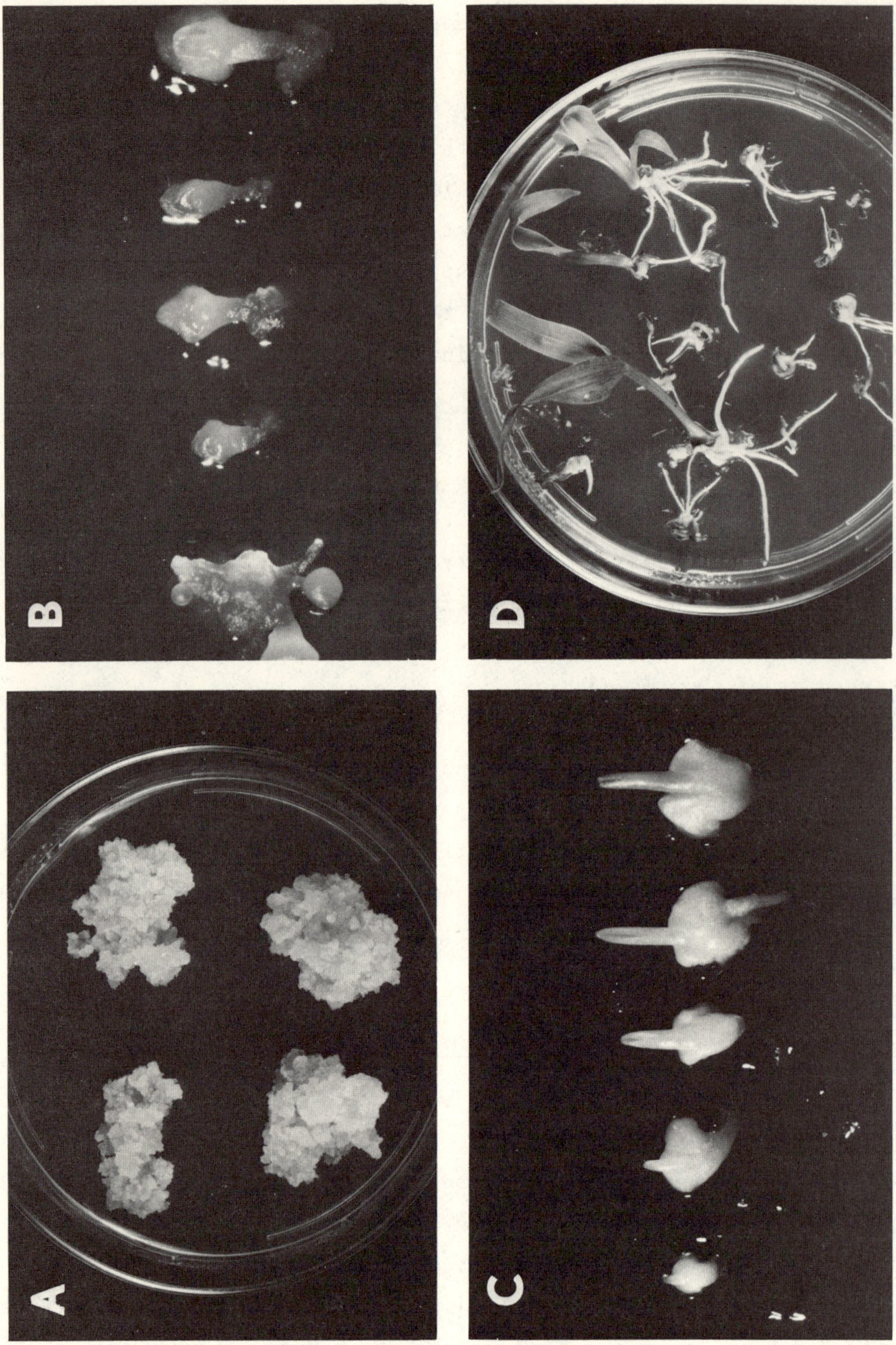
A
B
C
D

stage they are similar in size and shape to the mature embryos found in kernels. Their most prominant features include the scutellum and an embryonic axis in which the coleoptile appears to have begun to germinate. These embryos rapidly germinate and grow into plants when placed on medium containing 2% sucrose (Figure 3d). The plants are then established in soil and are grown to maturity.

One of the valuable attributes of the friable embryogenic cultures just described is that they are excellent for the initiation of suspension cultures. The resulting suspensions are composed of a mixture of cell types and aggregates which contain a range of approximately twenty to hundreds of cells per aggregate. These cultures grow actively but few somatic embryos are produced in the liquid medium. Embryogenesis is very active, however, when these cultures are plated on agar-based medium. Embryogenic suspension cultures have a variety of potential uses including mutant protoplasts [17]. Perhaps cultures of this type will produce protoplasts which can grow and undergo somatic embryogenesis to produce plants.

Mutant Selection

Among the various motives for developing tissue culture methods in plants has been the objective of using these methods to isolate mutants. Most mutant selection efforts to date have been carried out with model species, most notably tobacco (Nicotiana ssp.), where the various tissue culture methods are relatively well-developed. In cereals, the in vitro selection of mutants has not progressed rapidly, in part because the development of effective tissue culture

←

Fig. 3. Plant regeneration from friable callus cultures of corn by somatic embryogenesis. A = friable callus (1X); B = early stages of embryogenesis (40X); C = later stages of embryo maturation (1X); D = embryo germination to produce plants.

methods has been slow. A few mutants have been recovered, however, such as heritable resistance to Helminthosporium maydis race T pathotoxin in Texas cytoplasm tissue cultures of maize [1,4] and the selection of heritable resistance to lysine plus threonine which is also in maize [9].

Maize kernels, as well as the grain of other cereal crops, are deficient for certain amino acids essential for proper nutrition of non-ruminant animals. This fact led us to propose a positive selection system to recover overproducer mutants in cereal species which could synthesize increased amounts of lysine, threonine, or methionine [7]. The selection system is based on resistance to lysine plus threonine inhibition. The selections for resistance were carried out on diploid cultures initiated from immature embryos [9,10]. Studying the expression of overproducer mutants at the whole plant level reveals whether they can be employed to increase specific nutritionally limiting amino acids in such tissues as the grain and whether the increase is nutritionally significant.

Selection of 2mM lysine + threonine (LT) yielded the resistant lines, LT2, LT6, and LT19 after three selection cycles (three months) [9]. The LT19 line was highly resistant to LT while the other two lines were marginally resistant. Plants (R_0) were regenerated from LT2, LT6, LT19, and unselected control cultures. These plants were self-pollinated when possible or crossed to the inbred, A188. The R_1 and R_2 generation progeny from these crosses were analyzed using tissue culture or seedling bioassay methods to determine the inheritance of LT resistance. From these studies it was established that one line, LT19, possessed a transmissable resistance trait that was inherited as a dominant nuclear gene, Ltr*-19 [9].

The expression of LT resistance was observed in tissue cultures, initiated from immature embryos, of R_2 generation control and

LT19 plants in the presence of LT. Differences between the resistant cultures and the susceptible cultures were highly significant at LT concentrations higher than 1mM.

The effect of Ltr*-19 on seedling development was examined by growing mature embryos isolated from +/+ (susceptible) and hetero- and homozygous Ltr*-19 seed in the presence of LT [9]. Root and shoot development of susceptible seedlings was nearly completely inhibited at concentrations of 2mM LT and above. Roots and shoots of Ltr*-19/+ and Ltr*-19/Ltr*-19 seedlings grew much better than susceptible seedlings at all levels of LT tested.

Free amino acids were analyzed in tissue cultures initiated from immature embryos of susceptible and resistant plants [9]. The most significant change was a 6-fold increase in free threonine in resistant cultures over the level found in susceptible cultures. Except for a small increase (1.5-to 2-fold) in isoleucine, the remaining amino acids were unchanged between susceptible and resistant cultures grown at 0mM LT.

Analysis of free amino acids was also conducted on +/+, Ltr*-19/+, and Ltr*-19/Ltr*-19 kernels (Table 1) [9]. Of particular interest is the marked increase in the level of free threonine in Ltr*-19/+ and Ltr*-19/Ltr*-19 kernels as compared to normal. The 30-fold increase in free threonine in heterozygous kernels and the 77-fold increase in homozygous kernels illustrates the dominance and gene dosage effect of Ltr*-19. Amino acid analyses of other homozygous kernels have revealed increase in free threonine as high as 109-fold. Methionine, serine, and proline were increased 3-4 times in homozygous kernels but the free pools of the remaining amino acids were not changed appreciably.

The effect of threonine overproduction on total kernel threonine is shown in Table 2 [9]. These date indicate that kernel

Table 1

Free Amino Acids in Lysine + Threonine Hetero- (Ltr*-19/+) and Homozygous (Ltr*-19/Ltr*-19) Resistant and Susceptible (+/+) Seed

Amino acid	Genotypes* +/+	Ltr*-19/+	Ltr*-19/Ltr*-19	Ltr*-19/Ltr*-19 to +/+ ratio
	μmol/g dry weight			
Threonine‡	0.15 ± 0.01†	4.35 ± 0.35	11.15 ± 1.33	76.8
Serine	0.74 ± 0.10	0.81 ± 0.10	2.37 ± 0.25	3.2
Proline	0.35 ± 0.09	2.63 ± 0.80	1.39 ± 0.19	4.0
Methionine	0.10 ± 0.03	0.05 ± 0.01	0.36 ± 0.09	3.7
Lysine	0.15 ± 0.04	0.16 ± 0.03	0.19 ± 0.01	1.3
Arginine	trace	trace	trace	---
Total	6.74	12.08	19.70	
Total kernel	0.84	1.62	2.54	

* Ltr*-19/Ltr*-19 seed was obtained by self-pollination of a third generation Ltr*-19/Ltr*-19 plant which was also crossed to +/+ to produce the Ltr*-19/+ seed. +/+ seed was from an unselected regenerated control plant crossed to A188 and then backcrossed to A188 in the second generation.

† Each value represents the mean and standard error of the mean of 4 replications.

‡ Genotype had little affect on level of other amino acids assayed. Aspartic acid, 1.1-1.7; Glutamic acid, 1.0-1.6; Glycine, 0.23-0.35; Alanine, 0.35-0.63; Valine, 0.35-0.49; Isoleucine 0.10-0.19; Leucine, 0.07-0.08; Tyrosine, 0.18-0.21; Histidine, 0.16-0.27 μmol/g dry weight.

weight, total protein, and the threonine content of the protein were not altered appreciably between the +/+, Ltr*-19/+; and Ltr*-19/Ltr*-19 genotypes. The large increase in free threonine in homozygous Ltr*-19 kernels increased the total threonine by 33-59%.

In conclusion, a dominant mutation, Ltr*-19, conditions the overproduction of the nutritionally essential amino acid, threonine in tissue cultures and most importantly in the seed of regenerated plants and subsequent generations. The magnitude of threonine over-production in seed carrying Ltr*-19 suggests an important oppor-

Table 2

Effects of Free Threonine Overproduction in Various Genotypes on Total Threonine in Seed

	+/+		Ltr*-19/+	Ltr*-19/Ltr*-19	
	1	2	1	1	2
	mg				
Kernel weight	116 ± 5*	123 ± 9	154 ± 14	122 ± 9	134 ± 10
Protein/100 mg meal	9.4 ± 0.15	10.1 ± 0.18	8.9 ± 0.11	10.4 ± 0.14	10.2 ± 0.09
Threonine/100 mg protein	4.05 ± 0.49	3.95 ± 0.41	3.81 ± 0.29	3.99 ± 0.42	3.90 ± 0.44
Protein threonine/kernel	0.44 ± 0.05	0.49 ± 0.05	0.52 ± 0.06	0.51 ± 0.06	0.53 ± 0.04
Free threonine/kernel	<.01 ± ≪.01	<.01 ± ≪.01	0.07 ± 0.01	0.17 ± 0.02	0.31 ± 0.03
Total threonine/kernel	0.44	0.50	0.59	0.68	0.84
	%				
Free threonine as % of protein threonine	0.4	0.6	13	33	59

* Each value represents the mean and standard error of the mean of 3 replications.

tunity to isolate and use amino acid overproducer mutants to selectively increase the levels of specific nutritionally limiting amino acids in seeds. In light of these results, it is clearly desirable to isolate lysine, tryptophan, and methionine overproducer mutants in various crops.

REFERENCES

1. Brettell, R.I.S., E. Thomas, and D.S. Ingram. 1980. Reversion of Texas male-sterile cytoplasm maize in culture to give fertile, T-toxin resistant plants. Theor. Appl. Genet. 58:55-58.
2. Cummings, D.P., C.E. Green, and D.D. Stuthman. 1976. Callus induction and plant regeneration in oats. Crop Sci. 16:465-470.
3. Dunstan, D.I., K.C. Short, H.D. Dhalival, and E. Thomas. 1979. Further studies on plantlet production from cultured tissues of *Sorghum bicolor*. Protoplasms 101:355-361.

4. Gengenbach, B.G., C.E. Green, and C.M. Donovan. 1977. Inheritance of selected pathotoxin resistance in maize plants regenerated from cell cultures. Proc. Natl. Acad. Sci. (USA) 74:5113-5117.

5. Green, C.E. 1977. Prospects for crop improvement in the field of cell culture. Hort. Sci. 12:131-134.

6. Green, C.E. 1982. Friable callus cultures of maize; Somatic embryogenesis and plant regeneration (in preparation).

7. Green, C.E., and R.L. Phillips. 1974. Potential selection system for mutants with increased lysine, threonine, and methionine in cereal crops. Crop Sci.. 14:827-830.

8. Green, C.E., and R.L. Phillips. 1975. Plant regeneration from tissue cultures of maize. Crop Sci. 15:417-421.

9. Hibberd, K.A., and C.E. Green. 1982. Inheritance and expression of lysine plus threonine resistance selected in maize tissue culture. Proc. Natl. Acad. Sci. (USA) vol. 79 (in press).

10. Hibberd, K.A., C.E. Green, T.J. Walter, and B.G. Gengenbach. 1980. Characterization of a selected feedback insensitive tissue culture line of maize. Planta 148:183-187.

11. Kermicle, J. 1969. Androgenesis conditioned by a mutation in maize. Science 166:1422-1424.

12. Rhodes, C.A., and C.E. Green. 1982. Haploid tissue cultures of maize: Selection, initiation, and plant regeneration. (in preparation).

13. Shimoda, T. and Y. Yamada. 1979. Wheat plants regenerated from embryo cell cultures. Japan J. Genetics 54:379-385.

14. Steward, F.C., M.O. Mapes, K. Mears. 1958. "Growth and organized development of cultured cells." II Organization in cultures grown from freely suspended cells. Am. J. Bot. 43:705-708.

15. Steward, F.C., M.O. Mapes, A.E. Kent, and R.D. Holsten. 1964. Growth and development of cultured plant cells. Science 143:20-27.

16. Thomas, E.., P.J. King, and I. Potrykus. 1977. "Shoot and embryo-like structure formation from cultured tissues of _Sorghum_ _bicolor_. _Naturwissenschaften_ 64:587.

17. Vasil, V. and I.K. Vasil. 1980. Isolation and culture of cereal protoplasts. _Theor_. _Appl_. _Genet_. 56:97-99.

DRUGS AND ANTIBIOTICS: AN OVERVIEW
CHAIRMAN'S COMMENTS

Claude H. Nash, III
Sterling-Winthrop Research Institute
Rensselaer, New York 12144

Biotechnology provides exciting new approaches for the discovery and production of novel biologically active molecules. This technology is applicable to numerous stages involved in the discovery and development of new drugs. Drug discovery is a complex process requiring a diverse group of scientific talents. In general, the process starts with a proposal for the intervention in the course of a specific disease. The initial idea is followed by a period of exploratory research, culminating in the identification of a chemical compound with the desired biological activity. The active chemical is then further investigated in preclinical testing, toxicology, and clinical studies. If the biological activity is confirmed and the compound has an adequate margin of safety, then a manufacturing process is developed. Drug discovery is a labyrinth of hidden problems which must be resolved in order to achieve successful marketing of a new drug.

Research opportunities are identified and prioritized based on therapeutic need, market potential, and emerging biology. Significant disease areas that meet those criteria include: anti-infective agents (fungi and viruses), cancer, cardiovascular system, central nervous system, gastro-intestinal tract, arthritis, immunodeficiencies, and aging. Successful drug discovery depends on emerging biology which reveals novel sites for intervention in the course or onset of a disease.

Once the research objectives have been established, the next phase of the drug discovery process is to design and implement biological test systems. The initial test may utilize an animal model which mimics the disease, a tissue system, or a biochemical test which is based on a molecular mechanism of drug action. In general, a series of tests is used sequentially to characterize the biological activity of a potential drug. Unfortunately, in many diseases neither the etiology nor the molecular mechanism has been adequately elucidated for rational design of an experimental model. Recent advances in molecular biology and especially molecular genetics are beginning to provide insight into diseases such as immunological disorders, cancer, and intracellular infections.

After the experimental model has been validated, it is necessary to identify chemicals which elicit the desired activities. These compounds can be derived from natural sources such as plasma, microbes, plants, etc., from chemical synthesis based on structure-activity relationships, or from structure design. The design of specific inhibitors which bind at active sites of enzymes or at drug receptors is presently being explored by pharmaceutical and university laboratories. Successful drug design depends on an extensive knowledge about either the conformation of the drug receptor or a series of active compounds.

The pharmacological activity and pharmacokinetics of active compounds are further elucidated prior to drug metabolism and acute toxicity studies. If these studies demonstrate an adequate margin of safety (therapeutic index), the lead compound will be tested in Phase I human trials. Adequate tolerance of the new drug will permit further clinical testing in Phase II and III clinical studies which are designed to show efficacy and safety. Concurrent with these clinical studies, the compound will be tested in long-term toxicity tests and a satisfactory manufacturing process will be developed. After 8-15 years of research and development, the product could be introduced to the market.

Molecular biology provides new insight into the molecular basis of disease while biotechnology provides an efficient method for manufacturing complex molecules. These technologies, unfortunately, do not eliminate the complex process involved in drug discovery and development.

Examples of applications of biotechnology for the development of drugs and antibiotics include:

1) Manufacturing of commercially available products such as insulin, growth hormone, antibiotics, etc. These applications provide alternative manufacturing processes and, therefore, have the highest prospect of success. Once the product produced via biotechnology is proven to be biologically equivalent to existing products, it can be introduced to the market. Improved strains for production of antibiotics or steroid transformation would also be easily introduced as process improvements. The decision to initiate such a project is primarily economic.

2) Production of close analogs of existing products such as human insulin and subunit vaccines will require more extensive testing. These products also have a high probability of success.

3) Production of rare peptides with known biological activity for clinical testing, such as interferon, cytokines, and hormones. These materials provide an opportunity to learn

about cell-to-cell communication, but if used as a final product, they must be tested as any other new drugs and, therefore, will require several years for clearance.

4) Development of new diagnostic reagents such as monoclonal antibodies and sequence-specific diagnostics.

5) Synthesis of novel compounds such as hybrid antibiotics, hybrid peptides, and multi-antigenic subunit vaccines. This represents another source of potentially active compounds for testing and is an exciting application for biotechnology since these complex chemicals are not easily synthesized.

6) The elucidation of biological receptors or defining of the sequence of events involved in initiating a disease provides opportunity for the design of effective new drugs.

These are only a few possible applications of biotechnology relative to drug discovery and development. Additional applications will be discussed in other chapters of this volume.

DESIGN AND SYNTHESIS OF OPTICALLY-PURE COMPOUNDS USING MICROBIAL SYSTEMS

Charles J. Sih, Ching-Shih Chen, Gary Girdaukas, and Bing-Nan Zhou
School of Pharmacy
University of Wisconsin
Madison, Wisconsin 53706

INTRODUCTION

As the useful biological activities of most therapeutic agents are associated with only one enantiomer, the preparation of optically-pure compounds continues to be a major contemporary problem of synthetic organic chemistry. Because conventional chemical transformations generally give statistical mixtures of optical enantiomers, it is necessary to remove the unwanted antipode at the end of the reaction sequence by resolution using an asymmetric agent, which is often a natural product.

Microbial enzymes are excellent organic asymmetric reagents, capable of catalyzing a wide variety of reactions with a high degree of stereoselectivity under very mild conditions. Thus, a valuable approach to the total synthesis of complex natural products is to utilize microbial systems for either the preparation of chiral intermediates or the introduction of key chiral centers into the target molecule.

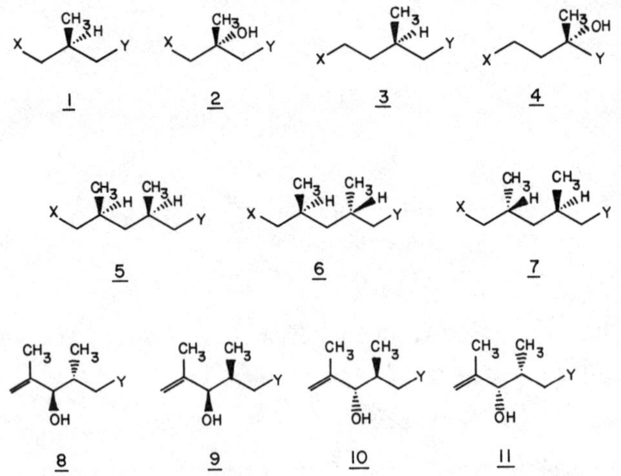

1 2 3 4

5 6 7

8 9 10 11

Fig. 1. Useful bifunctional chiral synthons for asymmetric synthesis.

One alternative approach to the construction of complex organic molecules with multiple chiral centers entails the successive assembly of a series of prefabricated, optically-active building blocks containing the desired stereochemical and functional features of the intended synthetic target. This strategy not only eases the design and execution of a total synthetic scheme but also can be applied to a wide variety of synthetic objectives. Hence, we have undertaken a program aimed at the systematic preparation of the following classes of bifunctional, chiral synthons where X and Y represent protected functions (Fig. 1). The synthetic utility of these chiral building blocks is illustrated in Fig. 2. It is evident that the carbon framework of highly functionalized molecules with multiple chiral centers such as erythronolide A [1], calcimycin [2], monensin [3], and α-tocopherol [4] may be more easily constructed via systematic assemblies of the appropriate chiral synthons as shown.

Although it is possible to reverse the latent and reactive properties of X and Y to obtain synthons of opposite chirality, in

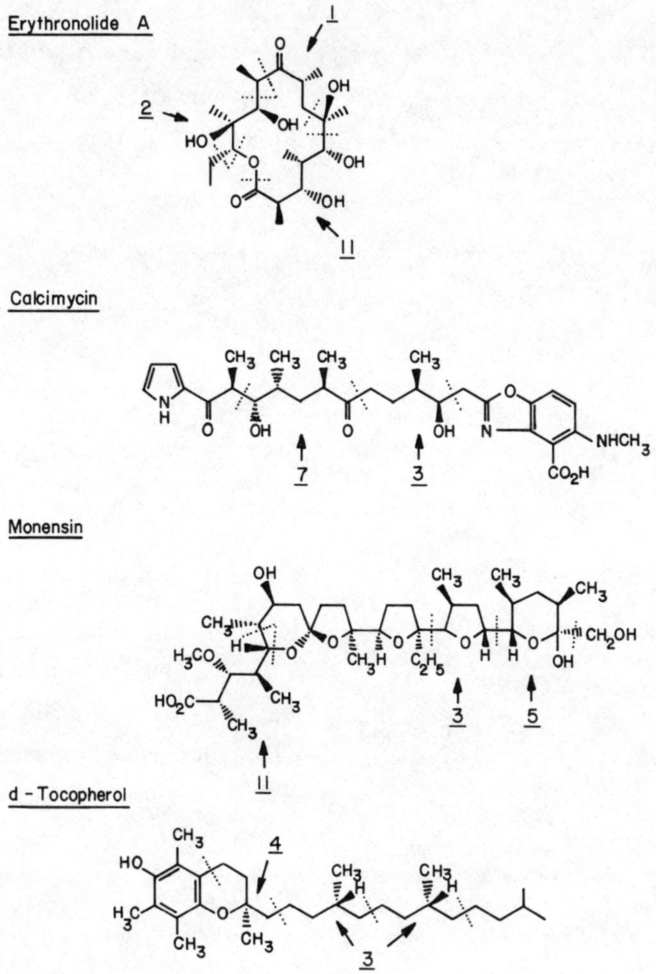

Fig. 2. Chiral synthons as possible precursors of complex natural products.

practice, this would often require the precipitous manipulation of protecting groups. Because both the R and S forms of these synthons are needed for synthetic applications, we have elected to accomplish this objective by means of biochemical kinetic resolutions of enantiomers.

Theory

Suppose that A and B are the fast and slow reacting enantiomers that compete for the same site on the enzyme. For a simple three-step kinetic mechanism assuming the reaction is virtually irreversible.

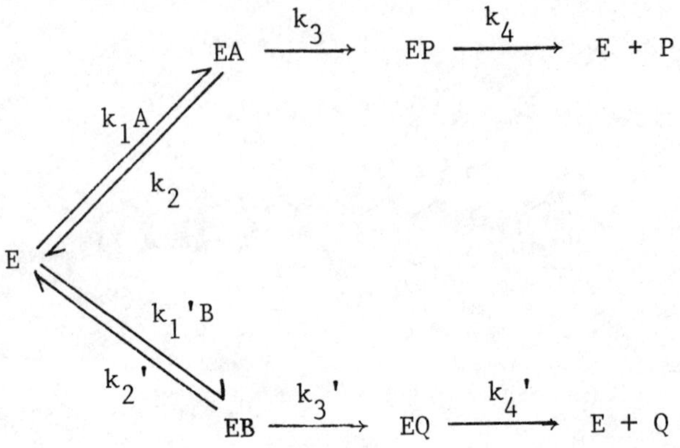

(1)

and there is no product inhibition, the ratio of the two partial reaction rates (v_a and v_b) may be shown by steady state kinetics to be

$$\frac{v_a}{v_b} = \frac{V_a}{V_b} \times \frac{K_b}{Ka} \times \frac{A}{B} \qquad (2)$$

where V_a, K_a and V_b, K_b denote maximal velocities and Michaelis constants of the fast and slow reacting enantiomers respectively.

Integration of eqn. 2 affords the homocompetitive equation 3, which reveals that the discrimination between two competing enantiomers (A and B) by enzymes is dictated by the ratios of V/K (specificity constants) [5] or E.

$$\frac{\ln (A/A_o)}{\ln (B/B_o)} = \frac{V_a/K_a}{V_b/V_b} = E \qquad (3)$$

In instances where kinetic resolution experiments are conducted by the selective destruction of one of the antipodes, e.g., D-amino acid oxidases [6] have been used to oxidize D-α-amino acids preferentially leaving most of the L-acids unchanged, the relationship between c (the extent of the reaction) and <u>ee</u>(S), enantiomeric excess, of the recovered substrate fraction [(B - A)/(A + B)] for various values of E (enantiomeric ratio) is governed by eqn. <u>4</u>.

$$\frac{\ln\{[1 - c][1 - \underline{ee}(S)]\}}{\ln\{[1 - c][1 + \underline{ee}(S)]\}} = \frac{V_a/K_a}{V_b/K_b} = E \qquad (4)$$

Eqn. <u>4</u> (Fig. 3) correlates the three interrelated variables, <u>ee</u>(S), c, and E. It should be borne in mind that under steady-state conditions, free enzyme is constantly being regenerated and competed for by A and B. Consequently, <u>E is dependent on the ratios of the specificity constants (V/K), and is independent of substrate concentrations.</u>

In kinetic resolution experiments using hydrolytic enzymes such as acylases [7] and carboxyesterases [8], it is also desirable to relate c and <u>ee</u>(P), enantiomeric excess, of the product fraction [(P-Q)/(P+Q)] to various values of E. This correlation may be achieved by converting eqn. <u>3</u> into a form (eqn. <u>5</u>) more compatible with experimental data and more suitable for graphical representation [9].

$$\frac{\ln\{1 - c[1 + \underline{ee}(P)]\}}{\ln\{1 - c[1 - \underline{ee}(P)]\}} = \frac{V_a/K_a}{V_b/K_b} = E \qquad (5)$$

It is evident that knowledge of any two of the variables allows the definition of the third. The graph (Fig. 4) clearly shows the abrupt decrease in <u>ee</u>(P) for values of c beyond 0.5. Consequently, to maximize values of <u>ee</u>(P) and c, one should not carry out the conversion beyond 50% irrespective of the value of E.

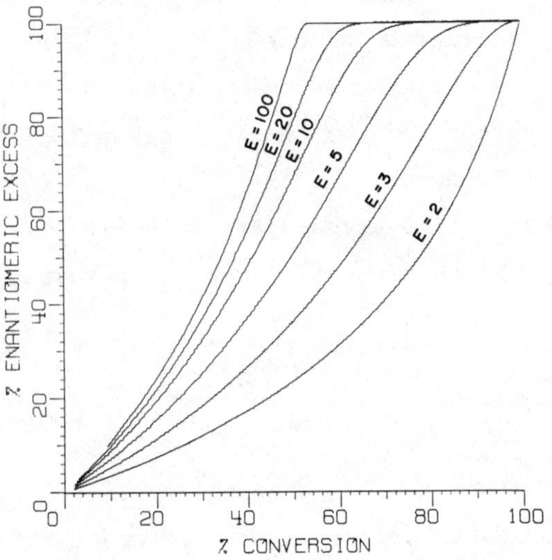

Fig. 3. Plot of percentage enantiomeric excess ee(S) as a function of the percentage conversion of various enantiomeric ratios (E).

In an idealized situation, one would like to conduct biochemical kinetic resolution experiments with E values of >100.

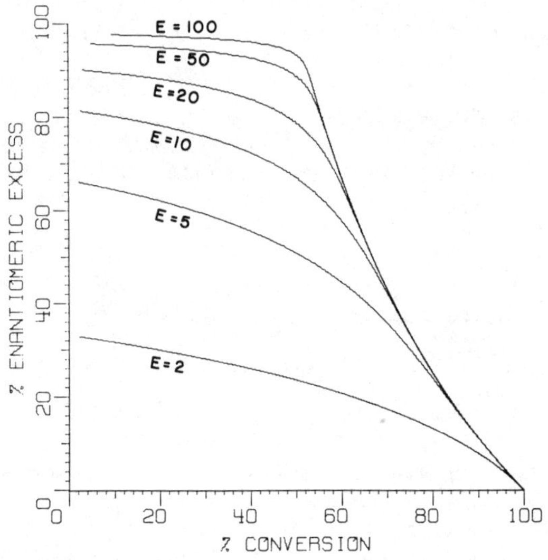

Fig. 4. Plot of percentage enantiomeric excess ee(P) as a function of the percentage conversion for various enantiomeric ratios (E).

Although in our experience the magnitude of E values observed for microbial carboxyesterases acting on a variety of racemic compounds ranged from 1 to >100, most of these possessed rather moderate E values of between 5 to 10. On the other hand, there are numerous advantages of using hydrolytic enzymes for kinetic resolutions of enantiomers, not the least of which are their broad substrate specificities, lack of coenzyme requirements, favorable equilibria . . . but rather the product may be easily reesterified and recycled [10] to further enhance the optical purities of the antipodal mixture. Hence, a new expression is needed to relate the variables c, E, ee_o (initial ee), and ee' (final desired ee).

If we consider one mole of an antipodal mixture with an initial ee of ee_o, this would contain $(1 + ee_o)/2$ mole of A_o (fast reacting) and $(1 - ee_o)/2$ mole of B_o (slow reacting). Whence, $A = (1 + ee_o)/2 - c[(1 + ee')/2]$ and $B = (1 - ee_o)/2 - c[(1 - ee')/2]$. Substitution of these terms into eqn. 3 affords eqn. 6.

$$\left[1 - c\left(\frac{1 + ee'}{1 + ee_o}\right)\right] = \left[1 - c\left(\frac{1 - ee'}{1 - ee_o}\right)\right]^E \qquad (6)$$

For recycling studies, when enzymes with modest E values of 5-10 are used, it is more advantageous to arrange the aforementioned variables into the format shown in Fig. 5. This graph now allows one to estimate the relationship between ee' and c at various fixed values of E and ee_o. For example, starting with an antipodal mixture with an ee_o of 0.67 and E of 10, the ee' obtainable after 80% conversion is 0.91. In principle, the product could be recycled an infinite number of times to achieve the ultimate goal of absolute optical purity (99.99...%). In reality, to prepare enantiomers with ee' values of >0.98, it would be more convenient to select biochemical systems with E values of $\geq$10 and subject the product to recycling not more than two times.

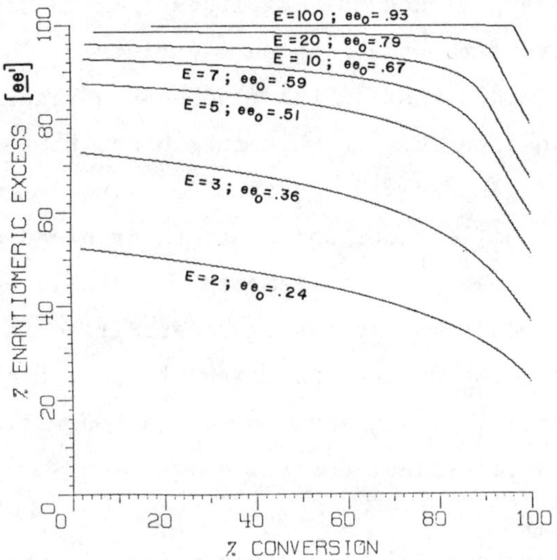

Fig. 5. The expression of the final percentage enantiomeric excess (ee') as a function of the percentage of conversion for various values of initial enantiomeric excess (ee_o) and enantiomeric ratio (E).

EXPERIMENTAL METHODS

Isolation of Microorganisms Containing Carboxyesterase

Nutrient agar petri-dishes containing phenol red (0.018 g/l), pH 7.4 were prepared. To one set of the plates was added (±)3, emulsified in Tween 80, to give a final concentration of 1 mg/ml. After diluting the soil samples to concentrations of 10^{-3}, 10^{-4}, and 10^{-5}, 1 ml of the diluted samples was added to each set of the plates. After incubation at 28°C for 16 hours, the control plates [without (±)3] showed colonies surrounded by yellow zones. By the second day the yellow zones disappeared. In contrast, growth on plates containing (±)3 generally did not appear until the second or third day. Colonies surrounded by yellow (acid) zones were picked and evaluated for the hydrolysis of (±)3. The control plates at the same dilution contained approximately twice the number of colonies as plates containing (±)3. Hence, this method not only allows one to select for colonies with yellow zones as an indication of ester hydrolysis but also eliminates the examination of organisms that are inhibited by (±)3.

Stereospecific Hydrolysis of (±)Methyl-4-benzyloxy-2-methyl butyrate (3)

Surface growth from a one week old agar slant of *Bacillus sp.*, grown on Difco nutrient agar, was suspended in 5 ml of an 0.85% saline solution. One ml portions of this suspension were used to inoculate a 250 ml Erlenmeyer flask (F-1 stage) each containing 50 ml of Difco nutrient broth. The flasks were incubated at 25°C on a rotary shaker (250 cycles/min - 2" radius) for 24 hours, after which a 10% by volume transfer was made to a 2 liter Erlenmeyer flask containing 600 ml of Difco nutrient broth. After 16 hrs, 600 mg of (±)methyl-4-benzyloxy-2-methylbutyrate (3) in 25 ml of 10% Tween 80 was added to the flasks resulting in a final substrate concentration of 0.1%. After incubating the F-2 stage flasks for an additional 96 hours under the conditions used in the F-1 stage, the reaction was terminated by the addition of 6N HCl until the pH of the medium was lowered to 2. The contents were filtered through a pad of celite and the filtrate was extracted with ethyl acetate (3 x 500 ml). The combined ethyl acetate extracts were dried over sodium sulfate and concentrated *in vacuo* to give a residue (900 mg). This residue was dissolved in 4 ml of a solvent mixture of Skelly B-ethyl acetate (15:1) and chromatographed over a silica gel column (MN Kieselgel 60, Brinkmann, 1.2 x 40 cm). The column was eluted with Skelly B-ethyl acetate (15:1) and 18 ml fractions were collected. Fractions 1-5 consisted of 199 mg of residual (+)methyl-4-benzyloxy-2-methylbutyrate, $[\alpha]_D^{25}$ +19.02° (c,2.3 $CHCl_3$); *ee* = 0.84; fractions 16-30 containted 200 mg of (-)4-benzyloxy-2-methylbutyric acid, which was converted to its methyl ester by methylation with CH_2N_2, $[\alpha]_D^{25}$ -18.55° (c, 2.1 $CHCl_3$); ee = 0.85.

The progress of the microbial hydrolysis of (±)3 was followed by thin-layer chromatographic analyses using Brinkmann 20 x 20 cm (EM) plates (0.25 mm thickness) of silica gel containing PF254 indicator. The solvent system was: ethyl acetate-hexane-acetic acid (50:50:2). R_f of ester = 0.50; R_f of acid = 0.29.

Determination of c and ee

Values of ee were determined by ^1H NMR spectroscopy (CCl_4) in the presence of $Eu(hfc)_3$ [10]. Values of c were obtained by two independent methods: a) The amount of residual ester was estimated by quantitative GLC analyses (5% QF-1 Chromosorb G HP columns, 6 ft, 175°); b) The value of c is related to the ee of the substrate [ee(S)] and ee of the product [ee(P)] by the following relationship:

$$(1 - c)\frac{1 - ee(S)}{2} + c\frac{1 + ee(P)}{2} = 1/2.$$

Hence, c may be computed from the equation,

$$c = \frac{ee(S)}{ee(S) + ee(P)}.$$

The enantiomeric ratio, E, may be calculated by substituting the values of c and ee (S) into eqn. 3 or c and ee(P) into eqn. 4.

RESULTS AND DISCUSSION

Before examining the validity of our theoretical considerations, one may raise some questions pertaining to possible variables that may influence the E value. Although one may envisage that variations in media composition, aeration, flask size, mixing, inoculum size, etc. can all affect cell growth rate, fortunately, the enantiomeric ratio, E, is independent of time and substrate concentrations. Consequently, good correlations of eqns. 4 and 5 with kinetic resolution data derived from intact cell experiments should be obtained for a given substrate when the pH and temperature are kept constant. Because transition states of enzymes are not well understood, it remains to be established as to whether changes in temperature would affect E values. It should also be borne in mind that E values may be altered by changes in pH if substrates possess ionizing groupings.

Another factor that merits consideration is that some microorganisms may possess more than one type of the same enzyme with different E values. However, the E value of each enzyme in a microorganism for a specified substrate is manifested in the experimental E_{app} value [11] where α is a proportionality constant for the different concentrations of each enzyme present.

$$E_{app} = \frac{\Sigma\ \alpha_1 \frac{V}{K}_1 + \alpha_2 \frac{V}{K}_2 \ldots \alpha_i \frac{V}{K'}\ n-1}{\Sigma\ \alpha_1 \frac{V}{K}_1 + \alpha_2 \frac{V}{K}_2 \ldots \alpha_1 \frac{V}{K'}\ n-1} \quad (7)$$

Having discussed some of the possible factors that may contribute to variations in E value determinations in intact cell experiments, we then turned our attention to testing the fidelity of our theoretical equations.

When (±)3 was exposed to Bacillus sp., a soil isolate, the (-) form was preferentially hydrolyzed. An E value of 14 ± 0.5 was established for this system and the experimental c and *ee* values were in good agreement with the predicted curves (Fig. 6) derived from eqns. 4 and 5. The remaining (+) ester (77% *ee*) was transformed (hydrogenation and acidification) into 2*S*-methylbutyrolactone, $[\alpha]_D 25 = -13.0$ (c = 1.6, ethanol) [reported $[\alpha]_D^{25} = +13.8$ for

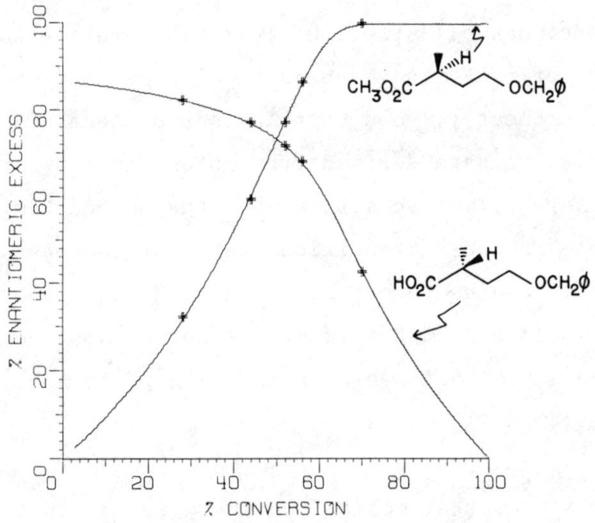

Fig. 6. The dependence of percentage enantiomeric excess (ee) on the percentage of conversion. The curves for E = 14 were computer generated from eqns. 4 (ester) and 5 (acid). # = Experimentally determined values of Bacillus sp.

2R-methylbutyrolactone (12)], thereby establishing that the R-isomer of 3 was preferentially attacked (Scheme 1). The resulting chiral acid was treated with diazomemethane, and reincubated with Bacillus sp. to enhance its optical purity. Fig. 7 clearly shows that there was little deviation of the experimentally determined ee' values from the predicted curve of eqn. 6.

By following a similar approach, we have prepared most of the desired bifunctional chiral synthons shown in Fig. 1. The E values and the biochemical systems used in effecting the stereospecific or enantioselective hydrolyses are summarized in Table 1.

In conclusion, we have developed basic equations and useful graphs for the unified treatment of biochemical kinetic resolution data. These expressions have now been verified experimentally and

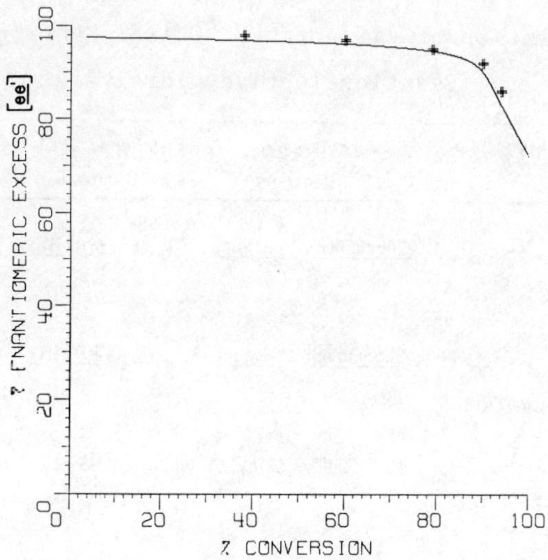

Fig. 7. Final percentage enantiomeric excess (ee') as a function of the percentage of conversion. The curve for E = 14 and ee_o = 0.72 were computer generated (eqn. 6). # = Experimentally determined values.

Scheme 1

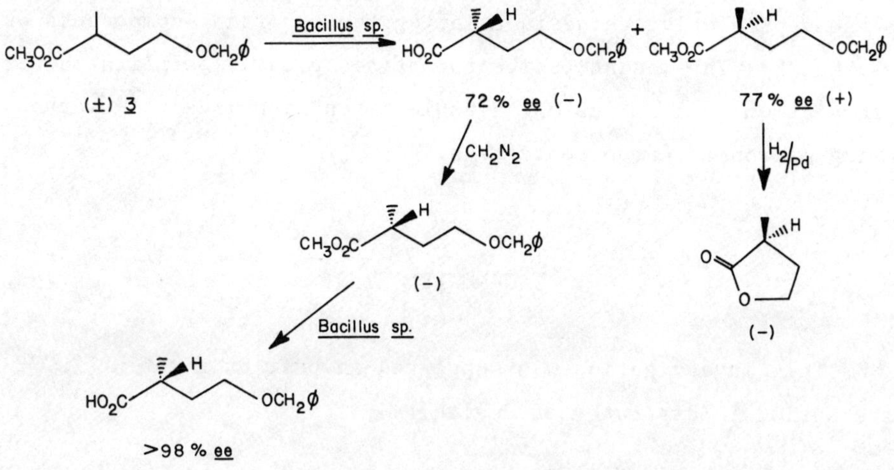

Table 1

Generation of Bifunctional Chiral Synthons via Enantioselective Hydrolyses

Substrate	Microorganism / Enzyme	Enantiomer Preferentially Cleaved	E
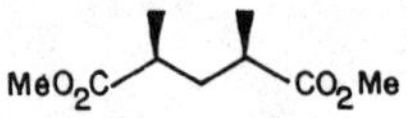	Gliocladium roseum	pro R	>100
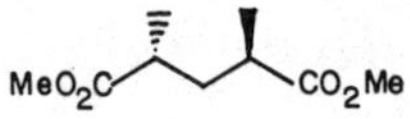	Gliocladium roseum	2R,4R	11
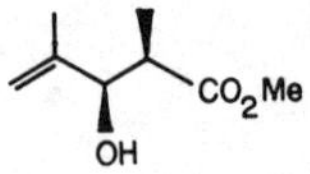	Gliocladium roseum	2S,3S	20
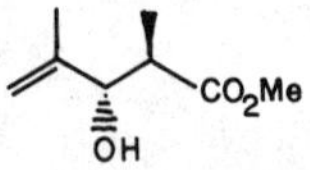	Pig liver esterase	2S,3R	9.7
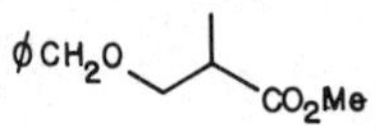	Enterobacter cloacae	R	>100
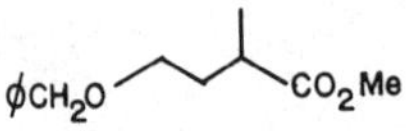	Bacillus sp.	R	14

possess predictive value in relating the important components of c, ee, and E. This quantitative format has greatly facilitated our preparation of a series of valuable bifunctional chiral synthons using microbial carboxyesterases.

ACKNOWLEDGEMENTS

This investigation was supported in part by grant HL 25772 of the National Institutes of Health.

REFERENCES AND NOTES

1. Corey, E.J., P.B. Hopkins, S. Kim, S.E. Yoo, K.P. Nambiar, and J.R. Falck. 1979. Total synthesis of erythromycins. V. Total synthesis of erythronolide A. J. Am. Chem. Soc. 101:7131-7134.
2. Evans, D.A., C.E. Sacks, W.A. Kleschick, and T.R. Taber. 1979. Polyether antibiotics synthesis. Total synthesis and absolute configuration of the ionophore A-23187. J. Am. Chem. Soc. 101:6789-6791.
3. Collum, D.B., J.H. McDonald III, and W.C. Still. 1980. Synthesis of the polyether antibiotic monensin. III. Coupling of precursors and transformation to monensin. J. Am. Chem. Soc. 102:2120-2121.
4. Cohen, N., W.F. Eichel, R.J. Lopresti, C. Neukom, and G. Saucy. 1976. Synthetic studies on (2R,4'R,8'R)-α-tocopherol. An approach utilizing side chain synthons of microbiological origin. J. Org. Chem. 41:3505-3511.
5. For a definition of V/K, see: Fersht, A. 1977. In Enzyme Structure and Mechanism. Freeman, San Francisco.
6. Meister, A., L. Levintow, R.B. Kingsley, and J.P. Greenstein. 1951. Optical purity of amino acid enantiomorphs. J. Biol. Chem. 1921:535-541.
7. Greenstein, J.P. and M. Winitz. 1961. Determination of optical and steric purity, p. 1734. In Chemistry of the Amino Acids, Vol. 2. Wiley, New York.
8. Krisch, K. 1971. Carboxylic ester hydrolases. In The Enzymes, Vol. 5; 3rd Ed., Academic Press, New York, Chapter 3.
9. Fig. 4 was computer generated by relating the variables c and ee(P) in eqn. 5 to a function of x for values of $\leq x \leq 1$; $c = 1 - x/2 - x/2 - x^E/2$ and $ee(P) = \dfrac{x - x^E}{2 - x - x^E}$. Implicit functions (eqns. 5 and 6) were solved by parametric representations. See: Buck, R.C. 1965. In Advanced Calculus; 2nd Ed. McGraw Hill, New York, p. 3-13.

10. Chen, C.S., Y. Fujimoto, and C.J. Sih. 1981. Bifunctional chiral synthons via microbiological methods. I. Optically active 2,4-dimethyl-glutaric acid monomethyl esters. J. Am. Chem. Soc. 103:3580-3582.

11. The E_{app} value may be affected by changes in substrate concentrations when the Michaelis constants of two or more enzymes are widely different.

12. Meyers, A.I. and E.D. Mihelich. 1975. An asymmetric synthesis of 2-substituted γ-butyrolactones and 2-substituted, 1,4-butanediols. J. Org. Chem. 40:1186-1187.

DISCUSSION

Q. R. SUBDEN (Univ. of Minnesota): I have a question for Dr. Sih. Instead of using the microorganisms for bioconversions of the sterols you described, would it not have been more efficient to construct a yeast strain that would make the desired sterol? Yeasts accumulate ergosterol as well as a number of other sterols, especially in mutants blocked in the sterol biosynthetic pathway. Could these sterols be starting material for formation of the desired compounds?

A. SIH: It is a matter of economics. I think the quantity of the sterol in yeast strains is very small when compared to the amount of saterols that can be obtained from soybeans or other plants. In addition, the sterol in yeast is primarily ergosterol rather than the most desired starting material for conversion.

Q. C. NASH (Sterling-Winthrop Res. Inst.): With regards to the computer models, is there a differece in the model for immobilized and soluble enzymes?

A. SIH: We haven't applied the theory to immobilized enzymes, but I think it should be the same because the E value doesn't change with time or substrate concentrations. It should behave the same.

MUTASYNTHESIS AND DIRECTED BIOSYNTHESIS FOR THE PRODUCTION OF NEW ANTIBIOTICS

Charles A. Claridge
Pharmaceutical Research and Development Division
Bristol-Myers Company
Syracuse, New York 13201

The fact that this Symposium on the Biological Basis of New Developments in Biotechnology is being held at this time is evidence of the increasing awareness throughout the world of the impact that modern microbiology is now having upon the production of antibiotics, new products in medicine, alternate sources of fuel for our world and the development of new and more efficient plants to feed our peoples. An example of the recognition of these developments was seen recently when Scientific American devoted an entire issue to "Industrial Microbiology".

I would like to address one small aspect of this field, that is the use of Mutasynthesis or Mutational Biosynthesis and of Directed Biosynthesis for the production of new antibiotics. I specify the title because I believe that there is good evidence that both processes can be applied successfully to the development of new antibiotics, both in the antiinfective field and in antitumor medicine.

Table 1

Deoxystreptamine Analogs Yielding New Antibiotics

Microorganism	Usual antibiotic	Deoxystreptamine analogues yielding new antibiotic	References
Streptomyces fradiae	Neomycin	streptamine 2-epi-streptamine 2,6-dideoxystreptamine 3-N-methyldeoxystreptamine streptidine 2,5-dideoxystreptamine 2-bromodeoxystreptamine 6-bromodeoxystreptamine	52 9 45
Streptomyces rimosus var. *paromomycinus*	Paromomycin	streptamine 2,6-dideoxystreptamine	54
Streptomyces kanamyceticus	Kanamycin	1-N-methyldeoxystreptamine 2-epi-streptamine	28
Streptomyces ribosidificus	Ribostamycin	streptamine 2-epi-streptamine 1-N-methyldeoxystreptamine 3',4'-dideoxyneamine	28
S. griseus	Streptomycin	2-deoxystreptidine	36
S. spectabilis	Spectinomycin	streptamine N-N'-dimethylstreptamine 2-epi-streptamine actinamine N-demethylactinamine	56
Bacillus circulans	Butirosin	streptamine streptidine 2,5-dideoxystreptamine 6'-N-methylneamine 3',4'-dideoxyneamine 3',4'-dideoxy-6'-N-methylneamine 3',4'-dideoxy-6'-C-methylneamine 6'-N-methylgentamine C_{1a} gentamine C_2 gentamine$_{1a}$ 1-deamino-2-deoxy-1-hydrostreptamine	57, 58, 59, 60 18
Micromonospora inyoensis	Sisomicin	streptamine 2,5-dideoxystreptamine 5-epi-deoxystreptamine 2-epi-streptamine 1-N-methyldeoxystreptamine N-methyl-2,5-dideoxystreptamine 1,3,5-triaminocyclohexane-4,6-diol	16 63
Micromonospora purpurea	Gentamicin	streptamine 2,5-dideoxystreptamine	10
Micromonospora sagamiensis	Sagamicin	2-deoxystreptamine streptamine	27

The impact of one process or the other on any commercial exploitation of an antibiotic development program frequently will depend upon the combined results obtained from a whole technological evaluation team that will include chemists, pharmacologists, toxicologists, and clinicians as well as fermentation microbiologists.

Mutasynthesis, or Mutational Biosynthesis, is a term originally defined by Rinehart and Stroshane [48] and by Nagaoka and Demain [36] for the concept that an exogenous moiety is needed for the synthesis of a secondary metabolite by a mutant of the producing organism. The mutant which requires this special nutrient to produce a product peculiar to that organism has been termed an "idiotroph" [36], in contrast to an "auxotroph" which is a mutant that is dependent upon an added nutrient for growth.

The success of such an approach to the development of new antibiotics was predicted in 1963 by Birch [4] when he suggested that it should be possible to mutate an organism so that it cannot complete the synthesis of an antibiotic unless given a normal precursor which the mutant cannot make but can utilize. If an altered intermediate can be utilized, then the mutant should be able to synthesize a new antibiotic. This prediction was confirmed by the work of Shier *et al*. [53] who showed the development of a new group of aminocyclitol antibiotics they called "hybrimycins" by the use of 2-deoxystreptamine idiotrophs of the neomycin-producing organism *Streptomyces fradiae*.

By Directed Biosynthesis, we mean the addition to the fermentation medium of an analog of a part of the antibiotic molecule which the organism is then capable of incorporating into its enzymatic processes to yield a modified antibiotic. This concept has wide application in the field of industrial antibiotic production, most notably in the penicillin fermentation.

The fact that both of these processes, Mutasynthesis and Directed Biosynthesis, lead to the formation of new antibiotic materials demonstrates that there is some low substrate specificity of antibiotic-committed enzymes to enable modified antibiotics to be produced.

There are, additionally, other genetic processes for the transfer and recombination of DNA among and between species that result in new antibiotics or increased production levels of ones already in use that are to be dealt with in other chapters.

Mutasynthesis

The major work employing the mutasynthesis process has been in the field of aminocyclitol antibiotics. Shier *et al*. [53] were able to develop a blocked mutant of *Streptomyces fradiae* that would not produce the normal neomycin antibiotics unless 2-deoxystreptamine (DOS) was added to the fermentation medium. When streptamine and *epi*-streptamine were substituted for DOS, new antibiotics termed "hybrimycins" were formed. Subsequently, other microorganisms that produce aminocyclitol antibiotics were mutated, and the resultant idiotrophic mutants were used to develop analogs of the parental antibiotic when various DOS analogues were added to the fermentation medium. A summary of the various aminocyclitol-producing organisms and the DOS analogs that lead to the development of new antibiotics is given in Table 1.

It should be noted, as has been pointed out by Rinehart [46], that it cannot be assumed that the DOS analog will be incorporated to yield a simple modification of the parental antibiotic, and that it is necessary to isolate and carefully characterize the new antibiotic. For example, when 2,5-dideoxystreptamine was fed to a DOS-requiring mutant of *Bacillus circulans* a new compound identified as 5-deoxy-6'-deamino-6'-hydroxybutirosamine was isolated in addition to the anticipated 5'-deoxybutirosamine [7].

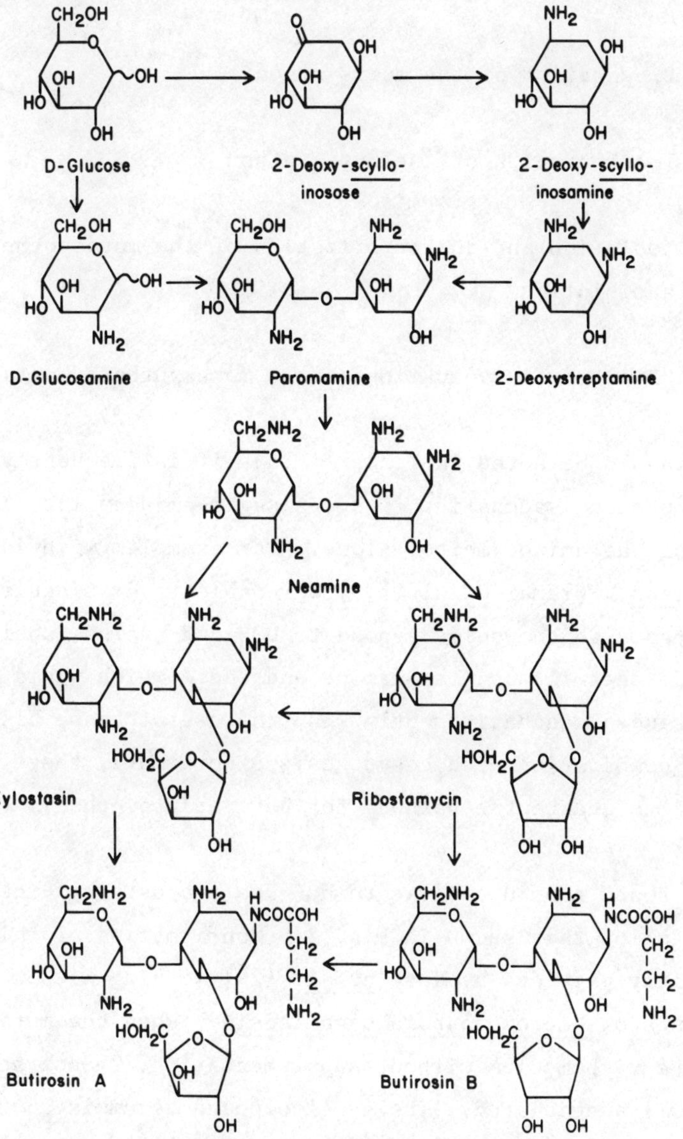

Fig. 1. Pathway of buitrosin biosynthesis.

The surrogate aminocyclitols fed to the idiotrophic mutants have been referred to by Rinehart as mutasynthons, and the new antibiotic as a mutasynthetic antibiotic. Thus, in a mutasynthesis experiment at least four distinct steps are required [45].

1. Preparation of the mutasynthon

2. Incorporation of the mutasynthon

3. Isolation and characterization of the mutasynthetic antibiotic

4. Biological evaluation of the mutasynthetic antibiotic

It should be noted in Table 1, that it is frequently possible to use a pseudodisaccharide (i.e., a sugar-aminocyclitol) moiety instead of the aminocylcitol alone. For example, with idiotrophs of *B. circulans*, Furumai *et al.* [19] were able to distinguish between those mutants which would respond to DOS and the pseudodisaccharides neamine and paromamine and those which would respond to the pseudodisaccharides only. By the use of these blocked mutants in combination with cosynthesis experiments, these workers were able to deduce the pathway for butirosin synthesis (Fig. 1).

The route from D-glucose to DOS was proposed by Rinehart *et al.* [47] to follow that shown in Fig. 2. Confirmation of this pathway was recently provided by Kase *et al.* [23] working with a DOS-requiring mutants of *Micromonospora sagamiensis*. When the mutant was grown in a rich medium without supplementation, 2-deoxy*scyllo*-inosoamine (DOI) accumulated. The same compound accumulated from one of the blocked mutants of *B. circulans* reported by Fujiwara *et al.* [17].

Thus, it may be concluded that in the biosynthesis of DOS, the amination of position 3 occurs first followed by oxidation-amination at position 1 as in pathway (a) of Fig. 2.

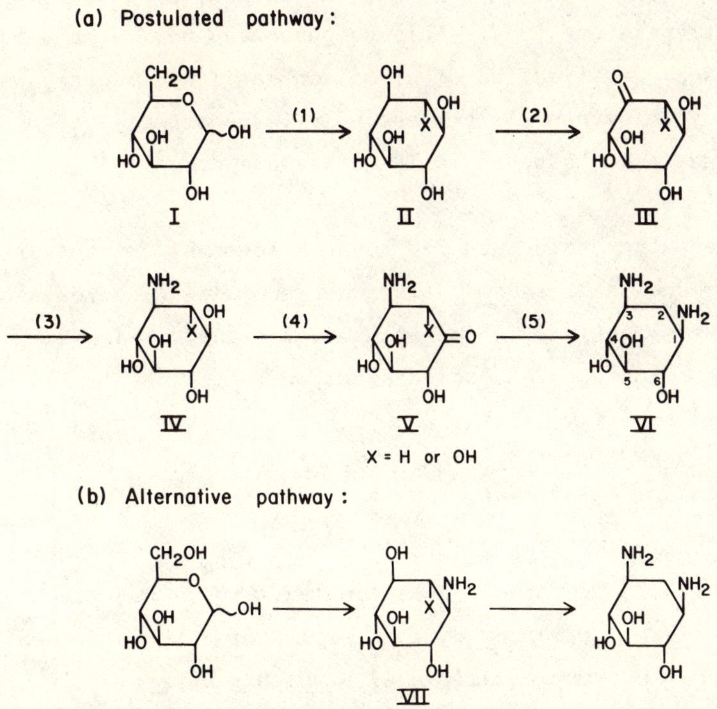

Fig. 2. Deoxystreptamine biosynthesis.

Although a large number of mutasynthetic antibiotics have been prepared, the great commercial success early envisaged after the initial development of the "hybrimycins" has not occurred. However, there have been compounds reported which appear superior. The 6-deoxyneomycins, prepared by feeding 2,6-dideoxy-streptamine to S. fradiae are more active than neomycin C against Escherichia coli, Proteus mirabilis, Staphylococcus aureus, and Salmonella typhimurium [9]. In addition, some of the new sisomicin derivatives produced upon feeding streptamine and 2,5-dideoxystreptamine to idiotrophs of M. inyoensis are more active than sisomicin against sisomicin- and gentamicin-resistant strains [61].

Perhaps the most important of these is 5-epi-sisomicin (or

MU-6) which was obtained by feeding the appropriate mutant 2-deoxy-5-epi-strepatamine [61]. This compound can now be made more readily by chemical modification of sisomicin but its discovery was by the mutational biosynthesis process. It is reportedly under extensive investigation as a potentially marketable drug [30].

When streptamine was fed to an idiotrophic mutant of the sagamicin-producing _M. sagamiensis_, the resulting 2-hydroxysagmicin produced was slightly less potent against sagamicin-sensitive strains but more potent against some sagamicin-resistant strains. Moreover, the acute toxicity of the mutasynthetic antibiotic was one-fourth to one-fifth that of sagamicin or the gentamicin C complex [27].

Recently, Kase _et al_. [24] have isolated a new series of antibiotics, designated the SU complex, from a DOS idiotroph of _M. sagamiensis_. One member of the complex of interest, SU-2 [55], is 1-deamino-1-hydroxygentamicin C_{1a}, which had previously been chemically synthesized from gentamicin C_{1a} [5]. This antibiotic was produced without supplementation, confirming that amination of the DOS precursor at position 3 occurs before position 1 and that a complete antibiotic can be synthesized without amination at position 1.

Another promising mutasynthetic antibiotic is Win 42122-2 or 2-hydroxy-gentamicin, produced by feeding streptamine to an idiotrophic mutant of _M. purpurea_ [49]. The new compound is generally less active than gentamicin against _Pseudomonas_ and many _Enterobacteriaceae_. However, Win 42122-2 is markedly less toxic than gentamicin in subacute nephrotoxicity studies in rats, ototoxicity in guinea pigs, and ataxia determination in cats [6].

An interesting variation of the mutasynthesis process has been applied by Oka _et al_. [37] who took advantage of the fact that most

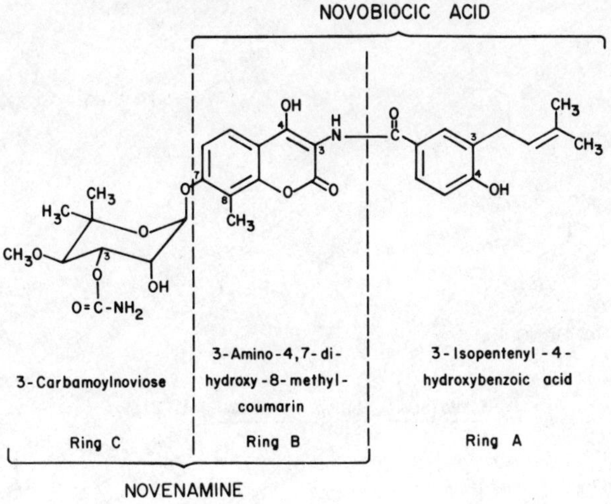

Fig. 3. Structure of novobiocin.

of the gentamicins produced by fermentations are 3',4'-dideoxy-compounds. When a non-producing idiotroph of a gentamicin-producing Micromonospora was fed kanamycin A or B, both of which are 3',4'-oxocompounds, a new series of antibiotics characterized by 4"-C-methylation as well as 3',4'-dideoxygenation of the kanamycin molecule was produced. These compounds were named combimicins, with B_2 being of particular interest because of its decreased toxicity when compared to gentamicin. It is reportedly undergoing clinical testing in Japan.

Sebek [51] has recently pointed out that aminoglycosides are generally good material for the study and investigation by the mutasynthesis procedure because most of them consist of three components, each formed separately and joined together only in the final stages of synthesis. However, other antibiotics constructed of more than one moiety are also suitable for such studies. In view of the large number of such antibiotics, it is perhaps surprising that outside the aminoglycoside field, the literature records only a few cases of this manipulation.

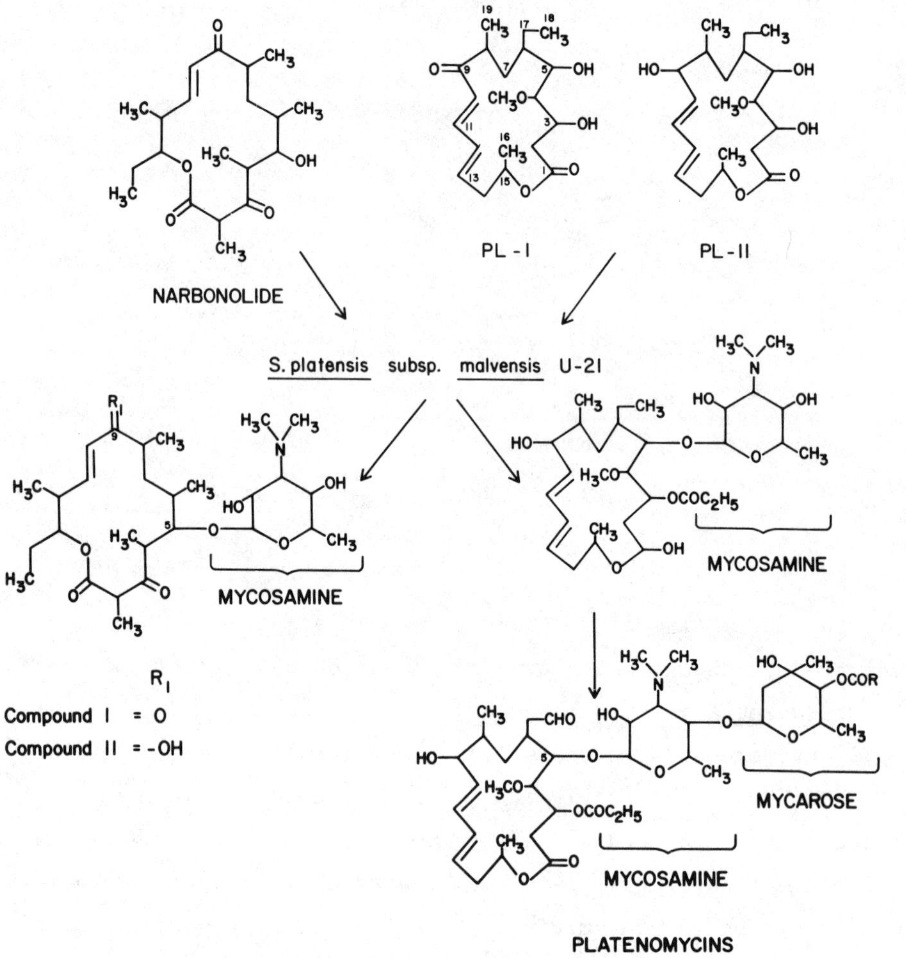

Fig. 4. Mutasynthesis of new macrolides.

Sebek [50] described an idiotrophic mutant of the novobiocin-producing strain of Streptomyces niveus that was blocked in the formation of ring B; antibiotic production was restored only when the medium was supplemented with ring B or novobiovic acid (Fig. 3). A new novobiocin analog was formed when a chlorine-containing derivative of ring B (8-demethyl-8-chloro-3-amino-4,7,-dihydroxycoumarin) was supplied. The antibacterial spectrum of this product was

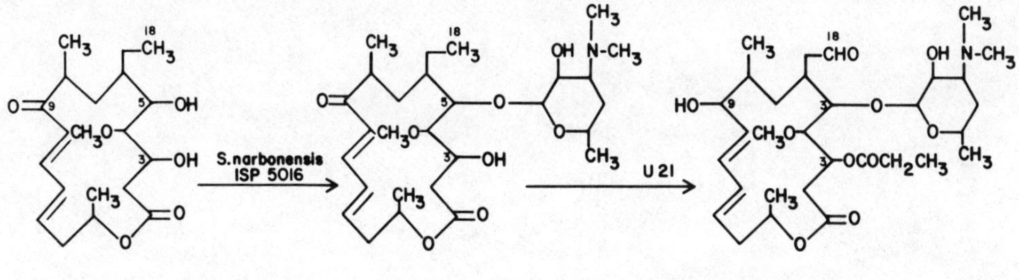

I II III

Fig. 5. Mutasynthesis with *S. narbonensis*. I = platenolide I; II = 5-0-desosaminylplatenolide I; III = 3-0-propionyl-5-0-desosaminyl-9-dihydro-18-oxo-platenolide I.

practically the same as that of novobiocin. Other modified coumarins were tested in the same fashion and new bioactive products were formed, but no additional data have been recorded [51].

The macrolide-producing culture *S. platensis* subsp. *malvensis* produces the 16-membered antibiotic platenomycin. An idiotrophic mutant was obtained which would snythesize antibiotics only in the presence of added platenolide I or II. If the 14-membered aglycone narbonolide was substituted, the mutant was able to glycosylate the aglycone forming compound I (Fig. 4), which, however, had only about 25% of the activity of narbomycin. Another product (compound II) in which the C9 ketone was reduced was also formed. However, this compound was almost devoid of activity [31].

In addition, these same workers reported that platenolide I would be glycosylated by the narbomycin-producing *S. narbonensis* resulting in the formation of 5-0-desosaminylplatenolide I. This compound is also devoid of antibiotic activity. If this compound is then fed to the U-21 mutant of *S. platensis* the antibiotically active 3-0-propinoyl-5-0-desosaminyl-9-dihydro-18-oxo-platenolide I is produced (Fig. 5)[32].

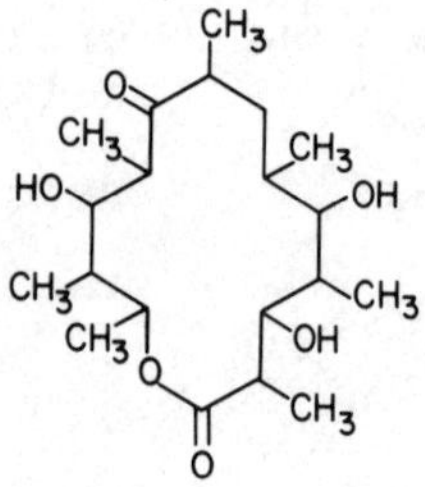

Fig. 6. 8,8α-deoxyoleandolide mutasynthon fed to S. erythreus.

When a blocked mutant of the erythromycin-producing organism S. erythreus, which would convert added erythronolide to erythromycin was fed 8,8a-deoxy-oleanodolide, the deoxyaglycone lactone of oleandomycin, a new antibiotic, was produced [33]. Although this new antibiotic was not isolated, it is reasonable to expect that it is glycosylated to form the erythromycin analog (Fig. 6).

An alternate procedure to mutasynthesis employing a specific inhibitor in place of the blocked idiotrophic mutant has been used by Omura et al. [43] to form a new macrolide antibiotic with a strain of Streptomyces. A schematic comparison of mutasynthesis with their process, which they call hybrid biosynthesis, is seen in Fig. 7.

The normal macrolide formed by this Streptomyces strain is picromycin. In the presence of the enzyme inhibitor cerulenin (which acts as an inhibitor of fatty acid and polyketide biosynthesis) and the unnatural macrolide aglycone protylonolide, the new macrolide antibiotic was formed.

There are some recent reports of anthracycline antibiotic-producing organisms that have been mutated to yield idiotrophic mutants. Fleck [16] obtained a mutant of the daunomycin-producing S.

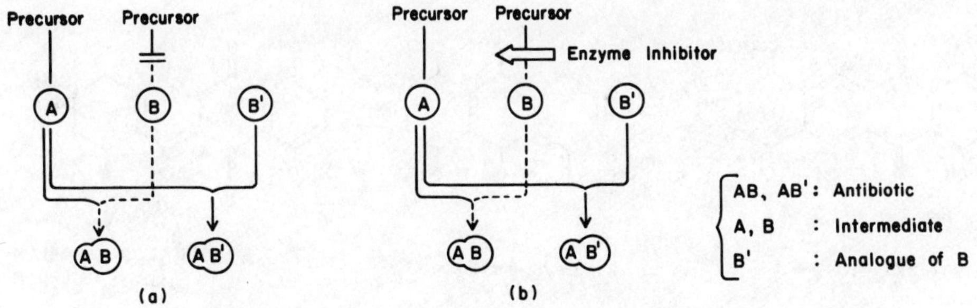

Fig. 7. Comparison of mutasynthesis and hybrid biosynthesis.

griseus that was blocked in the synthesis of the aglycone daunomycinone. When rhodomycinone or similar aglycones were incubated with this mutant, new antibiotics different from the parental type were formed. Similarly, Fleck [16] also reported blocked mutants of the violamycin-producing *S. violaceus* culture that behaved in the same manner. In addition, Claridge (unpublished experiments) has found that idiotrophic mutants of two anthracycline-producing cultures, *Actinosporangium* sp. that forms the bohemic acid complex, and a *Streptosporangium* sp. that produces the fiagoric acid complex, will produce new anthracyclines when fed aglycones not normally produced by these cultures.

More definitive studies with blocked mutants of the anthracycline-producing cultures have come from the laboratories of the Sanraku- Ocean Company in Japan. They have studied idiotrophic mutants of *S. coeruleorubidus* (which produces carminomycin and baumycin) and *S. galilaeus* (which produced aclacinomycin). Idiotrophic mutants of the first culture would produce the normal antibiotics when fed the aglycone aklavinone but if the unnatural aglycones ε-pyrromycinone or ε-isorhodomycinone were substituted, two new glycosides designated GPI and GPII were formed (Fig. 8)[69].

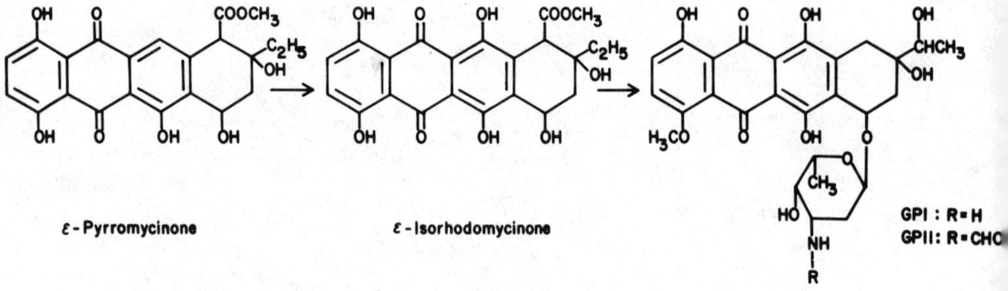

Fig. 8. Formation of GPI and GPII by S. coeruleorubidus.

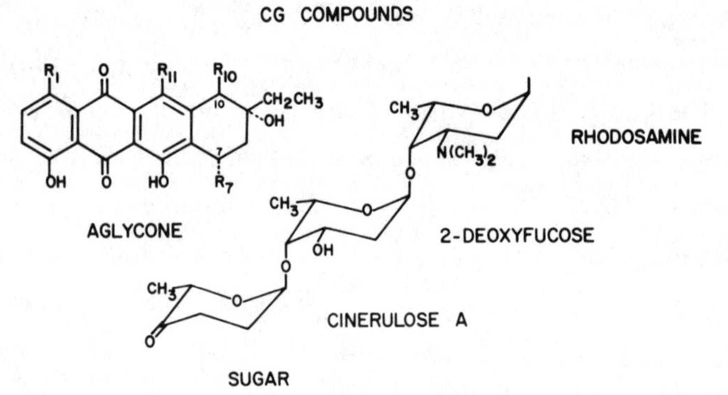

Compound	R_1	R_{11}	R_{10}	R_7
ACM (AKN-Sugar)	H	H	CO_2CH_3	O-Sugar
CG5 (ε-RMN-Sugar)	H	OH	CO_2CH_3	O-Sugar
CG 6 (ε-IsoRMN-Sugar)	OH	OH	CO_2CO_3	O-Sugar
CG 7 (β-RMN-Sugar)	H	OH	OH	O-Sugar
CG8 (γ-RMN-Sugar)	H	OH	O-Sugar	H

Abbreviation: ACM = Aclacinomycin A, AKN = Aklavinone, ε-RMN = ε-Rhodomycinone, ε-IsoRMN = ε-Isorhodomycinone, β-RMN = β-Rhodomycinone and γ-RMN = γ-Rhodomycinone

Fig. 9. Structures of CG compounds.

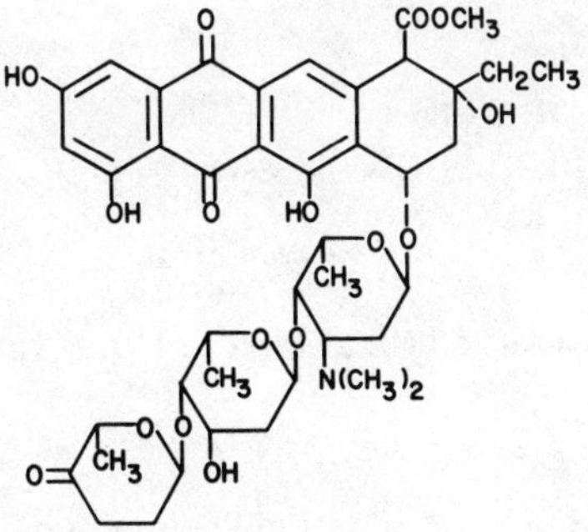

Fig. 10. Structure of 2-hydroxyaclacinomycin A.

With the aclacinomycin-producing strain S. galilaeus, the blocked mutants obtained an accepted number of unnatural aglycones to produce new anthracycline antibiotics. ε, α, and β rhodomycinones were incorporated to form new anthracyclines designated CG5 and CG8 and CG7, with ε-isorhodmycinone leading to the formation of CG6 [34,38]. These structures are seen in Fig. 9. Another blocked mutant from the same culture incorporated 2-hydroxyaklavinone to yield 2-hydroxyaclacinomycin A (Fig. 10). This new compound showed marked cytotoxicity against cultured L1210 cells and preferentially inhibited RNA synthesis. Against L1210 leukemia in CDF_1 mice, the effective dose range was much wider than aclacinomycin A [39].

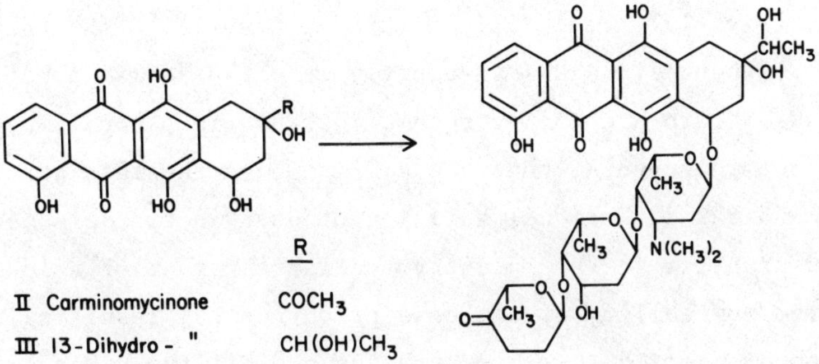

Fig. 11. Formation of trisarubicinol.

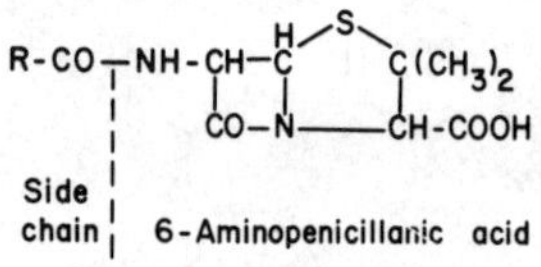

Fig. 12. Basic structure of penicillins.

Still another mutant of this culture has recently been reported [68] to incorporate carminomycinone and 13-dihydrocarminomycinone to form a new anthracycline called trisarubicinol (Fig. 11).

Directed Biosynthesis

1. Penicillins. Directed biosynthesis means that the direction of a fermentation can be controlled by the addition to the medium of a suitable precursor or inhibitor to cause the formation of a desired secondary metabolite. Most examples cite the formation of new antibiotics, where this technique has had its widest application Perhaps the most noted example of this procedure is in penicillin production, where in a normal fermentation it was early realized that several different penicillins were being produced in the same medium. These so-called "natural" penicillins were found to differ only in the acyl side chain attached to the 6-aminopenicillanic acid nucleus. (Fig. 12). Penicillin F (R=Δ^2-pentenyl), G (R-benzyl), X (R=p-hydroxybenzyl), and K (R-heptyl) were the normal penicillins formed. When corn steep liquor came into use in penicillin production, it was discovered that penicillin G was the main natural product and the intentional addition of phenylactic acid became standard practice in the industry. A large number of acids were tested for suitability of use as a precursor [3] resulting in the formation of over 100 new biosynthetic penicillins. One such biosynthetic penicillin which became commercially important was penicillin V formed by the addition of phenoxyacetic acid to the

Table 2

Natural and Biosynthetic Penicillins

Types of precursor	Penicillins obtained (examples)
Saturated and unsaturated aliphatic acids	penicillin F, dihydro F
Substituted or unsubstituted phenylacetic acids	penicillin G
Substituted or unsubstituted cyclic polycyclic or heterocyclic acetic acids	cyclopentymethyl penicillin
Substituted or unsubstituted mercapto-acetic and oxyacetic acids	phenoxymethyl penicillin

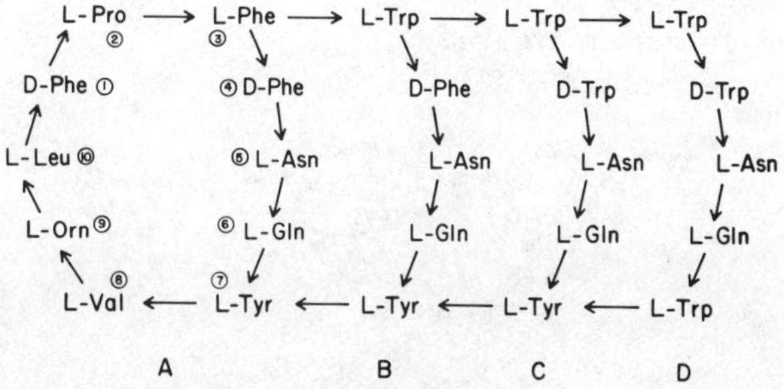

Fig. 13. Structures of tyrocidines. Left side of figure is common to all the structures. (From Katz and Demain, ref. 25, with the permission of Am. Soc. for Microb.)

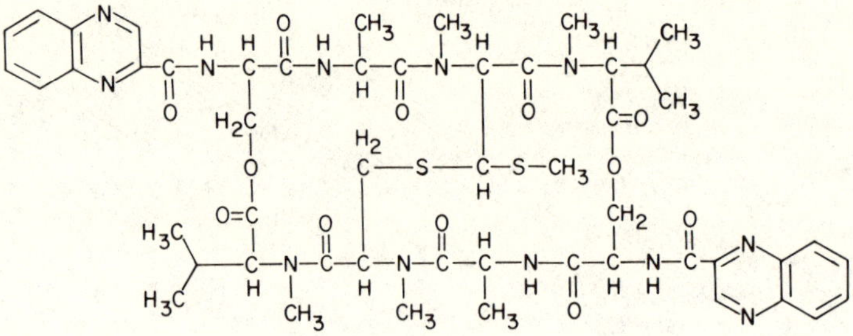

Fig. 14. Structure of actinomycin D.

medium. This pencillin became important because of its acid stability and thus suitable for oral administration. Examples of the natural and biosynthetic penicillins produced by fermentation are given in Table 2.

Not all acids are accepted by the Penicillium culture to form a biosynthetic penicillin. Those that were formed a class of compounds leading to the formation of "Behrens' rule", which states that the only compounds acceptable as a penicillin precursor would be monosubstituted acetic acid derivatives containing at least one free α hydrogen [3]. The limitation on the types of new penicillins was not overcome until 6-APA became available by either enzymatic or chemical splitting of penicillin G or V. 6-APA reacts with a wide variety of acylating agents to form the new penicillins that have been introduced in recent years.

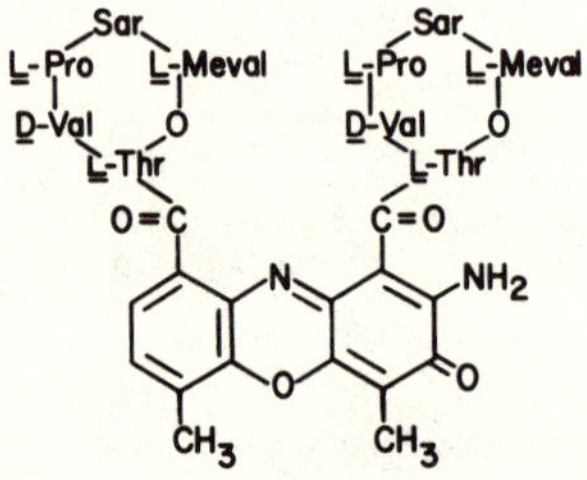

Fig. 15. Structure of echinomycin (Quinomycin A).

Table 3

Chromophore Analogs Leading to New Echinomycins

SUBSTITUENT CHROMOPHORE	STRUCTURE	REFERENCE
Quinazol-4-one-3-acetic acid	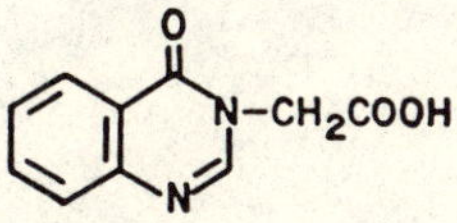	13
Quinaldinic acid	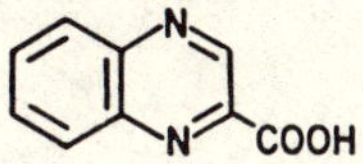	67
7-Chloroquinoxaline-2-carboxylic acid	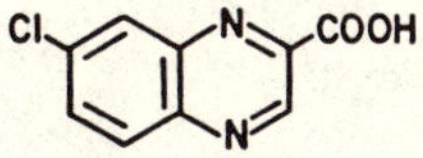	66
Thieno(3.2-b)pyridine-5-carboxylic acid	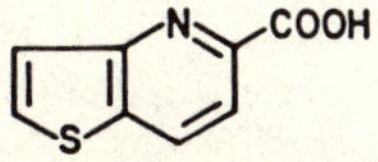	66
6-Methylquinoline-2-carboxylic acid	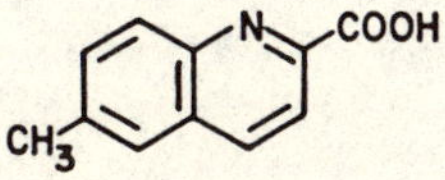	66

2. *Peptide Antibiotics*. A number of peptide antibiotic fermentations respond dramatically to the addition of various precursors to the culture medium. Those that are produced by the genus *Bacillus* were reviewed recently by Katz and Demain [25], who noted that due to the broad specificity of the antibiotic synthetases, amino acids structurally similar to those found in the antibiotic could replace certain amino acid residues normally present. As an example, the ratio of tyrocidines A, B, and C normally produced by *B. brevis* can be modified by the addition of other amino acids to the medium. With the addition of tryptophan, A and B are not produced, but C and a new tyrocidine, D, appear. If phenylalanine is added, only tyrocidines A and B are seen (Fig. 13). Other

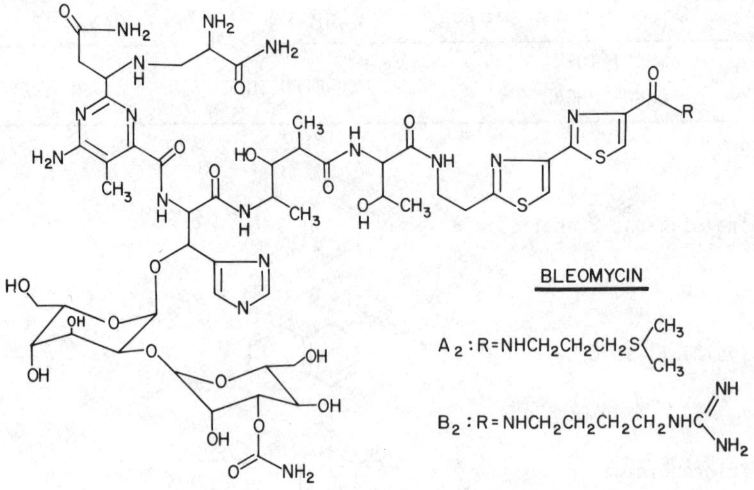

Fig. 16. Structure of bleomycins.

additions lead to further modifications of the tyrocidine molecule produced by the *B. brevis* culture.

The actinomycins produced by *S. antibioticus* represent another large class of peptide antibiotics that can be modified by precursor feeding (Fig. 14). The addition of sarcosine and hydroxyproline can alter the ratio of the natural actinomycins and the addition of valine to the medium increases markedly the proportion of actinomycin IV. New actinomycins have also been produced by the addition of proline analogues such as pipecolic acid; azetidine-2-carboxylic acid, 3-, 4-, 5-methyl proline; 4-fluoro-, bromo-, chloro-, or thioproline. Some of these new biosynthetic actinomycins have altered therapeutic indices and showed early promise in cancer chemotherapy but failed clinical trials for various pharmacological reasons.

Echinomycin (quinomycin) is a peptide antibiotic containing two quinoxaline carboxylic acid chromophores linked to a cross-bridged

Table 4

Some Amine Moieties of Natural and Biosynthetic Bleomycins

Natural	Biosynthetic
$-NH-(CH_2)_3-SO-CH_3$	$-NH-(CH_2)_3-NH_2$
$-NH-(CH_2)_4-NH_2$	$-NH-(CH_2)_3-NH-(CH_2)_3-OH$
$-NH(CH_2)_4-NH-\overset{NH}{\overset{\Vert}{C}}-NH_2$	$-NH-(CH_2)_3-N$ 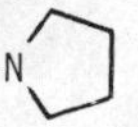
	$-NH-(CH_2)_3-NH-$ 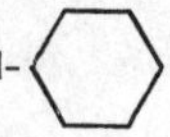

dilactone cylic peptide (Fig. 15). Analogs of the quinoxaline carboxylic acid have been fed to the producing culture resulting in new biosynthetic derivatives [13,66,67](Table 3). Because of the asymmetric nature of the molecule, each new chromophore addition leads to three new echinomycins. The newly described related antitumor antibiotic luzopeptin [29], produced by Actinomadura luzonensis, is probably capable of being biosynthetically modified in much the same manner.

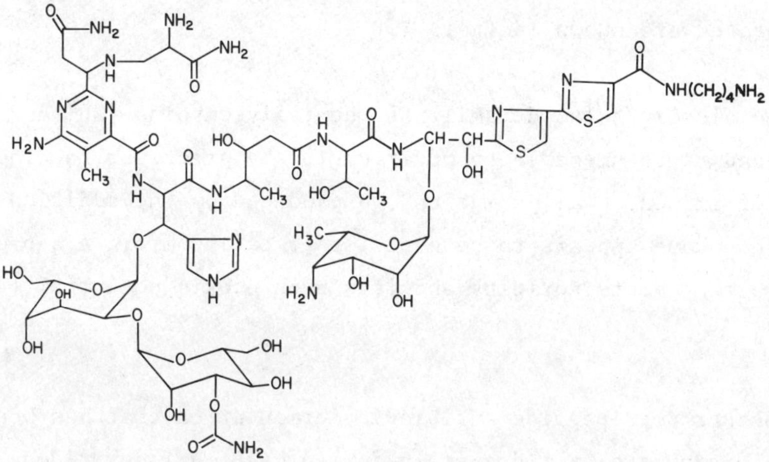

Fig. 17. Structure of tallysomysin $S_{10}b$.

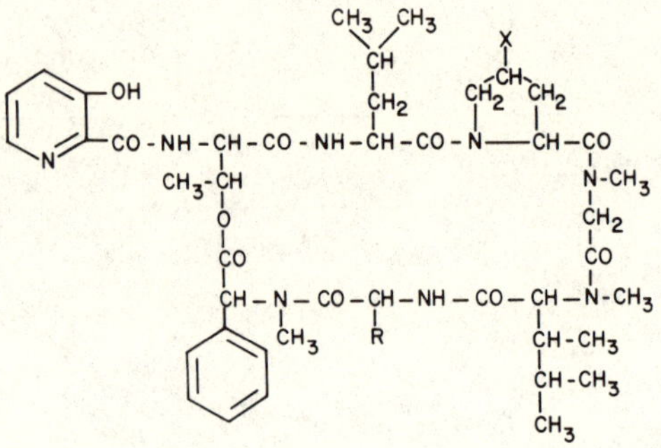

	R	X
Neoviridogrisein I	$-CH_2CH_3$	-H
Neoviridogrisein II	$-CH_3$	-H
Neoviridogrisein III	$-CH_2CH_3$	-OH
Neoviridogrisein IV (= Viridogrisein)	$-CH_3$	-OH

Fig. 18. Formation of new neoviridogriseins.

The bleomycins constitute a family of important peptide antibiotics of significant use in cancer chemotherapy [62](Fig. 16). A number of natural bleomycins are formed by S. verticillus, but this range can be broadened extensively by the addition to the medium of a number of amines. Some of the amines that are biosynthetically incorporated are shown in Table 4.

The closely related family of the tallysomycins [26] has also been found to be amenable to modification by precursor feeding of a number of amines. Tallysomycin $S_{10}b$ produced by the addition of 1, 4-diaminobutane appears to be superior to tallysomycin A because of less apparent acute toxicity and less nephrotoxic potential (Fig. 17) [35].

Another depsipeptide antibiotic fermentation that has been modified is that of viridogrisein formed by S. griseoviridus. The addition of the amino acids α-amino-n-butyric acid, proline, and methionine lead to the formation of new analogs (Fig. 18) labeled

Table 5

Precursors of New Novobiocins

(Reproduced with the permission of the Soc. Ind. Microbiol.)

NOVOBIOCIN

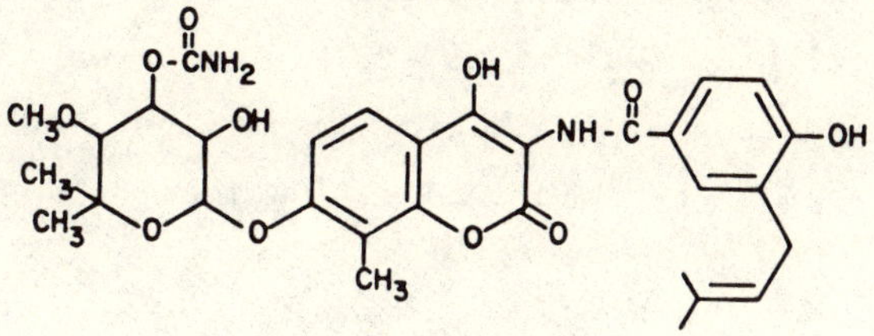

Precursors of Biosynthetic Novobiocins

3-hexyl-4-hydroxybenzoic acid

4-ethoxy-3(3-methyl-2-butenyl)benzoic acid

4-hydroxy-3(3-phenylpropyl)benzoic acid

3-isopentyl-4-methoxybenzoic acid

4-hydroxy-3-pentylbenzoic acid

4-hydroxy-3-isopentylbenzoic acid

4-acetoxy-3-isopentylbenzoic acid

4-methoxy-3(3-methyl-2-butenyl)benzoic acid

4-hydroxy-3-isobutylbenzoic acid

3-(2,3-dichloropropyl)4-methoxybenzoic acid

4-hydroxy-3-propylbenzoic acid

4-hydroxy-3-γ-methylallyl) benzoic acid

4-hydroxy-3-(2-methylallyl)benzoic acid

4-hydroxy-3-(α-methylallyl)benzoic acid

3-allyl-4-hydroxybenzoic acid

4-hydroxy-3-methylbenzoic acid

3-ethyl-4-hydroxybenzoic acid

4-amino-3-methylbenzoic acid

3-allyl-4-methoxybenzoic acid

neoviridogrisein I, II, and III. Neoviridogrisein II proved to be more active than the parent against gram positive bacteria and *Mycoplasma* species [40,41,42).

3. Novobiocins. Already mentioned has been the formation of new novobiocin analogs through the use of an idiotrophic mutant of the producing culture. Walton *et al*. [64] much earlier had succeeded in producing biosynthetic novobiocins by the addition to the medium of several benzoic acid derivatives. Those reported to be active are shown in Table 5.

4. Mitomycins. Claridge *et al*. [8] have recently reported on the formation of new analogs of mitomycin C by the addition of primary amines to the culture medium of the producing culture *S. caespitosus*. Two new mitomycin types were formed, one similar to mitomycin C with the added amine being substituted at position C7. The other was related to mitomycin B, having an OH at position C9a and a methyl group on the aziridine N with the added amine also appearing at C7. The amines tested and found to be active are shown in Table 6. The two classes of mitomycins were labeled I and II, with those closely related to mitomycin C (I) having greater activity than those of class II. Activity in a prophage induction test and against leukemia L1210 in mice is shown in Table 7. The impetus for this work was in response to the report by Iyengar *et al*. [22] that mitomycin analogs could be chemically synthesized with a number of them showing superiority over the parent when measured by various *in vivo* antitumor tests and leukopenic effects. However, the chemical synthesis route required a conversion of mitomycin C to mitomycin A prior to C7 substitution with overall yields being somewhat low. Nevertheless, the chemical method proved superior because the most desirable analogs could not be biosynthetically produced.

5. Other Antibiotics. *Streptomycins cacaoi* can be induced to synthesize unnatural polyoxins when either 5-fluoro, 5-bromo, or

Table 6

Structures of Compounds Isolated

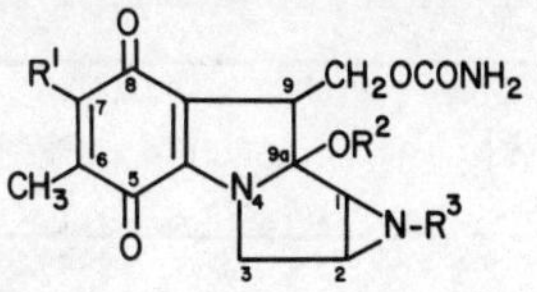

NSC NO.	COMPOUND	R^1	R^2	R^3
26980	MITOMYCIN C	NH_2	CH_3	H
75986	MITOMYCIN A	CH_3O	CH_3	H
75987	MITOMYCIN B	CH_3O	H	CH_3
56410	PORFIROMYCIN	NH_2	CH_3	CH_3
329086	METHYLAMINE I	CH_3NH	CH_3	H
329087	METHYLAMINE II	CH_3NH	H	CH_3
329085	ETHYLAMINE I	C_2H_5NH	CH_3	H
325313	ETHYLAMINE II	C_2H_5NH	H	CH_3
123115	n-PROPYLAMINE I	C_3H_7NH	CH_3	H
333059	n-PROPYLAMINE II	C_3H_7NH	H	CH_3
331126	PROPARGYLAMINE I	$HC\equiv CCH_2NH$	CH_3	H
331127	PROPARGYLAMINE II	$HC=CCH_2NH$	H	CH_3
332583	2-METHYLALLYLAMINE I	$CH_2=\underset{CH_3}{C}CH_2NH$	CH_3	H
332584	2-METHYLALLYLAMINE II	$CH_2=\underset{CH_3}{C}CH_2NH$	H	CH_3

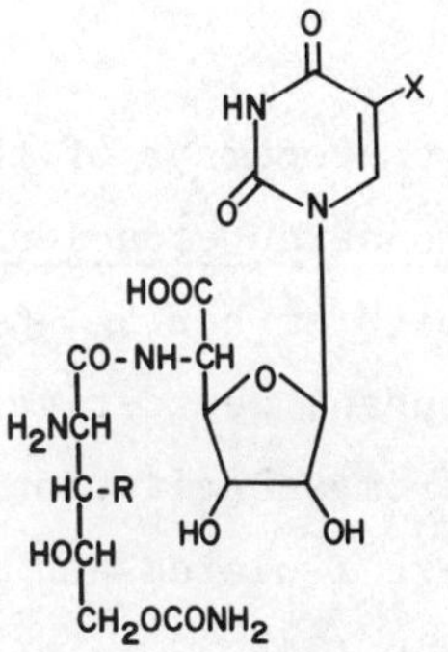

	X	R
Polyoxin L	-H	-OH
5-fluoropolyoxin L	-F	-OH
Polyoxin M	-H	-H
5-fluoropolyoxin M	-F	-H

Fig. 19. Structures of polyoxins.

Table 7

Prophase Induction Activity and

Activity Against Leukemia L1210 in Mice

COMPOUND	PROPHAGE INDUCTION ACTIVITY T/C AT 0.5 μG/ML	L1210 ACTIVITY T/C	DOSE MG/KG
MITOMYCIN C	22	160	6
MITOMYCIN A	34.6		
PORFIROMYCIN	8.9		
METHYLAMINE I	5.9	124	24
II	0.9	100	24
ETHYLAMINE I	8.7	142	24
II			
n-PROPYLAMINE I	8.1	166	6.25
II	1.0	100	24
PROPARGLYAMINE I	11.6	186	24
II	1.7	100	24
2-METHYALLYLAMINE I	2.5	126	24
II	1.4	100	24

6-azauracil is added to the fermentation medium [21]. These nucleoside antibiotics are extremely toxic to phytopathogenic fungi and are competitive inhibitors of chitin synthetase. Bacteria, plants, and animals are not inhibited by the polyoxins. However, the new fluorinated analogs are inhibitory to bacterial cells. Their structures are shown in Fig. 19.

D-tryptophan is known to be direct precursor of the antifungal agent pyrrolnitrin produced by <u>Pseudomonas aureofaciens</u>. When fermentation media were supplemented with either 5-, 6-, or 7-fluorotryptophan or 5-, or 7-methyl-tryptophan, new derivatives were formed [20]. Two derivatives, those from substitution with 6-fluorotryptophan and 7-methyltryptophan were isolated and shown to have activity similar to that of pyrrolnitrin (Fig. 20).

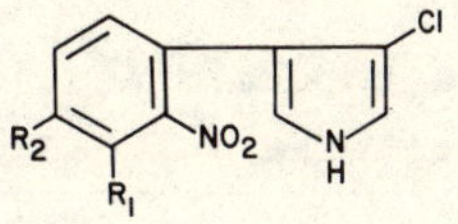

	R_1	R_2
Pyrrolnitrin	-Cl	-H
4'-fluoropyrrolnitrin	-Cl	-F
3'-methyl-3'-dechloropyrrolnitrin	$-CH_3$	-H

Fig. 20. Structures of pyrrolnitrins.

Dulaney *et al*. [15] some years ago reported that supplementation of the fermentation medium of *S. rimosus* with ethionine resulted in the production of the N-ethyl homolog of oxytetracycline as well as the normal oxytetracycline. It had been shown previously that 7-bromotetracycline could be formed by the addition of bromide ion to the medium of the chlorotetracycline producer [14].

Addition of ethionine to fermentations of *S. lincolnensis* grown in a complex medium resulted in the production of S-demethyl-S-ethyllincomycin [2]. On the other hand, when ethionine was added to

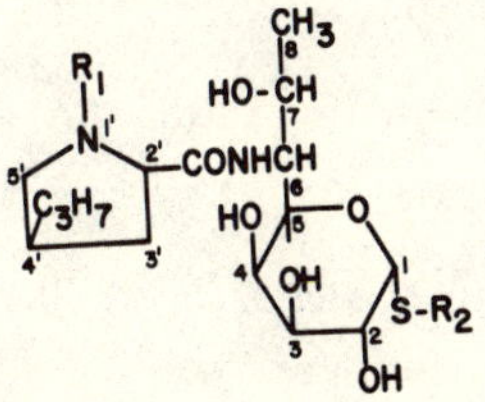

	R_1	R_2
Lincomycin	$-CH_3$	$-CH_3$
S-Demethyl-S-ethyllincomycin	$-CH_3$	$-C_2H_5$
N,S-Didemethyl-N,S-diethyllincomycin	$-C_2H_5$	$-C_2H_5$

Fig. 21. Structures of the lincomycins.

Table 8

Acids Added to the Fermentation Medium of

<u>Streptomyces caelestis</u>

medium of <u>Streptomyces caelestis</u>

1. 4-Aminosalicylic acid
2. Anthranilic acid
3. m-Aminobenzoic acid
4. p-Aminobenzoic acid
5. N-Methyl anthranilic
6. p-Dimethylaminobenzoic acid
7. p-Methylaminobenzoic acid
8. p-Acetamidobenzoic acid

cultures grown in a synthetic medium an additional new antibiotic, N,S-didemethyl-N,S-diethyl-lincomycin, was produced. (Fig. 21).

The closely related celestosaminide antibiotics produced by *S. caelestis* can be modified by the addition of aromatic acids to the culture medium (Table 8). The analog produced by the addition of 4-aminosalicyclic acid was isolated and characterized as desalicetin 2'-(4-aminosalicylate) [1]. Its antimicrobial spectrum is identical to that of celesticetin (Fig. 22).

Recently, Werner and Demain [65] have shown that new analogs of indolmycin can be produced by *S. griseus* upon supplementation of the growth medium with tryptophan derivatives substituted in the 5-position (Fig. 23). The new analogs showed some moderate increase in antimicrobial activity as compared to indolmycin, but did not markedly change the gram positive/gram negative ratio.

I have tried to show how many natural antibiotic fermentations can and have been modified to cause the formation of new secondary

	R
Celesticetin	-H
Desalicetin 2'-(4-amino-salicylate)	$-NH_2$

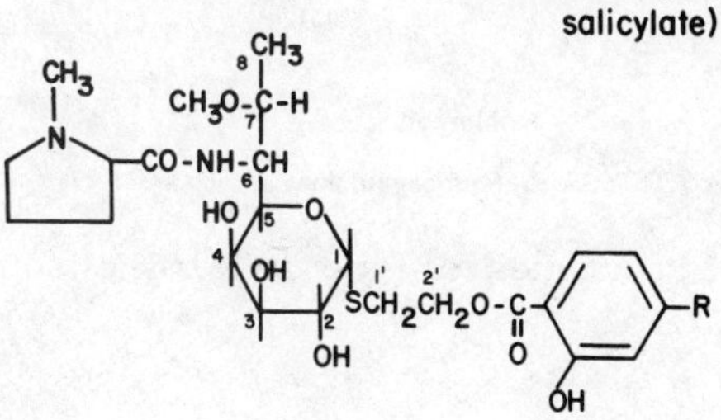

Fig. 22. Structures of the celesticetins.

metabolites. I do not believe that the full potential of these procedures has yet been exploited by many industrial laboratories. There are numerous other examples of secondary metabolite expression that can be cited as fruitful endeavors for the resourceful applied microbiologist.

Dr. Arnold Demain [12] has outlined in a recent review some of the directions that are needed for applied microbiology in the future. Better and safer antibiotics are needed to combat gram-negative infections. Truly non-toxic antifungal agents for systemic use have yet to be discovered. Agents active against protozoal infections are required. In the area of viral diseases and cancer, a real need exists for effective antiviral and antitumor agents.

As new lead compounds in all these areas become more difficult to find, microbial broths will have to fill the void. It is not wishful thinking to predict that microbial products will gain importance in therapy of non-microbial diseases. New opportunities exist for applied scientists who can devise simple tests for screening microbial broths for such activities. Perhaps more vigorous exploitation of mutasynthesis and directed biosynthesis will solve some of these problems.

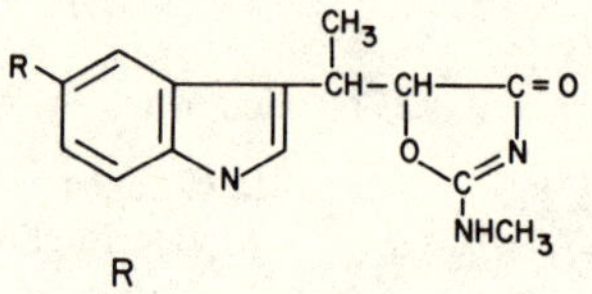

R	
H	Indolmycin
OCH_3	5-Methoxyindolmycin

Fig. 23. Structures of the indolmycins.

I am reminded of Dr. David Perlman's laws of applied microbiology which he promulgated in 1979 [44], but can just as readily be applied in 1982 (Table 9). I would like to leave these with you.

Table 9

Perlman's Laws of Applied Microbiology for 1982

1. The microorganism is {always right / your friend / a sensitive partner}
2. There are <u>no</u> stupid microorganisms
3. Microorganisms {can / will} do anything
4. Microorganisms are {smarter / wiser / more energetic} than chemists, engineers, etc.
5. If you take care of your microbial friends, they will take care of your future (and you will live happily ever after)

REFERENCES

1. Argoudelis, A.D., J.H. Coats, and L.E. Johnson. 1974. Directed biosynthesis of new celestosaminide antibiotics by *Streptomyces caelestis*. J. Antibiot. 27:738-743.
2. Argoudelis, A.D., T.E. Eble, and D.J. Mason. 1970. Studies on the biosynthesis of lincomycin V. Effect of ethionine on fermentation of *S. lincolnensis*. J. Antibiot. 23:1-8.
3. Behrens, O.K. 1949. Biosynthesis of penicillins, pp 657-679. *In* The Chemistry of Penicillin (H.T. Clarke, J.R. Johnson, and R. Robinson, Eds.),. Princeton Univ. Press, Princeton, New Jersey.
4. Birch, A.J. 1963. The biosynthesis of antibiotics. Pure and Applied Chemistry, 7:527-537.
5. Boxler, D.L., R. Brambilla, D.H., Davies, A.K. Mallams, S.W. McCombie, J.B. Morton, P. Reichert, and H.F. Vernay. 1981. Semisynthetic aminoglycoside antibacterials. 9. Synthesis of novel 1- and 3-substituted and 1- and 3-*epi* substituted derivatives of sisomicin and gentamicin from the 1- and 3-oxo-derivatives. J. Chem. Soc. Perkin I 1981. pp 2168-2185.
6. Came, P.E., J.R. O'Connor, R.A. Dobson, R.B. Wagner, and R.J. Fabian. 1979. Antibacterial activities, nephrotoxicity, and ototoxicity of a new aminoglycoside, Win 42122-2. Antimicrob. Agents and Chemother. 16:813-822.
7. Claridge, C.A. 1979. Amioglycoside antibiotics. pp 151-238. *In* Secondary products of metabolism (A.H. Rose, Ed.). Academic Press, London.
8. Claridge, C.A., J.A. Bush, T.W. Doyle, D.E. Nettleton, J.E. Mosley, and D. Kimball. 1982. New mitomycin analogues produced by directed biosynthesis. Abstracts of the Annual Meeting of the Am. Soc. for Microbiology. Abstract 028.
9. Cleophax, J., S.D. Gero, J. LeBoul, M. Akhtar, J.E.G. Barnett, and C.J. Pearce. 1976. A chiral synthesis of D-(+)-2,6-dideoxystreptamine and its microbial incorporation into novel

antibiotics. J. Am. Chem. Soc. 98:7110-7112.

10. Daum, S.J., D. Rosi, and W.A. Goss. 1977. Mutational biosynthesis by idiotrophs of Micromonospora purpurea. II Conversion of non-amino containing cyclitols to aminoglycoside antibiotics. J. Antibiot. 30:90-105.

11. DeFuria, M.D., and C.A. Claridge. 1976. Aminoglycoside antibiotics produced by the genus Bacillus. pp 427-436. In Microbiology - 1976 (D. Schlessinger, Ed.). American Society for Microbiology, Washington, D.C.

12. Demain, A.L. 1981. Applied microbiology - A personal view. pp 1/1-1/31, In Essays in applied microbiology (J.R. Norris and M.H. Richmond, Eds.), John Wiley and Sons, Ltd.

13. Dhar, M.M., C. Singh, A.W. Khan, A.J. Arif, C.M. Gupta, and A.P. Bhaduri. 1971. Studies on the cell-free synthesis of echinomycin and an echinomycin analogue. Pure Appl. Chem. 28:469-473.

14. Doershuk, A.P., J.R. D. McCormick, J.J. Goodman, S.A. Szumski, J.A. Growich, P.A. Miller, B.A. Bitler, E.R. Jensen, M.A. Petty, and A.S. Phelps. 1956. The halide metabolism of Streptomyces aureofaciens mutants. The biosynthesis of 7-chloro, 7-chloro^{36}-, and 7-bromotetracycline and tetracycline. J. Am. Chem. Soc. 78:1508-1509.

15. Dulaney, E.L., I. Putter, D. Drescher, L. Chaiet, W.J. Miller, F.J. Wolf, and D. Hendlin. 1962. Transethylation in antibiotic biosynthesis. I. An ethyl analogue of oxytetracycline. Biochim. Biophys. Acta. 60:447-449.

16. Fleck, W.F. 1979. Genetic approaches to new streptomycete products. pp 117-122. In Genetics of Industrial Microorganisms (O.K. Sebek and A.I. Laskin, Eds.), American Society for Microbiology, Washington, D.C.

17. Fujiwara, T., Y. Takahashi, K. Matsumoto, and E. Kondo. 1980a. Isolation of an intermediate of 2-deoxystreptamine biosynthesis from a mutant of Bacillus circulans. J. Antibiot. 33:824-829.

18. Fujiwara, T., Y. Takahashi, K. Matsumoto, and E. Kondo. 1980b.

Production of a new aminoglycoside antibiotic by a mutant of Bacillus circulans. J. Antibiot. 33:836-841.

19. Furumai, T., K. Takeda, A.Kinumaki, Y. Ito, and T. Okuda. 1979. Biosynthesis of butirosins II. Biosynthetic pathway of butirosins elucidated from co-synthesis and feeding experiments. J. Antibiot. 32:891-899.

20. Hamill, R.L., R.P. Elander, J.A. Mabe, and M. Gorman. 1970. Metabolism of tryptophan by Pseudomonas aureofaciens III. Production of substituted pyrrolnitrins from tryptophan analogues. Appl. Microbiol. 19:721-725.

21. Isono, K., and R.J. Suhadolnik. 1976. The biosynthesis of natural and unnatural polyoxins by Streptomyces cacaoi. Arch. Biochem. Biophys. 173:141-153.

22. Iyengar, B.S., H.-J. Lin, L. Cheng, W.A. Remers, and W.T. Bradner. 1981. Development of new mitomycin C and profiromycin analogues. J. Med. Chem. 24:975-981.

23. Kase, H., T. Iida, Y. Odakura, K. Shirahata, and K. Nakayama. 1980. Accumulation of 2-deoxy-scyllo-inosamine by a 2-deoxystreptamine-requiring idotroph of Micromonospora sagmiensis. J. Antibiot. 33:1210-1212.

24. Kase, H., S. Kitamura, and K. Nakayama. 1982. Production of antibiotic SU-2 complex by a 2-deoxystreptamine idiotroph of Micromonospora sagamiensis. J. Antibiot. 35:385-390.

25. Katz, E., and A.L. Demain. 1977. The peptide antibiotics of Bacillus: Chemistry, biogenesis and possible functions. Bacteriol. Rev. 41:449-474.

26. Kawaguchi, H., H. Tsukiura, K. Tomita, M. Konishi, K. Saito, S. Kobura, K. Numata, K. Fujisawa, T. Miyaki, M. Hatori, and H. Koshiyama. 1977. Tallysomycin, a new antitumor antibiotic complex related to bleomcin I. Production, isolation and properties. J. Antibiot. 30:779-788.

27. Kitamura, S., H. Kase, Y,. Odakura, T. Iida, K. Shirahata, and K. Nakayama. 1982. 2-Hydroxysagamicin: A new antibiotic produced by mutational biosynthesis of Micromonospora

sagamiensis. J. Antibiot. 325:94-97.

28. Kojima, M., and A. Satoh. 1973. Microbial semi-synthesis of aminoglycosidic antibiotics by mutants of S. ribosidificus and S. kanamyceticus. J. Antibiot. 26:784-786.

29. Konishi, M., H. Ohkuma, F. Sakai, T. Tsuno, H. Koshiyama, T. Naito, and H. Kawaguchi. 1981. BBM-928, a new antitumor antibiotic complex. III. Structure determination of BBM-928A, B, and C. J. Antibiot. 34:148-159.

30. Leitner, F., and K.E. Price. 1982. Aminoglycosides under development, pp 29-64. In The Aminoglycosides (A. Whelton and H.C. Neu, Eds.),. Marcel Dekker, Inc. New York.

31. Maezawa, I.A., A. Kinumaki, and M. Suzuki. 1976. Biological glycosidation of macrolide aglycones. I. Isolation and characterization of 5-0-micaminosyl narbonolide and 9-dihydro-5-0-mycaminosyl narbonolide. J. Antibiot. 29:1203-1208.

32. Maezawa, I.A., A. Kinumaki, and M. Suzuki. 1978. Biological glycosidation of macrolide aglycones. II. Isolation and characterization of desosaminyl-platenolide I. J. Antibiot. 31:309-318.

33. Martin, J.R., R.S. Egan, A.W. Goldstein, S.L. Mueller, E.A. Hirner, and R.S. Stanaszek. 1974. 8,8a-Deoxyoleandolide: Elaborated by a blocked mutant of the erythromycin-producing organism Streptomyces erythreus. J. Antibiot. 27:570-573.

34. Matsuzawa, Y., A. Yoshimoto, T. Oki, H. Naganawa, T. Takeuchi, and H. Umezawa. 1980. Biosynthesis of anthracycline antibiotics by Streptomyces galilaeus II. Structure of new anthracycline antibiotics obtained by microbial glycosidation and biological activity. J. Antibiot. 33:1341-1347.

35. Miyaki, T., K. Numata, Y. Nishiyama, O. Tenmyo, M. Hatori, H. Imanishi, M. Konishi, and H. Kawaguchi. 1981. Tallysomycin, a new antitumor antibiotic complex related to bleomycin. V. Production characterization, and antitumor activity of Tallysomycin $S_{10}b$, a new biosynthetic tallysomycin derivative.

J. Antibiot. 34:665-674.

36. Nagaoka, K., and A.L. Demain. 1975. Mutational biosynthesis of a new antibiotic, Streptomutin A, by an idiotroph of Streptomyces griseus. J. Antibiot. 28:627-635.

37. Oka, Y., H. Ishida, M. Morioka, Y. Numasaki, T. Yamafuji, T. Osono, and H. Umezawa. 1981. Combimicins, new Kanamycin derivatives bioconverted by some Micromonosporas. J. Antibiot. 34:777-781.

38. Oki, T., A. Yoshimoto, Y. Matsuzawa, T. Takeuchi, and H. Umezawa. 1980. Biosynthesis of anthracycline antibiotics by Streptomyces galilaeus. I. Glycosidation of various anthracyclines by an aclacinomycin-negative mutant and biosynthesis of aclacinomycins from aklavinone. J. Antibiot. 33:1331-1340.

39. Oki, T., A. Yoshimoto, Y. Matsuzawa, T. Takeuchi, and H. Umezawa. 1981. New anthracycline antibiotic, 2-hydroxy-aclacinomycin A. J. Antibiot. 34:916-918.

40. Okumura, Y. K. Okamura, T. Takei, K. Kuono, J. Lein, T. Ishikura, and Y. Fukagawa. 1979. Controlled biosynthesis of neoviridogriseins, new homologues of viridogrisein, I. Taxonomy and fermentation. J. Antibiot. 32:575-583.

41. Okumura, Y. T. Takei, M. Sakamoto, T. Ishikura, and Y. Fukagawa. 1979. Controlled biosynthesis of neoviridogriseins, new homologues of viridogrisein. II. Production, biological properties and structure of neoviridogrisein II. J. Antibiot. 32:584-592.

42. Okumura, Y., T. Takei, M. Sakamoto, T. Ishikura, and Y. Fukagawa. 1979. Controlled biosynthesis of neoviridogriseins, new homologues of viridogrisein. III. Production, structures, and biological properties of neoviridogriseins I and III. J. Antibiot. 32:1002-1010.

43. Omura, S., H. Ikeda, H. Matsubara, and N. Sadakane. 1980. Hybrid biosynthesis and absolute configuration of macrolide antibiotic M-4365G_1. J. Antibiot. 33:1570-1572.

44. Perlman, D. 1980. Some problems on the new horizons of applied microbiology. Dev. Indust. Microb. 21:xv-xxii.

45. Rinehart, K.L., Jr. 1977. Mutasynthesis of new antibiotics. Pure and Appl. Chem. 49:1361-1384.

46. Rinehart, K. L., Jr. 1980. Biosynthesis and mutasynthesis of aminocyclitol antibiotics, pp 335-370. In Amino-cyclitol antibiotics (Rinehart, K. L., Jr. and T. Suami Eds.), ACS Symposium Series No. 125. American Chemical Society, Washington, D.C.

47. Rinehart, K.L., Jr., J.M. Malik, R.S. Nystrom, R.M. Stroshane, S.T. Truitt, M. Taniguchi, J.P. Rolls, W.J. Haak, and B.S. Ruff. 1974. Biosynthetic incorporation of [1-^{13}C] glucosamine and [6-^{13}C] glucose into neomycin. J. Am. Chem. Soc. 96:2263-2265.

48. Rinehart, K. L., Jr., and R. M. Stroshane. 1976. Biosynthesis of aminocyclitol antibiotics. J. Antibiot. 29:319-353.

49. Rosi, D., W.A. Goss, and S.J. Daum. 1977. Mutational biosynthesis by idiotrophs of Micromonospora purpurea. I. Conversion of aminocyclitols to new aminoglycoside antibiotics. J. Antibiot. 30:88-97.

50. Sebek, O.K. 1974. On the biosynthesis and biomodification of novobiocin. Abstr. 2nd Int. Symp. Genet. Ind. Microorg. Academic Press, London.

51. Sebek, O.K. 1979. Novobiocin and other antibiotics as potential mutasynthetic models pp 318-321. In Microbiology-1979 (D. Schlessinger, Ed.). American Society for Microbiology, Washington, D.C.

52. Shier, W.T., S. Ogawa, M. Hitchens, and K. L. Rinehart, Jr. 1973. Chemistry and biochemistry of the neomycins. XVII. Bioconversion of aminocyclitols to aminocyclitol antibiotics. J. Antibiot. 26:551-561.

53. Shier, W.T., K.L. Rinehart, Jr., and D. Gottlieb. 1969. Preparation of four new antibiotics from a mutant of Streptomyces fradiae. Proc. Natl. Acad. Sci. U.S.A. 63:198-204.

54. Shier, W.T., P.C. Shaefer, D. Gottlieb, and K.L. Rinehart, Jr.

1974. Use of mutants in the study of aminocyclitol antibiotic biosynthesis and the preparation of the hybrimycin C complex. Biochemistry 13:5073-5078.

55. Shirahata, K., H. Kase, S. Kitamura, and T. Iida. 1982. The structures of aminoglycoside antibiotics SU-1, 2 and 3. J. Antibiot. 35:520-523.

56. Slechta, L., and J.H. Coats, 1974. Studies of the biosynthesis of spectinomycin. Abstracts 14th Interscience Conference on Antimicrobial Agents and Chemotherapy No. 294. San Francisco, California.

57. Takeda, K., A. Kinumaki, T. Furumai, T. Yamaguchi, S. Oshima, and Y. Ito. 1978a. Mutational biosynthesis of butirosin analogs. J. Antibiot. 31:247-249.

58. Takeda, K., A. Kinumaki, H. Hayasaka, T. Yamaguchi, and Y. Ito. 1978b. Mutational biosynthesis of butirosin analogs. II. 3',4'-dideoxy-6'-N-methylbutirosins, new semisynthetic aminoglycosides. J. Antibiot. 31:1031-1038.

59. Takeda, K., A. Kinumaki, S. Okuno, T. Matsushita, and Y. Ito. 1978c. Mutational biosynthesis of butirosin analogs. III. 6'-N-methylbutirosins and 3'-4'-dideoxy-6'C-methylbutirosins, new semisynthetic aminoglycosides. J. Antibiot. 31-1039-1045.

60. Takeda, K., S. Okuno, Y. Ohashi, and T. Furumai. 1978d. Mutational biosynthesis of butirosin analogs. I. Conversion of neamine analogs into butirosin analogs by mutants of *Bacillus circulans*. J. Antibiot. 31:1023-1030.

61. Testa, R.T., G.H. Wagman, P.J.L. Daniels, and M.J. Weinstein. 1974. Mutamicins: Biosynthetically created new sisomicin analogues. J. Antibiot. 27:917-921.

62. Umezawa, H. 1976. Bleomycin: Discovery, chemistry and action, pp 3-36. *In* Fundamental and Clinical Studies Bleomycin (S.K. Carter, T. Ichikawa, G. Mathe, and H. Umezawa, Eds.), University of Tokyo Press, Tokyo, Japan.

63. Waitz, J.A., G.H. Miller, E. Moss, Jr., and P.J.S. Chiu. 1978. Chemotherapeutic evaluation of 5-episisomicin (Sch 22591), a

new semisynthetic aminoglycoside. Antimicrob. Agents and Chemother. 13:41-48.

64. Walton, R.B., L.E. McDaniel, and H.B. Woodruff. 1962. Biosynthesis of novobiocin analogues. Dev. Ind. Microbiol. 3:370-375.

65. Werner, R.G., and A.L. Demain. 1981. Directed biosynthesis of new indolmycins. J. Antibiot. 34:551-554.

66. Williamson, M.P., D. Gauvreau, D.H. Williams, and M.J. Waring. 1982. Structure and conformation of fourteen antibiotics of the quinoxaline group determined by ^{1}H NMR. J. Antibiot. 35:62-66.

67. Yoshida, T., Y. Kimura, and K. Katagiri. 1968. Novel quinomycins: Biosynthetic replacement of the chromophores. J. Antibiot. 21:465-467.

68. Yoshimoto, A., Y. Matsuzawa, Y. Matsushita, T. Oki, T. Takeuchi, and H. Umezawa. 1981. Trisarubicinol, new antitumor anthracycline antibiotic. J. Antibiot. 34:1492-1494.

69. Yoshimoto, A., Y. Matsuzawa, T. Oki, H. Naganawa, T. Takeuchi, and H. Umezawa. 1980. Microbial conversion of ε-pyrromycinone and ε-isorhodomycinone to 1-hydroxy-13-dihydrodaunomycin and N-formyl-1-hydroxy-13-dihydrodaunomycin and their bioactivities. J. Antibiot. 33:1150-1157.

DISCUSSION

Q. P. ROGERS (Minnesota): In using directed biosynthesis or the mutasynthesis technique, you add potential substitutes to intact cells. The compounds must get into the cell if it is going to finally end up in a new antibiotic. Two problems that interest me are: 1) the transport problem. Have you had experience with types of compounds that can't be transported into the streptomycetes? The other problem involves the inhibition of the host cell by the new antibiotic. In other words the new antibiotic would be toxic to the producing microbes. Has any work been done on these two problems?

A. CLARIDGE: The uptake of new substrate added to cells is always a problem. I think it's something that Reinhardt addressed in his original work where the mechanism of discovery of a new antibiotic was based strictly on antibiotic activity. In this instance, when the mutasynthon is added to the cells, it results in a product that is not an antibiotic, so it is necessary to isolate the product. The second problem of whether the new antibiotic is going to kill the host organism that you're working with, is a common problem in any antibiotic fermentation. One of the ways of getting around this is to develop mutants of the producing organisms that are resistant to its own product. This is a well-established process in antibiotic research directed toward the development of mutants that are superior antibiotic-producing strains.

HOST/VECTOR SYSTEMS FOR ACTINOMYCETES AND APPLICATIONS TO STRAIN DEVELOPMENT

Janet Westpheling
Biological Laboratories
Harvard University
Cambridge, Massachusetts 02138

INTRODUCTION

Of the over 3000 known antibiotics, more than 2000 are produced by Actinomycetes. In fact, over 85% of the species which produce antibiotics are Actinomycetes, including *Nocardia*, *Streptosporangium*, *Micromonospora*, *Actinoplanes*, and *Streptomyces* [23,32], Table 1 shows how these are divided [3,26].

Not only are the Streptomycetes responsible for the vast majority of antibiotics in terms of the total number but also in terms of the number of commercially important compounds. The Streptomycetes also produce many β-lactam antibiotics including penicillins and cephalosporins but are not used industrially for the production of these compounds.

The term "antibiotic" is used to describe a variety of compounds which are structurally and functionally diverse, and the 70 commercially important *Streptomyces* antibiotics are examples of this diversity. They include compounds of interest because of the way in which they interrupt specific metabolic processes, which facilitates

Table I

Antibiotic Producers

	Total	Commercial
Actinomycetes:		
Streptomyces	1922	70
Nocardia	45	2
Micromonospora	41	2
Other bacteria:		
Bacillus	167	5
Pseudomonas	82	2
Fungi:		
Penicillium	123	3
Cephalosporium	20	1

the study of these processes, and of course for their importance in clinical medicine and agriculture [11]. The tetracyclines, erythromycin, the aminoglysosides (streptomycin, neomycin, kanamycin, gentamicin, and others), chloramphenicol, and lincomycin are examples of clinically important antibiotics. Other compounds which are invaluable tools for research in molecular biology and biochemistry, because they perturb biosynthetic processes in specific ways, include mitomycin C (DNA synthesis); actinomycin D, streptolydigin and rifamycin (transcription); puromycin, chloramphenicol and the aminoglycosies (translation); and cerulenin (fatty acid synthesis). Another significant use of Streptomycete antibiotics is as feed additives for livestock. In addition to their antimicrobial activities, antibiotics lead to more efficient weight gain; however, the increase in plasmid-borne, drug resistance transmissible to human pathogenic bacteria is a serious problem. The diversity of Streptomycete products has proven useful in the development of animal feed additives which are not clinically useful and not select for organisms cross-resistant to clinically important antibiotics; monensin is a notable example [29].

For the most part, these compounds are secondary metabolites in that they are produced at the end of vegetative growth as the cells are entering stationary phase. The occurence of these secondary metabolites coincides with the time of morphological differentiation.

The Streptomycetes show a complexity of morphological organization unique among bacteria in that they resemble fungi in growing as multinucleate branching hyphae which form a mycelial mass. Figure 1 is a diagram of the *Streptomyces* life cycle.

Spores germinate, giving rise to substrate mycelium which in turn develops aerial hyphae which coil and undergo septation to produce spores. A variety of developmental mutants has been isolated and characterized by Chater. These include *bld* (bald) mutants, blocked very early (they failed to produce aerial mycelium), and a variety of *whi* (white) mutants blocked at a number of stages in the process of spore formation. Streptomycetes do not produce endospores, but members of another Actinomycete genus, *Thermoactinomyces*, as well as the bacilli do: *Streptomyces* spores are very different structurally and they are not heat resistant.

The Streptomycetes exhibit a complex system of both biochemical and morphological differentiation. At the molecular level, these changes are characterized by changes in the pattern of protein and RNA synthesis. This process of cell differentiation and development differs from the temporal adaptations cells undergo in response to changing environmental conditions. Sets of genes are expressed in an ordered temporal sequence resulting in a new cell type such as a spore, or a secondary metabolite such as an antibiotic.

One may consider the two events - biochemical differentiation and morphological differentiation - as parallel developmental pathways, each requiring a mechanism of regulation for the expression of

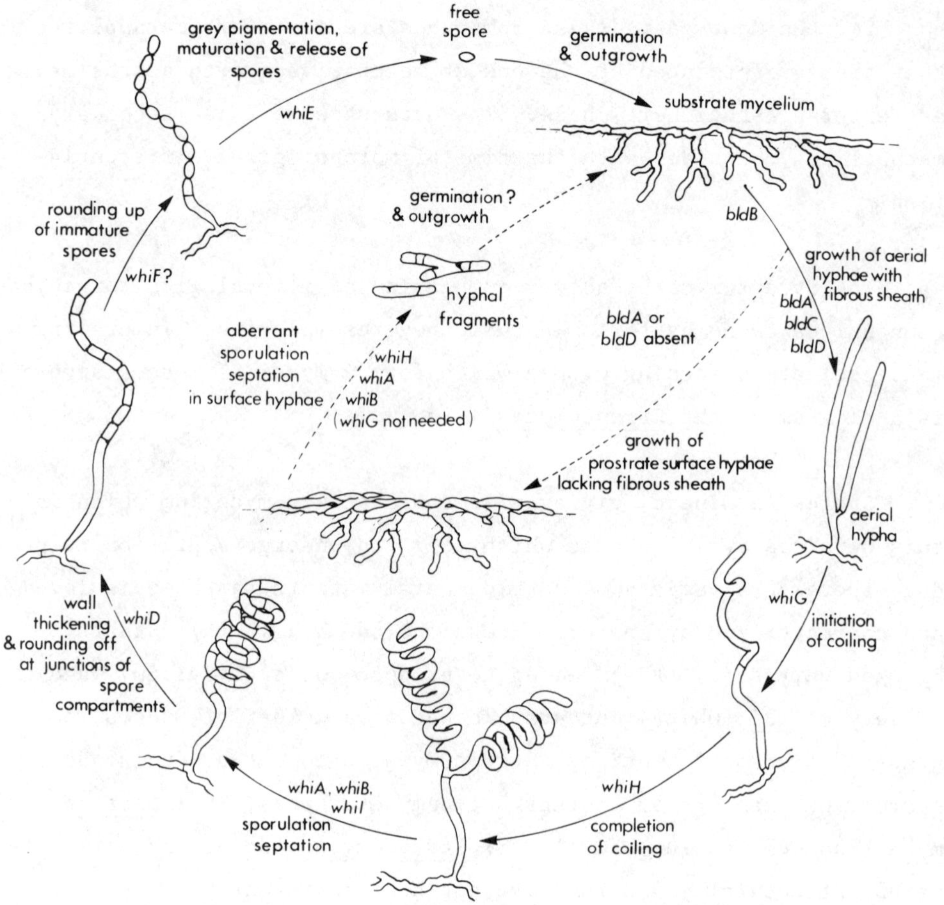

Fig. 1. The developmental life cycle of Streptomyces coelicolor, an aerobic Gram-positive soil bacterium which grows vegetatively as mycelium (from Chater and Merrick, ref. 7).

sets of genes in an ordered temporal sequence. In order to understand the complex regulatory mechanisms involved in the production of secondary metabolites, and eventually to manipulate these pathways, a basic understanding of the biological system involved is necessary. For example, any description of the location or organization of antibiotic production genes requires some knowledge of the general genetic makeup of the producing organism.

The best studied genetic system among the Actinomycetes is that of Streptomyces coelicolor [12]. A wide variety of genetic markers has been mapped using the plasmid mediated conjugal mating system in this organism. Auxotrophic and morphologic mutations as well as antibiotic production clusters and phage attachment sites have been identified.

Table 2 contains most of what is known about the genetics of antibiotic production.

Unfortunately, the list is painfully short. What is missing is a fundamental understanding of the genetics of most industrially important strains. Any serious investigation of antibiotic production at the molecular level requires the development of a workable

Table 2

Genetics of Streptomyces Antibiotics

Organism	Antibiotic	Genetic Control
S. coelicolor A3(2)	methylenomycin	at least 5 structural genes on the SCP1 plasmid (c. 170 kb; Westpheling, 1980; Kirby and Hopwood, 1977; Kirby et al., 1975)
S. coelicolor A3(2)	actinorhodin	at least 7 structural genes in a chromosomal cluster Rudd and Hopwood, 1979)
S. coelicolor A3(2)	undeclprodigiosin	at least 5 structural genes in a chromosomal cluster(Rudd, 1978)
S. fradiae	tylosin	a plasmid carries some structural genes (Richard Baltz, personal communication)
S. reticuli	leucomycin	a 75 kb plasmid needed for production (Schrempf and Goebel, 1979)
S. venezuilae	chloramphenicol	at least 3 structural genes in a chromosomal cluster; a plasmid probably involved in high level production (Akagawa et al, in press; Okanishi and Umezawa, 1978)

genetic system. Once this has been accomplished, the tools of molecular biology may be applied to full advantage.

Genetic manipulation in Streptomyces involves one or a combination of the following: 1) plasmid mediated conjugation; 2) protoplast fusion; 3) protoplast transformation using plasmid DNA or transfection using phage DNA; or 4) protoplast-liposome fusion for the introductin of DNA or biochemical precursors.

Protoplast preparation in Streptomyces is not a particularly complicated procedure. Mycelium are treated with lysozyme and washed, and for protoplast-protoplast fusion, cells are mixed in the presence of 50% PEG and plated on a suitable medium for regeneration [2,15]. There are several very important features of protoplast fusion: (A) protoplast fusion can be used to generate very high recombination frequencies for all regions of the chromosome, 10^{-1} as compared to 10^{-5} to 10^{-7} in conjugal mating (up to 30% when one or both parents are UV irradiated before fusion) [14]; (B) multiple cross-over classes are very frequent, 25% as compared to 2% in mating [13]; and (C) multiple parent recombinants are quite frequent, often 3 or more (up to 4 have been reported) parental types can contribute to the generation of single recombinants as compared with the usual 2 in mating [13].

Several aspects of protoplast fusion are industrially important. It allows for maximum genetic mixing, which is highly desirable in a strain selection program. For example, even if the structural genes for a given antibiotic are clustered, they are probably not the only ones involved in a high producing phenotype. Therefore, in order to generate recombinants which bring together all alleles involved, crossing over between all areas of the chromosome is desirable, or one can fuse high producers with wild type strains to eliminate deleterious mutations introduced during the course of a selection program, or to bring together alleles from divergent cell lines.

Another very important use of protoplasts is for plasmid DNA transformation [5]. In this case, mycelium is treated with lysozyme, washed and mixed with plasmid or phage DNA in the presence of 20% PEG, and plated on a suitable medium for regeneration. Plasmid transformation is very efficient in *Streptomyces*. Up to 80% of regenerated protoplasts are transformed by covalently closed circular (ccc) supercoiled plasmid DNA at saturating DNA concentrations, or about 10^7 transformants/μg DNA under non-saturating conditions. The frequency does not suffer dramatically, as is the case with *E. coli*, when one uses open circular (oc) or religated ccc non-supercoiled DNA. Religated plasmids have a 10 - 20% transformation frequency.

Another interesting aspect of *Streptomyces* plasmid transformation is a phenotype exhibited by *Streptomyces* plasmids which in some ways resembles lethal zygosis in *E. coli* [4]. Figure 2 illustrates this phenotype.

The phenotype is associated with plasmid transfer [16] and can be used to detect 1 in 10^9 transformants, which is very useful for detecting transformants in the absence of selectable markers on the plasmid.

There are several plasmid cloning vectors available in *Streptomyces*. I will discuss two of them in particular because, in addition to being useful cloning vectors, they have other interesting biological properties.

SLP1 is a *Streptomyces coelicolor* plasmid first isolated by Bibb [4] from *Streptomyces lividans* after an interspecific mating

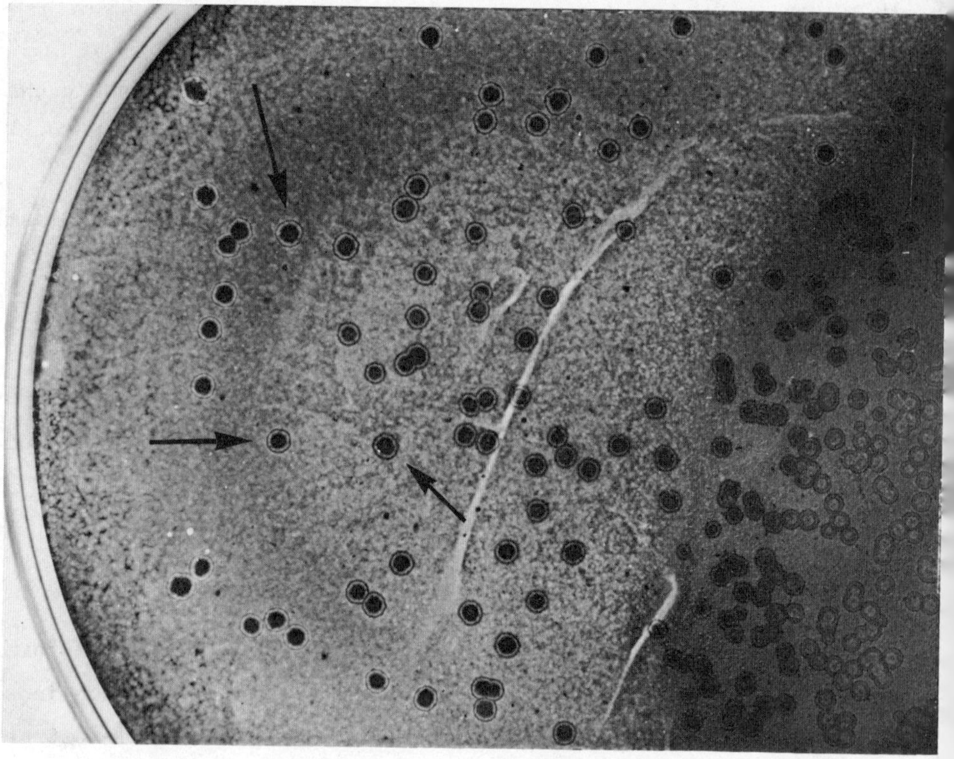

Fig. 2. This is a plate of regenerated protoplasts after transformation. The arrows point to colonies which have arisen from transformed cells. Cells which have received plasmid DNA inhibit the lawn of cells which have not received plasmid DNA and this area of inhibition is called a "pock".

with Streptomyces coelicolor. The DNA sequence of this plasmid is present in the S. coelicolor genome but is occasionally able to be isolated as an autonomous replicon. When it comes out of the DNA where it resides it apparently takes a portion of this DNA with it. The largest member of this family of plasmids contains a sequence of DNA absent in the smallest member and intermediate sized members have various lengths of this sequence. Any restriction sites within this dispensible region of DNA are therefore available for cloning [6].

One of these plasmids, SLP1.2 has been engineered as a cloning vector, pIJ41. Neomycin and thiostrepton resistance have been cloned into this plasmid and a portion was deleted leaving a unique *BamH1* site within the neo^R gene. One may clone a DNA fragment into this unique *BamH1* site and obtain hybrid plasmids by selecting thiostrepton resistance and screening for neomycin sensitivity [8].

pIJ101 is a small, high copy (40-300 copies/chromosome) plasmid and is notable in that this 9 kb of DNA acts as a self-replicating, self-transmissible sex factor which promotes chromosome recombination at a frequency of 10^{-3}. Kieser *et al.*, have generated a functional map of this plasmid identifying regions involved in plasmid transfer and replication. Another important feature of this plasmid is its large host range. It is able to be mated or transformed into a wide variety of *Streptomyces* species [16].

In addition to providing a way of getting plasmids into a strain, protoplasting also allows for their elimination. Protoplasting has been shown to be an excellent way of "curing" plasmids and, except for the elimination of the plasmid DNA, is a totally nonmutagenic treatment. In *S. coelicolor* up to 25% of regenerated protoplasts are cured of SCP1 plasmid DNA (Hopwood, personal communication).

Another use of protoplasting, which is very important in strains which do not sporulate or sporulate very poorly, is to obtain single cells allowing for genome segregation after mutagenesis or mating.

Makins and Holt have shown that *Streptomyces* proptoplasts can be fused with artificially prepared protoplast-like structures called lysosomes. Liposomes can be used to package protein precursors for the study of biosynthetic pathways or fragments of DNA. *Streptomyces* linear DNA has no transforming activity but by packaging DNA fragments in lyposomes one can achieve up to 10% transformation for single chromosomal markers [21] or, using phage DNA, obtain enhanced transfection frequencies of up to 5% (Chater, personal communication).

The basic tools now exist in *Streptomyces* which allow for the manipulation of this organism to improve fermentation efficiency, to generate new strains with desirable phenotypes, and to study its complex mechanisms of regulation at the molecular level (reviewed by Chater *et al*., ref. 8).

Westpheling and Losick have attempted to address the question of how development - both morphological and biochemical - is regulated in *Streptomyces*.

Losick and his coworkers have focused for several years on development in *Bacillus subtilis*, another example of complex prokaryotic differentiation. *Bacillus* is in some ways very similar to *Streptomyces* and in some ways very different. Superficially, the two organisms are morphologically similar and at the molecular level their 3' 16S rRNA sequences involved in ribosome binding are the same, each differing from those of *E. coli* [ref. 9; M.J. Bibb, personal communication.]

Structural genes are preceded by DNA sequences (promoter sequences) which attract RNA polymerase and direct the initiation of transcription. There is a subunit of RNA polymerase (the sigma subunit) which is responsible for recognition of this promoter sequence by the polymerase. Losick and his co-workers found rather unexpectedly that in the process of endospore formation in *Bacillus* different classes of genes are turned on at different times in development by different forms of RNA polymerase [19,20].

In *Bacillus* there are classes of genes, each class having its own promoter sequence which differs from the sequences of other classes of genes. These different classes of promoters are recognized by different forms of RNA polymerase which differ in their sigma subunit, the subunit which confers promoter recognition specificity. Therefore, these different forms of RNA polymerase have different promoter recognition specificities [22].

The model for temporal expression then is that vegetative genes are transcribed by vegetative polymerase. At the onset of sporulation, new sigmas become associated with the polymerase which change the recognition specificity and therefore the type of promoter recognized by the RNA polymerase. Early sporulation genes are transcribed by one sigma, later genes by yet another, and so on. It occurred to us that Streptomyces might be similar to Bacillus in this respect in having such a mechanism for gene regulation.

Our approach was to isolate a cell fraction from Streptomyces which contains RNA polymerase activity and test this activity in an in vitro transcription assay, called a run-off assay. DNA, cut at a restriction site downstream from a known promoter, is incubated in the presence of RNA polymerase and a transcript is generated from the start point to the end of the DNA fragment. In this way RNA of defined lengths is produced which can be sized by polyacrylamide gel electrophoresis. Several promoters have been cloned and characterized in Bacillus subtilis which are known to be developmentally regulated. The two used in this study were veg and spoVC. The veg gene is transcribed during vegetative growth in Bacillus and the spoVC is transcribed during an early stage of sporulation. The spoVC promoter is not recognized or transcribed by the vegetative RNA polymerase (containing σ55) but is transcribed by a novel form of RNA polymerase containing σ37 [25].

Using the run off assay, we have found that Streptomyces coelicolor contains activities which are able to recognize and transcribe both the veg and spoVC promoters and that these transcripts are very specific. The most likely explanation for these data is that there are two forms of RNA polymerase in Streptomyces: one which transcribes the veg promoter, and another which transcribes the spoVC promoter. In fact, in one experiment we have been able to separate these transcription activities, the veg transcribing fraction from the spoVC transcribing fraction, by salt gradient elution from a heparin column. We are in the process of purifying these enzymes to identify their subunits. These experiments were done with Bacillus promoter templates because they were well defined and the run off transcripts generated by various forms of RNA polymerase had been characterized. Recently, several Streptomyces genes have been cloned by Thompson et al. [31] and we have used one such cloned fragment from S. vinaceus in a transcription run-off assay. A unique transcript of 90 bp is generated by Streptomyces coelicolor extract. Neither σ55 nor σ37 RNA polymerases from Bacillus is able to transcribe this fragment, indicating the presence of a third form of RNA polymerase in Streptomyces, and we expect that there are many more.

Tools are now available in Streptomyces which allow for the manipulation of this organism not only for the improvement of its antibiotic-producing abilities but also for study at the molecular level of its developmental mechanisms of regulation.

REFERENCES

1. Akagawa, H., M. Okanishi, and H. Umezawa. Journal of Antibiotics (Japan), (in press).
2. Baltz, R.H., (1978). Genetic recombination in Streptomyces fradiae by protoplast fusion and cell regeneration. J. Gen. Microbiol. 107:93-102.

3. Berdy, J. (1974). Recent developments of antibiotic research and classification of antibiotics according to chemical structure. Adv. in Appl. Microb. 18:309-406.
4. Bibb, M.J. (1978). Genetic and physical studies of a *Streptomyces coelicolor* plasmid. Ph.D. Thesis, University of East Anglia, Norwich.
5. Bibb, M.J., J.M. Ward and D.A. Hopwood, (1978). Transformation of plasmid DNA into *Streptomyces* at high frequency. Nature 274:398-400.
6. Bibb, M.J., J.M. Ward, T. Kieser, S.N. Cohen, and D.A. Hopwood, (1981). Excision of chromosomal DNA sequences from *Streptomyces coelicolor* forms a novel family of plasmids detectable in *Streptomyces lividans*. Mol. Gen. Genet. 184:230-240.
7. Chater, K.F., and M.J. Merrick, (1979). "Streptomycetes" *In* Developmental Biology of Prokaryotes. (J.H. Parish, Ed.). Blackwell Scientific Publications, Oxford, pp 93-114.
8. Chater, K.F., D.A. Hopwood, T. Kieser, and C.J. Thompson (1982). Gene Cloning in *Streptomyces* *In* Current Topics in Microbiology and Immunology, Vol. 96:69-95 (W. Henle, P.H. Hofschneider, H. Koprowski, F. Melchers, R. Rott, H.G. Schweiger, and P.K. Vogt, Eds.). Springer-Verlag Berlin Heidelberg.
9. Fox, G.E. E. Stackebrandt, R.B. Hespell, J. Gibson, J. Maniloff, T.A. Dyer, R.S. Wolfe, W.E. Balch, T.A. Tanner, L.J. Magrum, L.B. Zablen, R. Blakemore, R. Gupta, L. Bonen, and C.R. Woese (1980). The phylogeny of prokaryotes. Science 209:459-463.
10. Hopwood, D.A. (1979). Genetics of antibiotic production by actinomycetes, Journal of Natural Products 42:596-602.
11. Hopwood, D.A. (1980). Actinomycete genetics and antibiotics. Current Advances in Plant Science 31:467-481.
12. Hopwood, D.A., K.F. Chater, J.E. Dowding, and A. Vivian. (1973). Advances in *Streptomyces* genetics. Bacteriol. Rev. 37:371-405.

13. Hopwood, D.A., and H.M. Wright (1978) Bacterial protoplast fusion: Recombination in fused protoplasts of Streptomyces coelicolor. Mol. Gen. Genet. 162:307-317.

14. Hopwood, D.A., and H.M. Wright (1979) Factors effecting recombinant frequency in protoplast fusions of Streptomyces coelicolor. J. Gen. Micro. 111:137-143.

15. Hopwood, D.A., H.M. Wright, M.J. Bibb, and S.N. Cohen. (1977). Genetic recombination through protoplast fusion in Streptomyces. Nature 268:171-174.

16. Kieser, T., D.A. Hopwood, H.M. Wright and C.J. Thompson (1982). pIJ101, a multi-copy broad host-range Streptomyces plasmid: Functional analysis and development of DNA cloning vectors. Mol. Gen. Genet. 185:223-238.

17. Kirby, R., L.F. Wright, and D.A. Hopwood (1975). Plasmid-determined antibiotic synthesis and resistance in Streptomyces coelicolor A3(2). Nature 254:265-267.

18. Kirby, R. and D.A. Hopwood, (1977). Genetic determination of methylenomycin synthesis by the SCP1 plasmid of Streptomyces coelicolor A3(2). Journal of General Microbiology 98:239-252.

19. Losick, R. (1981). Sigma factors, stage 0 genes, and sporulation. (H.S. Levinson, A.L. Sonenshein, and D.A. Tipper, Eds.). American Society for Microbiology, Washington, D.C.

20. Losick, R. and J. Pero. (1981). Cascades of sigma factors. Cell 25:582-584.

21. Makins, J.F. and G. Holt. (1981). Liposome-mediated transformation of Streptomycetes by chromosomal DNA. Nature 293:671-673.

22. Moran, C.P., N. Lang, C.D.B. Banner, W.G. Haldenwang, and R. Losick. (1981). Cell 25:783-791.

23. Nara, T., I. Kawamoto, R. Okachi and T. Oka. (1977). J. Antibiotics 30:S-174.

24. Okanishi, M. and H. Umezawa. (1978). Plasmids involved in antibiotic production on Streptomycetes. In Genetics of the Actinomycetes (E. Freerksen, I. Tarnok, and J.H. Thumin, Eds.), pp. 19-138, Stuttgart, New York: Gustav Fischer Verlag.

25. Ollington, J.E., W.G. Haldenwang, T.V. Huynh, and R. Losick, (1981). Developmentally regulated transcription in a cloned segment of the Bacillus subtilis chromosome. Journal of Bacteriology 147:432-442.

26. Perlman, D. (1977). The fermentation industries. ASM News 43:82-89.

27. Rudd, B.A.M. (1978). Genetics of pigmented secondary metabolites in Streptomyces coelicolor A3(2). Ph. D. Thesis, University of East Anglia, Norwich.

28. Rudd, B.A.M., and D.A. Hopwood, (1979). J. Gen. Microbiol. 114:45.

29. Stark, W.M. (1977). Lilly contributions to fermentation products. Dev. Ind. Microbiol. 18:27-37.

30. Schrempf, H. and W. Goebel. Functions of plasmid genes in Streptomyces reticuli In Plasmids of Medical Environmental and Commercial Importance (K.N. Timmis, Ed.), Amsterdam: Elsevier/North Holland, pp 259-268.

31. Thompson, C.J., J.M. Ward, and D.A. Hopwood. (1980). DNA cloning in Streptomyces: Resistance genes from antibiotic-producing species. Nature 286:525-527.

32. Umezawa, H. (1967). Index of Antibiotics from Actinomycetes, Baltimore, University Park Press.

33. Westpheling, J. (1980). Physical studies of Streptomyces plasmids. Ph.D. Thesis, University of East Anglia, Norwich.

SUICIDE ENZYME INACTIVATORS

Robert H. Abeles
Department of Biochemistry
Brandeis University
Waltham, Massachusetts 02156

I'd like to discuss some of our efforts towards the design of highly specific enzyme inactivators, which can be used in vivo. We hope that such inactivators can be useful as pharmacological agents.

First is a brief outline of the kind of inactivators we are attempting to develop. We call these "Suicide Enzyme Inactivators." All of you are undoubtedly familiar with active site directed inactivators, such as TPCK (tosyl-L-phenylalanine chloromethyl ketone), an activator of chymotrypsin. The active site directed inactivators are relatively reactive molecules that have attached to them a structure which the enzyme recognizes. Due to this recognition, this molecule goes to the active site, and since it is intrinsically chemically active it covalently labels a nucleophile at the active site and inactivates the enzyme. These molecules have been enormously important in studying the structure of active sites and elucidating enzyme mechanisms. They have applications in pharmacology as well. We wanted to improve this approach and to design molecules that are chemically as unreactive as possible, and will function as inactivators. The principle is the following: we design a molecule that looks like the substrate of the enzyme. This molecule will go to the active site, because the enzyme thinks that it is a substrate. The enzyme begins to operate on it as though it were a substrate. But, what the enzyme does not know is that, as a consequence of this operation - such as breaking of a carbon-hydrogen bond - the molecule will rearrange at the active site of the enzyme to form a reactive entity, which will covalently label the enzyme. An important property of our inactivator is that the inactivating species are never released into solution. These inactivators are also called mechanism based inactivators.

I should also point out that a suicide inactivator can also be a substrate. In many cases the suicide inactivators act as a substrate most of the time; i.e., they are converted to a product most of the time, and occasionally react covalently at the active site.

I am going to describe four kinds of inactivators which we have worked with over the years. Before discussing the actual inactivators, I would like to tell you a little about how we devise these inactivators. Initially, we design a molecule which we believe should inactivate a target enzyme. We then synthesize the molecule and test it against the target. If it does inactivate, a question arises: "Does it really inactivate for the reasons we had thought it should?" To obtain an answer to this question is frequently difficult, and takes considerable time. Sometimes it turns out that the inactivation does not occur by the mechanism which had originally lead us to synthesize the molecule. I am going to talk about some inactivators today for which we have not established the precise mechanism of inactivation.

Initially, I shall discuss an example of one of the oldest suicide inactivators: acetylenic compounds. This was the first type of inactivator designed and it is based on the following principle

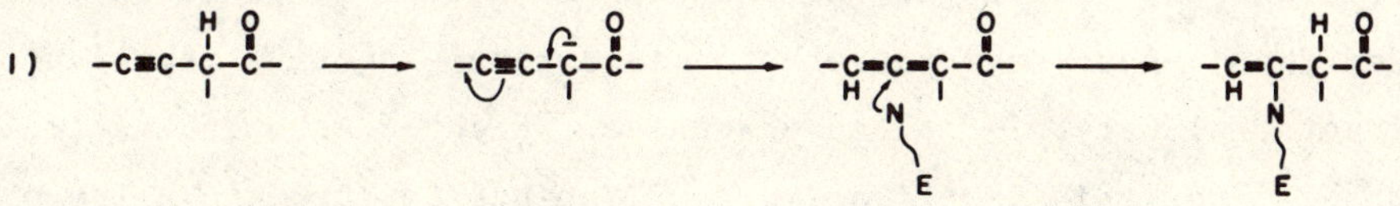

Fig. 1. Mechanisms of action of acetylinic inactivators.

(Fig. 1): the target enzyme abstracts a proton in the course of the reaction; in other words, it generates a carbanionic intermediate as follows. An acetylenic group is situated next to the group where the carbanion is generated. The resulting molecule resembles the substrate of the enzyme and will, therefore, be bound at the active site. The enzyme then removes a proton, as in the normal catalytic process. This results in the formation of a carbanion α to an acetylenic group. This carbanionic species rearranges to an allene, which is conjugated to a carbonyl group and is very susceptible to nucleophilic attack. Nucleophilic attack of a functional group at the active site leads to covalent bond formation and inactivation. Acetylenic substrate analogs are one of the most useful kinds of suicide inactivators. A large number of compounds have been designed on this principle.

I shall now discuss an example of this type of inactivator which we have recently designed. We are interested in the mechanisms of oxidations catalyzed by flavoproteins. There are some flavoproteins which introduce double bonds into CoA esters of fatty acids, and we believe this proceeds by way of a carbanion mechanism (Fig. 2). Based on what I have said, it becomes apparent that a β-γ

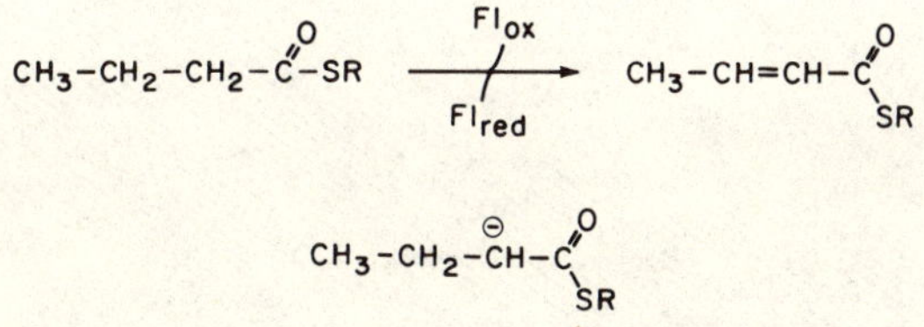

Fig. 2. Butyryl-CoA dehydrogenase.

acetylenic fatty acid CoA ester should be a suicide inactivator. We found that 3-pentynoyl-pantetheine is a very effective inactivator of bacterial butyryl-CoA dehydrogenase. Figure 3 shows a minimal mechanism for this inactivation. "P" stands for protein. The group which interacts with the suicide substrate is a carboxyl group of a glutamic acid residue. We postulate that this group is involved in the abstraction of a proton which leads to allene formation. After the allene is formed, the carboxyl group adds, and a covalent adduct is formed. In Fig. 3, we summarize some of the experimental evidence supporting formation of this covalent adduct. Reduction with $NaBH_4$ leads to the formation of pentane-1,3-diol. Reaction with hydroxylamine generates protein-hydroxamic acid. Base treatment releases a keto acid.

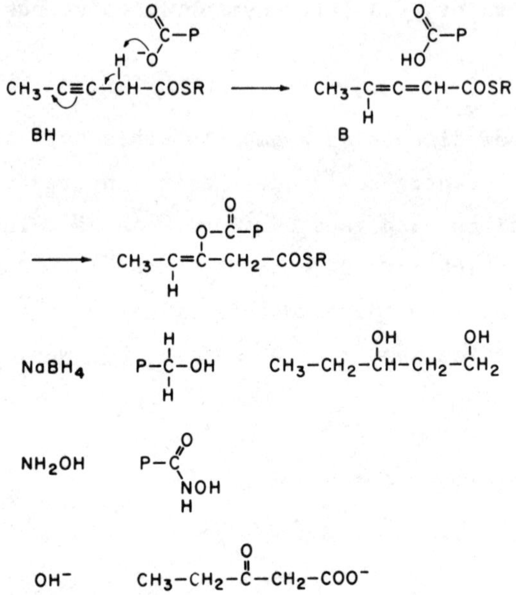

Fig. 3. Inactivation of Butyryl-CoA dehydrogenase.

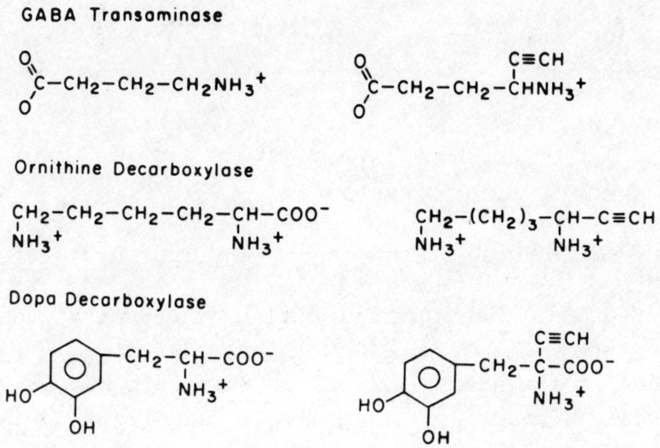

Fig. 4. Acetylinic inactivators.

Figure 4 shows several acetylenic suicide inactivators that have been synthesized by other investigators. They are directed against targeted enzymes which are of considerable biological interest.

So far, we have been most successful in designing suicide inactivators for enzymes that operate through carbanion mechanisms. A number of very effective approaches are not available for the inactivation of such enzymes. We, therefore, decided to focus on a different category of enzymes: hydrolytic enzymes, specifically serine proteases. These, of course, are of considerable pharmacological interest. We chose chymotrypsin as the first target enzyme. We chose that enzyme because much is known about it and it is available in large quantities. Our strategy is to design a core molecule that inactivates serine proteases. Eventually we plan to attach structures to the core molecule which will give it specificity. As you shall see, we have considerable indications that this is going to work. Before discussing specific inactivators, I want to remind you of the mechanism of action of chymotrypsin (Fig. 5). There is a

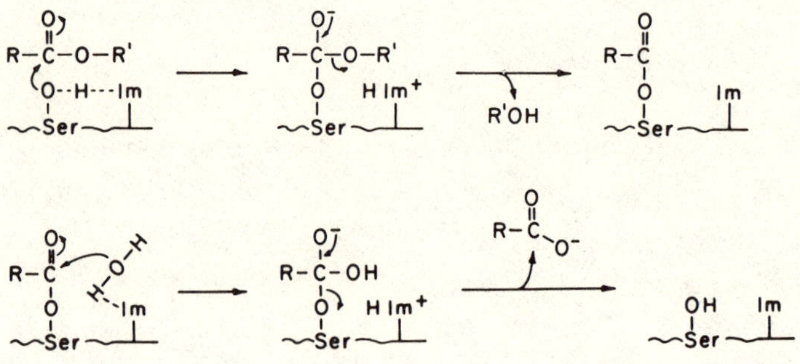

Fig. 5. Mechanism of action of chymotrypsin.

serine residue at the active site of chymotrypsin and an imidazole immediately adjacent to the serine. The imidazole is a general base which activates serine towards attack on the carboxyl group to form a tetrahedral intermediate. The alcohol then leaves from this tetrahedral intermediate aided by a proton from the imidazole-H^+. This results in the formation of an acyl-enzyme. The next phase of the reaction involves the attack of water on the acyl-enzyme, and finally hydrolysis. The two phases of the reaction, acyl-enzyme formation and acyl-enzyme hydrolysis, are quite analogous processes.

There appear to be two strategies for the inactivation of serine proteases: one could employ a compound which, after acyl-enzyme formation, unmasks a reactive species that could react with the imidazole. This would lead to enzyme inactivation since the incoming nucleophile would no longer be activated towards reaction with the acyl-enzyme. Alternatively, a substrate could be employed that generated an acyl-enzyme, which hydrolyzes at a very slow rate. That may have some advantages. For pharmacological purposes, it might be more desirable to inactivate an enzyme for a period of time rather than to inactivate it forever. I will give examples of both kinds of strategies.

Before describing our own work, I shall briefly review a few examples of work done previously by others. Figure 6 shows a

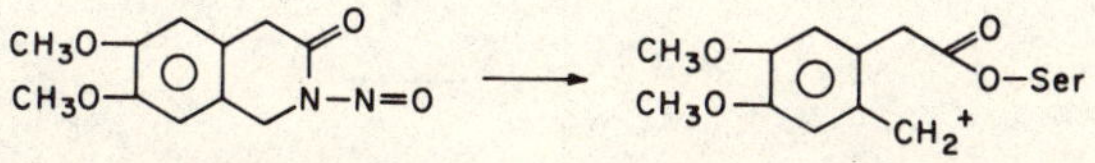

Fig. 6. Inactivation of chymotrypsin. White, E.H., et al. JACS 97:2290 (1975).

compound made by White. The compound resembles an amide. Formation of the acyl-enzyme leads to formation of a carbonium ion which is, of course, very reactive and tends to react with anything at the active site. This is a very nice idea. Unfortunately, this compound is unstable and therefore not useful in physiological systems. Figure 7 shows another approach devised by a French group. The inactivator resembles an ester. Attack by serine results in ring opening and bromide elimination. This generates a Michael acceptor, which reacts with the histidine at the active site and inactivates the enzyme.

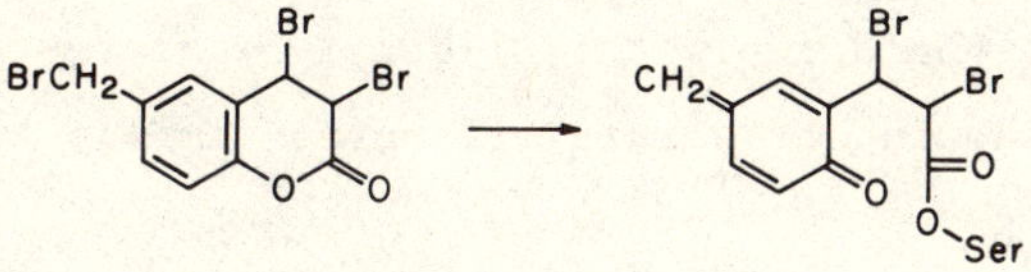

Fig. 7. Inactivation of chymotrypsin. Bechet, J.J., et al. E.J. Bioch. 35:527 (1973).

I shall now discuss some of the inactivators which we have developed. We have synthesized 6-chloro-2-pyrone shown in Fig. 8. This is a relatively stable molecule, its half-life, at pH 7, is about 26 hours. We hoped it would inactivate through the mechanism

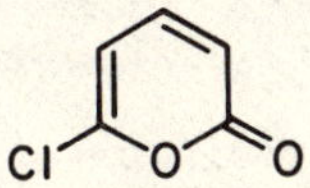

Fig. 8. Chloro-2-pyrone.

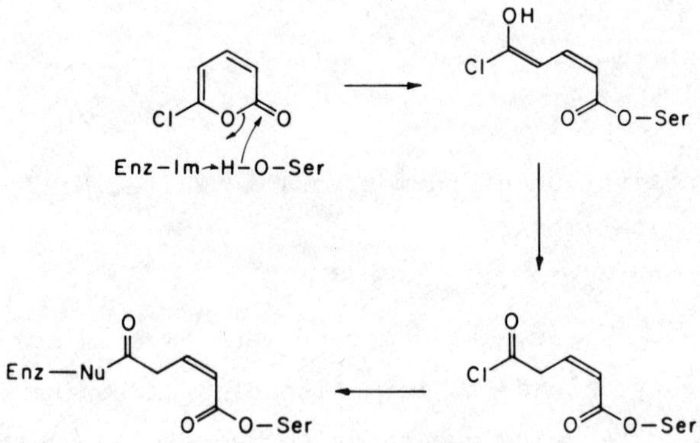

Fig. 9. Proposed mechanism of inactivation.

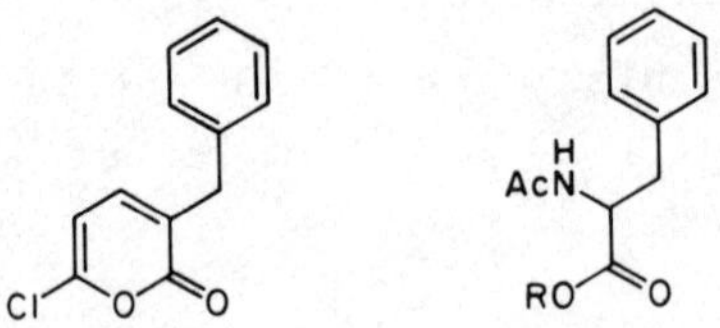

Fig. 10. Chymotrypsin inhibitor, 3-benyl-6-chloro-2-pyrone on the left showing structural features similar to a substrate on the right.

shown in Fig. 9. Attack of the active site, serine, leads to ring opening. The resulting compound can do one of two things: chloride can be expelled to form a ketene, or after protonation, an acid chloride will be formed. In either case, a sufficiently reactive species if formed, which can react with another nucleophile at the active site. The inactivator would then become attached at two points, which could result in enzyme inactivation. Actually, this compound did not react; however, the molecule does not really resemble a substrate for chymotrypsin. We therefore decided to attached a benzyl group as shown in Fig. 10. This compound now has many of the properties of a chymotrypsin substrate and it inactivates chymotrypsin in a time-dependent process. Clearly, the benzyl group makes a large contribution.

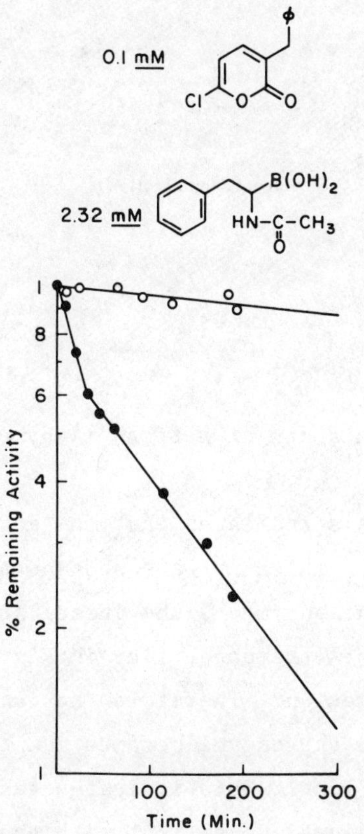

Fig. 11. Inactivation by chymotrypsin by 3-benzyl-6-chloro-2-pyrone, full circles. When the competitive inhibitor N-acetyl-α-borono-phenylethylamine was present, the enzyme was protected, open circles.

How does it really work? At this point we don't know. I shall tell you a little bit about what we know about the properties of this inactivator. Figure 11 shows the kinetics of the inactivation. The kinetics are biphasic due to the fact that chymotrypsin is not homogeneous. There are two forms of chymotrypsin which are inactivated at a different rate. Each one of these rates is a first order process. It is important to note that there is no lag period initially and no gradual increase in rate of inactivation as the

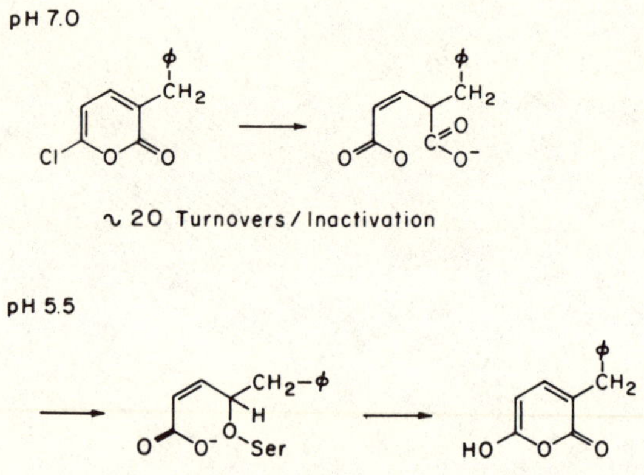

Fig. 12. Mechanism of action of chymotrypsin.

reaction proceeds. This indicates that the enzyme does not generate an inactivating species which is released and then reacts from solution. If we expose the enzyme to the inactivator in the presence of a competitive inhibitor (the upper line in Fig. 11), then there is essentially no inactivation. Therefore the inactivator reacts at the active site. When the enzyme becomes inactivated, the spectrum of the inactivator is lost. This indicates that upon inactivation the pyrone ring has opened, consistent with the proposed mechanism. The inactivator is also a substrate for the enzyme (Fig. 12). In one out of 20 turnovers, the enzyme is inactivated. This behavior is explained on the basis that the acid chloride derived from the opening of the pyrone ring can do one of two things: it can react either with water or with a nucleophile on the enzyme. Most of the time it reacts with water; when it does that, no inactivation occurs. If one lowers the pH to 5.5 another product, an anhydride, is formed (Fig. 12). This anhydride is formed through intramolecular reaction of the carboxylate with the serine ester. In other words, the reaction product is released from the enzyme when the carboxyl attacks serine, rather than by hydrolysis. It is reasonable that this should happen at low pH. At low pH the imidazole, which promotes hydrolysis by activating a water molecule, is protonated and cannot activate water.

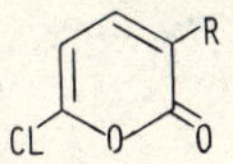

0.5 mM

R	CHYMOTRYPSIN	ELASTASE	ACH ESTERASE
-H	-	-	-
$-CH_3$	27.90	0.9	-
$-CH_2\phi$	30.80	?	45

NO INACTIVATION: LACTATE DEHYDROGENASE, PAPAIN, TRYPSIN
CARBOXYPEPTIDASE A, CREATINE KINASE

Fig. 13. Inactivation rates ($T_{1/2}$).

Figure 13 shows how the pyrone reacts with other enzymes. It is a reasonably specific inactivator of chymotrypsin. One can replace the benzyl group by a methyl group and maintain activity. Replacement by H results in loss of activity. The methyl compound also activates elastase. The pyrone is also an inactivator of acetylcholine-esterase. Acetylcholine-esterase is a serine protease. It should be noted that neither papain, trypsin, nor carboxypeptidase are affected by this inactivator. The mechanism of action of papain resembles that of chymotrypsin, except the active serine is replaced by cysteine.

What would happen if the benzyl group is moved from the 3 to the 5 position of the pyrone ring (Fig. 14)? This compound is also an inactivator, but it works by a different mechanism. We know this from spectroscopis data. As indicated above, chymotrypsin inactivated with 3-benzyl-6-chloro-2-pyrone does not have a spectrum characteristic of the pyrone system. On the other hand, when the benzyl group is in the 5 position, the inactivated enzyme does have the spectrum of the pyrone ring system. The spectrum has shifted approximately 10 nanometers towards the visible. Figure 14 shows what we think happens. With the 3-benzyl substituted compound, the serine attacks at position 2, whereas with the 5-benzyl substituted

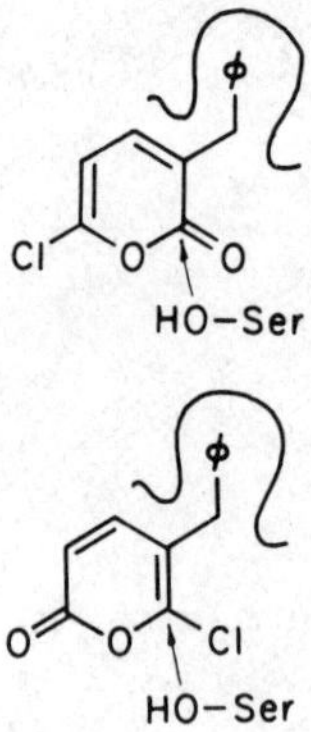

Fig. 14. Interaction of inactivator with the active site.

compound, serine attacks at position 6. The benzyl group determines the orientation of the inactivator at the active site.

We now have an inactivator which acts on a serine protease and is reasonably specific. We hope to make this compound much more specific by attaching appropriate structures to the ring. Our target enzymes will be elastase and trypsin.

Figure 15 shows some other molecules which we have synthesized which are structurally similar to the compounds discussed above. They do not inactivate; therefore, the halogen is absolutely necessary for inactivation.

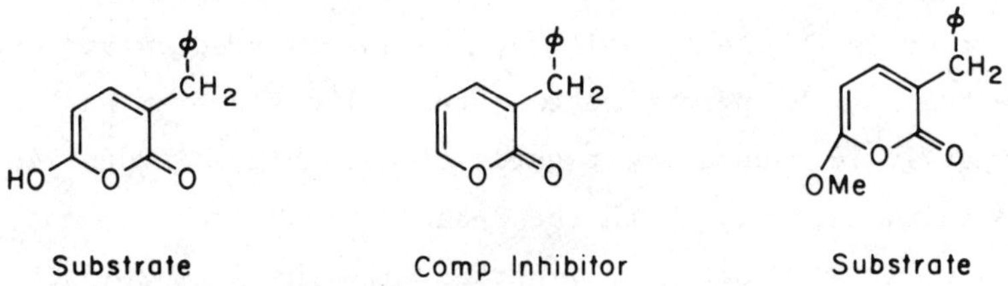

Fig. 15. Inactivator analogs.

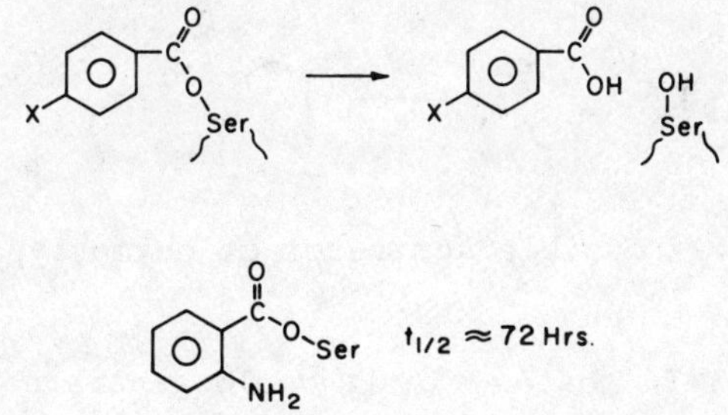

Fig. 16. Hydrolysis of substituted benzoyl chymotrypsin.

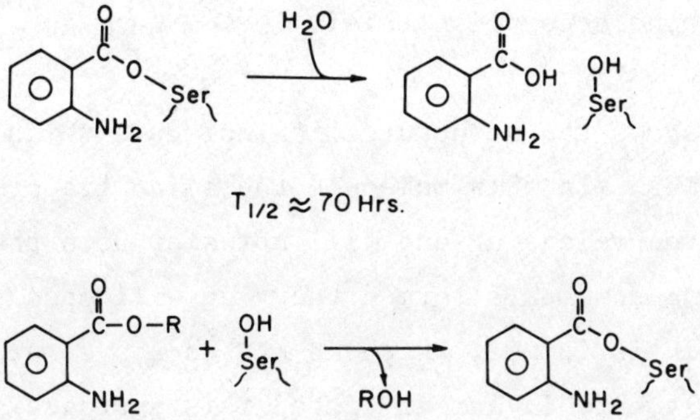

Fig. 17. Possible inactivators.

I shall now discuss an entirely different approach to the same problem. Some time ago Jencks studied the rate of hydrolysis of substituted benzyl chymotrypsin. He determined σ-p correlations. From his data one could calculate the o- or p-amino benzoyl chymotrypsin would hydrolyze with a half-time of approximately 72 hours (Fig. 16). Therefore, if one could generate o- or p-aminobenzoyl chymotrypsin, one would, for all practical purposes, inactivate chymotrypsin.

One might think that this is relatively simple (Fig. 17). One simply makes an ester of anthranilic acid and allows it to react

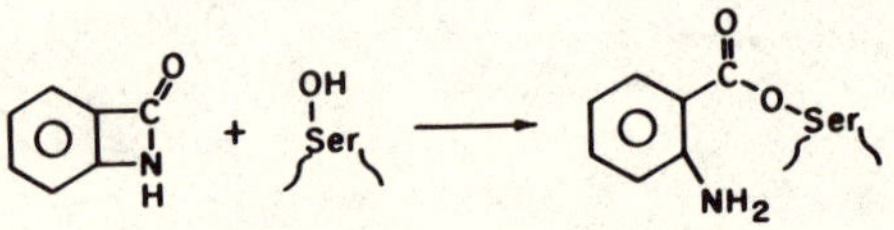

Fig. 18. Possible activator of chymotrypsin.

with chymotrypsin. If that works it would generate the desired o-amino-benzoyl chymotrypsin. This approach is unsatisfactory. the acylation process is exactly analogous to the deacylation process, and therefore, the factors which make the hydrolysis of the acyl-enzyme slow also make the acylation process slow. The following needs to be done: the amino group has to be masked until the acyl-enzyme is formed, and acyl-enzyme formation unmasks the amino group. How can one accomplish this?

Figure 18 shows the structure of a molecule which has the desired properties. In this molecule the amino group is acylated. It is not electron releasing and will not slow down the acylation. But once the acyl-enzyme is formed the ring will open and anthranoyl-chymotrypsin is formed, which as stated above, will hydrolyze slowly. Actually, Dr. T. Kaiser tested this approach a few years ago. He synthesized the compound shown in Fig. 18 with a t-butyl group on the nitrogen. It inactivates chymotrypsin but the inactivator is very unstable. We have used the compound shown in Fig. 19, isatoic anhydride. That compound is an excellent inactivator of chymotrypsin. It reacts stoichiometrically with chymotrypsin, and the inactivation proceeds rapidly. At 4°, $t_{\frac{1}{2}}$ for recovery of activity is in excess of 200 hours.

Figure 20 shows the mechanism by which we think it inactivates. The serine of chymotrypsin adds to the carbonyl group. This leads to ring opening and formation of carbamate, from which, after decarboxylation, anthranoyl-chymotrypsin is formed. Anthranoyl-chymotrypsin can be generated by other means, and its visible and

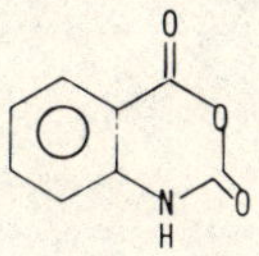

	CONC. μM	$T_{1/2}$ MIN	
α CHYMOTRYPSIN	12.5	1.3	
PANC. ELASTASE	125	<.25	REACTIVATES 49 MIN
TRYPSIN	125	2.0	REACTIVATES 145 MIN
PAPAIN	12.5	48	

NO INACTIVATION ($T_{1/2}$ >270 MIN, 1250 μM)

YEAST ALCOHOL DEHYDROGENASE, YEAST ALDEHYDE DEHYDROGENASE, ACETYLCHOLINE ESTERASE, CARBOXYPEPTIDASE A, PIG LIVER ESTERASE CREATINE KINASE

Fig. 19. Specificity of inactivation.

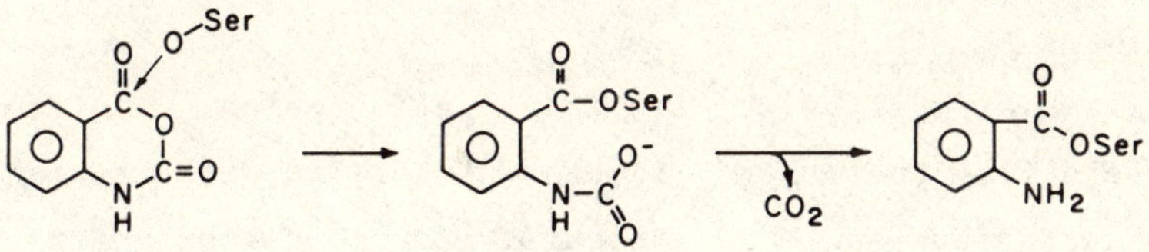

Fig. 20. Mechanism of inactivation by isatoic anhydride.

fluorescent spectrum is known. The adduct generated from isatoic anhydride has the same spectrum.

Isatoic anhydride is not a useful inactivator of elastase. It does inactivate, but the inactivatd complex regains catalytic activity rapidly. This is probably so because the deacylation step with elastase is very rapid. It is so rapid that although it is slowed down by the amine it still comes back too fast for our purposes. Figure 19 also shows data to illustrate the specificity

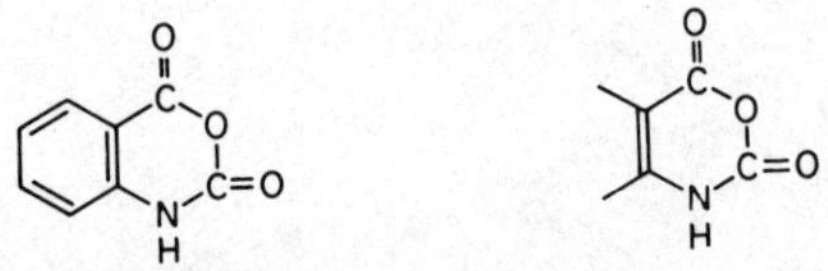

Fig. 21. Isatoic anhydride (left) with structural analog (right) which inactivates chymotrypsin and elastase.

of isatoic anhydride. Figure 21 shows a molecule which we have synthesized, the structure of which is based upon that of isatoic anhydride. This molecule inactivates chymotrypsin and elastase. In this case, inactivated elastase does not reactivate rapidly. At this point we do not know the mechanism of inactivation.

Next, we wished to establish at what position of the oxazine we should attach substituents which would impart specificity. From activity studies we found that substituents should be attached at position 4.

The last example of suicide inactivation which I want to discuss differs from the others, in that no covalent interaction between inactivator and enzyme occurs. Before discussing the inactivator I shall discuss the mechanism of action of the target enzyme, S-adenosine homocysteinase (Fig. 22). This enzyme is widely distributed and also occurs in mammalian systems. The enzyme hydrolyzes S-adenosine homocysteine (SAH). This enzyme is important because SAH is a very powerful inhibitor of many biological methyla-

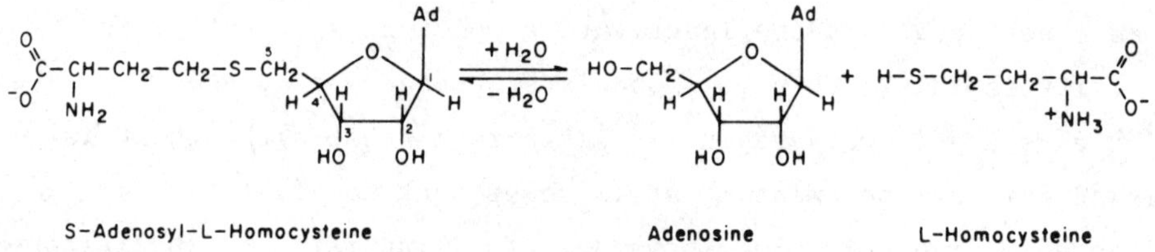

Fig. 22. S-adenosylhomocysteinase. Ad=Adenine.

tion reactions. The equilibrium of the reaction is towards biosynthesis, but under biological conditions adenosine is removed so that the enzyme works in the direction of hydrolysis. The reaction catalyzed by this enzyme is unlikely from a chemical point of view. Consider the reaction in the synthetic direction. An OH group is replaced by an SH group. Such a displacement is very unlikely. Figure 23 shows how the enzyme gets around this difficulty. NAD(DPN) is very tightly bound at the active site and it oxidizes the substrate in the 3 position. Subsequently, an α/β elimination reaction occurs. This elimination reaction leads to the formation of a Michael-acceptor. Water, then adds through a Michael addition. The resulting 3' keto-adenosine is then reduced and the reaction is complete. The enzyme has converted a very difficult S_N2 reaction to an addition-elimination process. In general, biological systems try to avoid S_N2 processes. Because this enzyme is physiologically so important, we wanted to design a suicide inactivator for this enzyme.

We synthesized 5', 5', 5'-trifluoro-5' deoxadenosine and hoped that it would be a suicide inactivator for SAHase (Fig. 24). Trifluoro-methyl groups are the basis of a group of suicide inactivators, which I have not discussed here. This compound did not inactivate. At about that time, Hirshfield reported that 2'-deoxyadenosine inactivates SAHase. A mechanism of inactivation suggested itself and is shown in Fig. 25.

The inactivator 2'-deoxy-adenosine is initially treated like the normal substrate, i.e., it is oxidized at C-3'. Moffatt has shown that 3-keto sugars are extremely unstable and eliminate adenine. The trans-elimination is preferred. The normal substrate, adenosine, cannot undergo a trans-elimination. However, 2'-deoxyadenosine can undergo a trans-elimination. This elimination leads to the formation of a keto-sugar, adenine, and the reduced form of the enzyme. The keto sugar dissociates from the enzyme and adenine

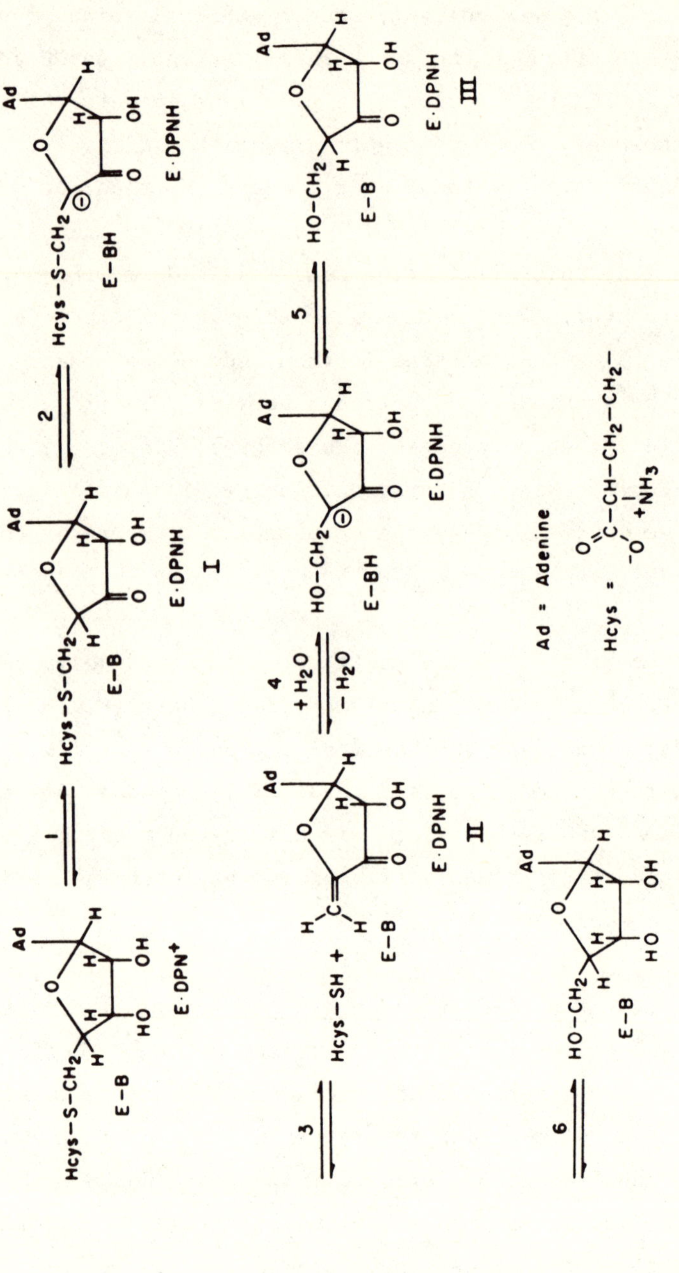

Fig. 23. The mechanism of action of S-Adenosylhomocysteinase.

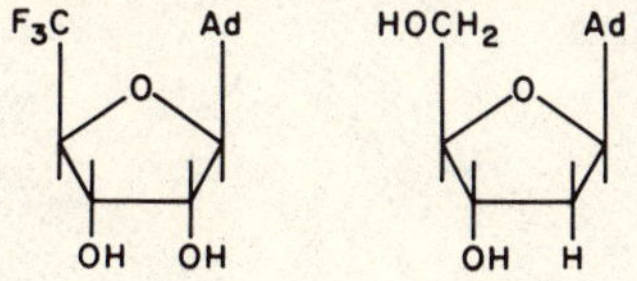

Fig. 24. Possible inactivators of S-adenosylhomocysteinase.

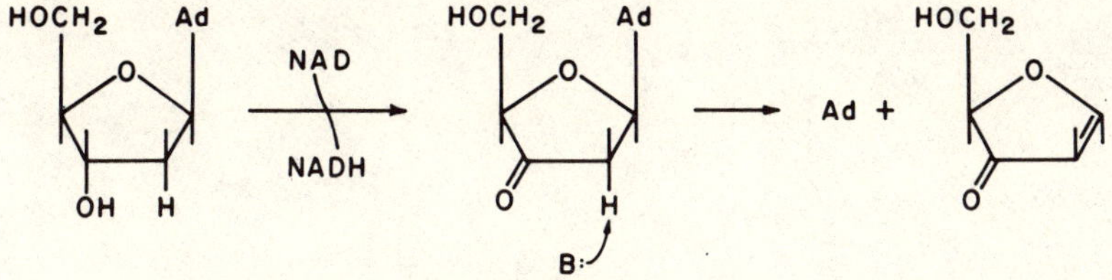

Fig. 25. Mechanism of inactivation by 2'-deoxyadenosine.

remains tightly bound. As you will recall, the normal catalytic process requires NAD in the initial step. However, the enzyme is now in the reduced form and is, therefore, catalytically inactive. This, then, provides an example of "suicide-inactivation" without covalent modification.

The investigations described herein were done by several workers. Gabriel Fendrich did the experiments with acetylenic inactivators, and those with inactivators for proteolytic enzymes were done by Drs. Allen Moorman and Rick Westkaemper. Dr. John Palmer and Miss Sue Fish did the work on SAH.

PROSPECTS FOR CHEMICALS AND FUELS PRODUCTION BY FERMENTATION

Charles L. Cooney
Biochemical Engineering Laboratories
Department of Chemical Engineering
Massachusetts Institute of Technology
Cambridge, Massachusetts 02139

THE CHEMICAL PROCESS INDUSTRY

The chemical industry or, more specifically, the organic chemical industry is characterized as a large volume converter of inexpensive feedstocks into both commodity and specialty chemical products. The chemical process industry, in 1981, produced over 175 billion pounds of organic chemicals which are primarily accounted for by the top 29 organics listed in Table 1 [1]. In addition, 22 inorganic chemicals accounted for 373 billion pounds of production. Total chemical sales for 1981 was $114 billion [1]. The primary feedstocks for the chemical industry are currently derived from petroleum and natural gas resources. It is interesting to consider the "typical" chemical process from a manufacturing cost point of view: 60-75% of the manufacturing costs are feedstock cost and 10-20% is capital-related. From Figure 1, which relates selling price to production volume, the price range for commodity chemicals is 10-50¢/lb. The capital investment for construction of a new chemical plant is approximately $0.25-0.30 per annual pound of product produced. The expected capital spending in the chemical

Table 1

U.S. Production of Organic Chemicals for 1981

Chemical	Production[5] (10^9 lb)	Price[4] (¢/lb)
Ethylene	29	25
Propylene	14	24
Toluene	10	21
Benzene	9.9	23
Ethylene dichloride	9.2	14
Methanol	8.4	11
Ethyl benzene	7.9	30
Vinyl chloride	6.7	22
Styrene	6.6	38
Xylene	6.4	21
Terephthalic acid	6.4	
(Formaldehyde[1])	(5.9)	(9)
Ethylene oxide	5.1	45
Ethylene glycol	4.1	33
p-Xylene	3.7	28
Cumene	3.3	23
Butadiene[2]	3.1	38
Acetic Acid	2.7	26
Phenol	2.6	36
Formaldehyde	2.2	29
Acetone	2.2	32
Aerylonitrile	2.0	46
Vinyl acetate	1.9	37
Propylene oxide	1.8	44
Cyclohexane	1.8	24
Isopropanol	1.6	32
Acetic anhydride	1.3	41
Adipic acid	1.2	57
Ethanol[3]	1.2	27

[1] Formaldehyde, 37% by weight

[2] Butadiene, rubber grade

[3] Ethanol, synthetic only

[4] Chemical Marketing Reporter, May 3, 1982

[5] Chemical and Engineering News, May 3, 1982

industry for 1982 is $14.7 billion [2]. Over the period 1971 to 1981, the annual growth in organic chemicals production has proceeded at 4.5%. More recently, however, softening of the economy, particularly in large markets for products such as housing

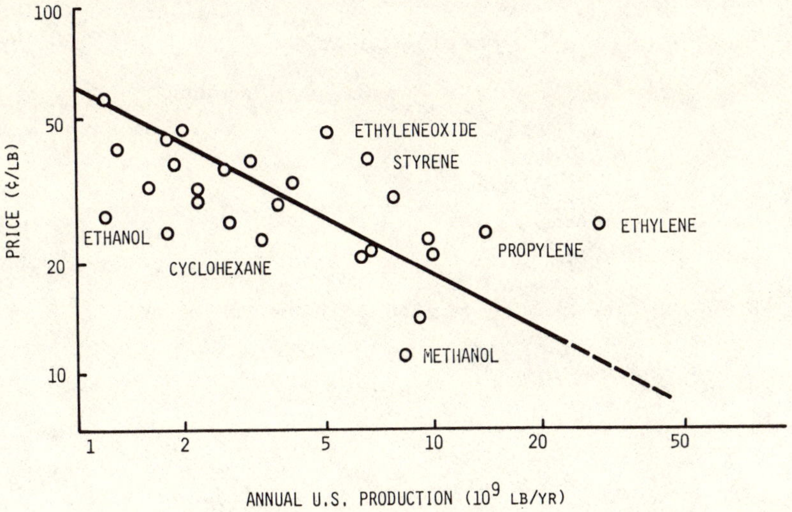

Fig. 1. Selling price related to production volume of a variety of chemicals.

construction, automobiles, and fibers has slowed growth in this industry so that for 1981, it was -0.6% [1]. As a consequence, the current utilization of production capacity is in the region of 50-70% as illustrated for some of the major commodity chemicals in Table 2 [3]. This is substantially lower than the 80-90% range which is desired for an acceptable return on investment.

Over the past couple of years, there has been considerable discussion about the role of biotechnology in the chemical industry and a number of projections have suggested that, by the year 2000, biotechnological processes will account for in excess of $10 billion a year. In light of these projections and estimates, it is useful to take a look at some of the changes that are currently taking place in the chemical process industry (Table 3) and examine how biotechnology might play a role. In addition, consideration is given to

Table 2

Operating Capacity[1]

	Capacity (10^9 lb/yr)	Operating Rate (%)
Ethylene	41	71
Propylene	22	66
Benzene	19	52
Phenol	4	65
Methanol	10	84
Styrene	9	76

Desired operating rate for acceptable ROI, 80-90%.

[1] Adopted from (3)

Table 3

Problems in the Chemical Industry

- Dependence of cost on feedstock
- Volatile feedstock cost
- Overcapacity
- High energy cost
- Environmental and safety regulations

identifying the problems that limit the application of biotechnology to the chemical process industry (CPI). An understanding of these problems can provide a basis for delineating research directions important to the development of a biochemical process industry (BPI).

CHANGES IN THE CHEMICAL PROCESS INDUSTRY

The major cost in the manufacture of organic chemicals is the feedstock cost. It is not surprising that this is likely to be the most sensitive area for change. Rising costs for both petroleum and natural gas feedstocks has caused chemical manufacturers to look for new sources of traditional feedstocks as well as novel and alternative feedstocks. Seeking new sources of traditional feedstocks is more likely to lead to a redistribution of manufacturing capacity worldwide with many of the petroleum and gas producing countries looking to vertically integrate their industries and take advantage of the value added in chemicals manufacture. Consideration of alternate sources for feedstocks has given rise to thoughts of using coal and biomass as a basis for building a chemical industry. The utilization of coal for a chemical industry is not new; however, it is hampered by the high cost of transporting and processing coal to make it suitable for chemicals production. In addition, process technology for utilization of coal is very capital-intensive and large plants are required in order to take advantage of the economy of scale. Biomass, on the other hand, is considered attractive as a renewable resource that is available at relatively low cost throughout many regions of the country.

As a consequence of the declining demand for chemicals and the increasing cost of capital, the capital intensivity, measured as dollars of capital investment per annual pound of product is of increasing concern to the chemical industry and alternative processes which would permit reduced capital requirements take on increasing interest.

Lastly, over the past couple of decades, there has been a dramatic change in environmental, social, and legal constraints that place increasing pressure on the chemical process industry. An increasing number of products and feedstocks are considered to be hazardous from an environmental, as well as a process point of view. As a consequence, there is increasing incentive to develop process technology using existing or alternative feedstocks that are more environmentally and socially acceptable.

THE ROLE OF BIOTECHNOLOGY IN THE CHEMICAL PROCESS INDUSTRY

The opportunities for biotechnology in the chemical process industry fall under several categories as summarized in Table 4.

First, and perhaps foremost, biotechnology can provide access to alternative feedstocks to decrease the dependence on petroleum and natural gas resources. Biomass may provide a lower cost feedstock, either because of its price per pound or because it is uniquely available in a local situation that makes it more attractive than petrochemical feedstocks. Alternative feedstocks are often useful in providing "swing capacity" with an alternative process for producing a product in a situation where there is a fluctuating demand. An example of this type of situation occurs in acetone manufacture. Through biotechnology, it may be possible to construct processes with lower pollution problems, less environmental and operating hazards by using less hazardous chemicals and operating conditions. Other possibilities where biotechnology may contribute relate to improved selectivity which leads to better product conversion yields from feedstocks and to easier purification. Decreased energy consumption, through operation at lower temperatures and pressures may also provide cost savings. Thus, there are problems in the CPI which might be solved through biotechnology. The difficulty, however, is developing low cost products!

An example of a commodity chemical often considered as a candidate for product by fermentation is acetone. Considered here from the CPI's viewpoint, is how biotechnology may play a role in acetone production. Currently, acetone is produced by two routes as shown in Figure 2. The first is as a coproduct from the oxidation of cumene to phenol and the second is the dehydrogenation is isopropanol. The numbers in parentheses are the 1981 production of each compound; there is a one to one stoichiometric relation between acetone and phenol as co-products from cumene. However, the demand for

Table 4

Opportunities for Biotechnology in

The Chemical Process Industry

Access to alternative feedstocks

- lower cost
- local situation
- swing capacity
- low pollution
- less hazardous

Improved selectivity

Decreased energy consumption

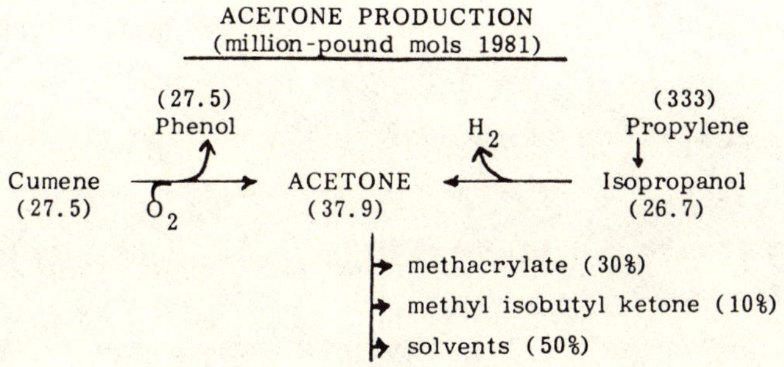

Fig. 2. Two routes of acetone production. The numbers in parenthesis are the 1981 production yields.

acetone is greater than the demand for phenol, as a consequence, some acetone is derived from isopropanol which is produced from propylene. The conversion of propylene to isopropanol represents a small portion of the total propylene available and the dehydrogenation of isopropanol to acetone is about 10 million pound-mols per year.

When considering the possibility of producing acetone by fermentation, the problem cannot be addressed in isolation. Unless a

Table 5

Problems in Development of

Biotechnology for the CPI

Unproven and/or volatile pricing for biomass
Low volumetric productivity
Unproven technology
Capital intensive processes
High water requirements
Coproduct processes

new route to phenol is developed, it is unlikely that acetone as a coproduct can be displaced. Likewise, if major amounts of acetone were produced from biomass feedstocks, there are going to be dislocations in the ispropanol industry. The economics of acetone production from isopropanol are not as attractive as from cumene so that the isopropanol route provides increasing capacity. Thus, there may be an opportunity for biotechnology if the economics are substantially better than from isopropanol but the market penetration is only a fraction of the total acetone market. By altering biochemical pathways, we can alter the enzyme compliment of the cell and possibly cause it to produce products that it did not produce before and by using gene amplification and to increase the amounts of key enzymes, either new ones or rate limiting enzymes in metabolic pathways, it may be possible to create better biocatalysts that are more effective in terms of rate and conversion yield than before. Yes, there are opportunities, but the difficulty remains that it is necessary to use low cost solutions to production of large volume, low margin products.

In summary, when one looks at what the problems in developing a Biochemical Process Industry there are several things which hold it back (Table 5). For the most part, there is unproven and volatile pricing for biomass. What will lignocellulosic biomass sell for?

We do not really know! Generally, biochemical processes have a low volumetric productivity. In the chemical industry one wants to see one to two moles of product per liter per hour. Often biochemical processes are less than 10% of this value. Unproven technology, particularly in regard to scale-up, the capital intensivity of biological processes compared to many chemical routes, a high water requirement in biological processing, and the fact that in biochemical processes one often has co-product processes, particularly when you are dealing with heterogeneous materials such as lignocellulosic biomass all present limitations to entry into the commodity chemical industries.

Using this example, I have tried to pinpoint some of the problems in the chemical industry that must be addressed by biotechnologists try to enter this business. Another area with potential for impact is in process development. The problem in process development falls into several categories: biocatalysis - the rate of catalysts, the stability of the catalyst, heat and mass transfer, conversion yields, and problems in product recovery. An interesting question to ask here is, how can genetic engineering and recombinant DNA be applied to solving these problems? There are four things that can be done with genetic engineering. One is to introduce foreign DNA into new organisms, two is to amplify that DNA to increase specific protein synthesis, three is to alter biochemical pathways, and four is to alter plant and animal metabolism. In addressing solving the problems of the chemical process industry, it is the second and third that are most significant. The chemical industry has problems. Efforts in biotechnology should be focused on solving these problems and not, as is often the case, focused on developing solutions to unidentified problems and then later seeking problems for the solutions.

REFERENCES

1. Anonymous, 1982. Chemical and Engineering News May 3, p. 10.

2. Anonymous, 1982. Chemical Week, May 19, p. 12.

3. Anonymous, 1982. Chemical Week, April 7, p. 44.

THE UTILIZATION OF INORGANIC PYROPHOSPHATE, TRIPOLYPHOSPHATE, AND TETRAPOLYPHOSPHATE AS ENERGY SOURCES FOR THE GROWTH OF ANAEROBIC BACTERIA

Harry D. Peck, Jr.[a], Chi-Li Liu[b], A. K. Varma[c], L. G. Ljungdahl[a], M. Szulczynski[d], F. Bryant[a], and L. Carreira[a]

ABSTRACT

Inorganic pyrophosphate (PP_i) has been shown to be utilized as a source of energy for the growth of a number of pure cultures of anaerobic bacteria and isolates from marine and fresh water environments. The microorganisms generally require a source of fixed carbon such as yeast extract for growth but with some of the sulfate reducing bacteria, acetate and sulfate were also required. Growth, as determined by optical density, cell numbers, or protein, is proportional to the concentration of PP_i over a limited range and growth is always accompanied by the hydrolysis of PP_i to orthophosphate. PP_i was also demonstrated to modify fermentations without

a: Department of Biochemistry, University of Georgia, Athens, GA

b: Exxon Research, P.O. Box 45, Linden, N.J. 07036

c: Jawaharlal Nehru University, New Delhi-110057, India

d: A. Mickiewicz University, Poznan, Poland

effecting growth Thus, methane formation by Methanosarcina barkeri from acetate, methanol or H_2 plus CO_2 is stimulated 2-3 fold in the presence of PP_i and, with the latter two substrates, an accumulation of acetate is observed without a significant increase in growth. Enrichment cultures have been obtained using tripolyphosphate and tetrapolyphosphate and it is evident that these polyphosphates can also be utilized as a source of energy for the growth of anaerobic microorganisms. An enzyme has been purified from Thermoanaerobacter ethanolicus which exhibits both PP_i:acetate kinase and ATP:acetate kinase activities and it is suggested that this kinase may be responsible for the widespread ability among anaerobic bacteria to utilize PP_i as a source of energy.

INTRODUCTION

Inorganic pyrophosphate (PP_i) is formed by biological systems in a large variety of biosynthetic reactions including amino acid activation, the biosynthesis of nucleic acids, formation of acyl CoA esters and the activation of carbohydrates by uridyl transferases [15]. The PP_i is generally believed to be hydrolyzed to orthophosphate (P_i) by inorganic pyrophosphatase (PPase) in order to "pull" these biosynthetic reactions in a thermodynamically unfavorable direction so that energy of the PP_i bond is essentially wasted. For the last 25 years, it has been speculated that PP_i might replace adenesine triphosphate (ATP) in some biosynthetic reactions but it is only in the last 10 years that such reactions have been reported [36,47]. From the energetic aspects, there is no reason to exclude PP_i as a source of energy and it has been proposed that PP_i is an evolutionary precursor of (ATP)(20]. However the bond energy of PP_i is dependent on the concentration of divalent cations such as Mg++. In the absence of divalent cations, the free energy of hydrolysis is the same as that of ATP (-7.60 Kcal/mole) [17] but in the presence of divalent cations, the energy of hydrolysis becomes less negative. This is due to the fact that P_i does not chelate divalent cations as strongly as does ADP. Thus, in the presence of mM Mg++ the free energy of hydrolysis of ATP to ADP and P_i is -7.6 Kcal/mole while that of PP_i is -5.27 Kcal/mole.

The first indirect evidence that PP_i could serve as a source of energy was the observation of Baltscheffsky and von Stedink [4] that PP_i synthesis is coupled to electron transfer in the photosynthetic bacteria. It was later demonstrated that PP_i could replace ATP as a source of energy in transhydrogenase, cytochrome c reduction, and the succinate-linked reduction of NAD [5]. More recently it has been reported that membrane-bound pyrophosphatase functions as a coupling factor for election transport driven pyrophosphate formation in plants and animals [16,25,37] in a fashion similar to membrane bound ATPase. A number of new enzymes which utilize PP_i in a biosynthetic fashion have been described and it is clear that PP_i serves as an energy source in the fermentation of carbohydrates by *Entamoeba histolytica* [36] and *Propionibacterium shermanii* [48]. These new enzymes involving PP_i and their reactions are as follows:

1. Carboxytransphosphorylase [39]

$$PP_i + \text{oxaloacetate} \rightarrow \text{P-enolpyruvate} \quad P_i + CO_2$$

2. Pyruvate: phosphate dikinase [10, 11, 33]

$$PP_i + \text{AMP} + \text{P-enolpyruvate} \rightarrow \text{pyruvate} + \text{ATP} + P_i$$

3. PP_i:phosphofructokinase [26,34]

$$PP_i + \text{fructose-6-phosphate} \rightarrow \text{fructose-1,6 bis P} + P_i$$

4. PP_i:serine kinase [7]

$$PP_i + \text{serine} \rightarrow \text{P-serine} + P_i$$

5. PP_i: acetate kinase [35]

$$PP_i + \text{acetate} \rightarrow \text{acetyl-P} + P_i$$

The PP_i:phosphofructokinase has recently been demonstrated in a number of plants [8] and photosynthetic bacteria [21,24,31].

We have recently found a third fermentation in the sulfate-reducing bacteria belonging to the genus Desulfotomaculum, in which PP_i serves as a major source of energy [2]. The sulfate-reducing bacteria, Desulfovibrio and Desulfotomaculum, oxidize a variety of compounds such as lactate, formate, H_2, ethanol, and utilize sulfate as their terminal electron acceptor with the formation of large amounts of H_2S [32]. Sulfate is not reduced as such but first must react with ATP in the presence of the enzyme, ATP sulfurylase, to yield equimolar amounts of adenylyl sulfate (APS) and PP_i [1]. The APS is directly reduced to sulfite by the enzyme, APS reductase. As the equilibrium of the reaction lies in the direction of ATP and sulfate, it has been believed that the PP_i was hydrolyzed by PPase to "pull" the reaction in the direction of APS and PP_i formation [29,45]. This conclusion is supported by the observation that extracts of Desulfovibrio contain high levels of PPase and the enzyme has been purified and characterized [2]. On the other hand, negligible amounts of PPase were found in Desulfotomaculum, and PPase appears to be replaced by high levels of PP_i:acetate kinase activity. Conversely, PP_i:acetate kinase activity was not detected in extracts of Desulfovibrio; however, the activity may have been "masked" by the high levels of PPase present in these extracts. Both

PPase and PP_i:acetate kinase activities are reductant activated [21,41] and appear to have analogous functions in removing PP_i formed during the activation of sulfate. Thus, each of these genera have different mechanisms for the overall formation of APS and these can be summarized as follows:

Desulfovibrio

$$ATP + SO_4^{2-} \rightarrow APS + PP_i$$

$$PP_i + H_2O \rightarrow 2\ P_i$$

Desulfotomaculum

$$ATP + SO_4^{2-} \rightarrow APS + PP_i$$

$$PP_i + acetate \rightarrow acetyl - P + P_i$$

$$acetyl\text{-}P + ADP \rightarrow ATP + acetate$$

From a consideration of these two mechanisms, it can be concluded that the bioenergetics of sulfate reduction in *Desulfovibrio* and *Desulfotomaculum* are completely different [28] in that two high energy phosphate groups are consumed for sulfate reduction by *Desulfovibrio* while only one is utilized for sulfate reduction by *Desulfotomaculum*. Thus, conservation of the bond energy of PP_i eliminates the necessity of invoking electron transfer coupled phosphorylation to account for the growth of *Desulfotomaculum* on organic substrates plus sulfate and explains many of the biological and biochemical differences between *Desulfovibrio* and *Desulfotomaculum*. This calculation and the absence of significant electron transfer coupled phosphorylation in *Desulfotomaculum* was confirmed by growth studies with *D. vulgaris* and *Dt. orientis* on lactate plus sulfate. Employing data from studies on growth yields of

Desulfovibrio [3] to indicate the number of moles of ATP produced by electron transfer phosphorylation coupled to the reduction of sulfate, it can be calculated that Desulfovibrio should produce three times as much ATP as Desulfotomaculum and this has been demonstrated by relative growth yields of these organisms growing on lactate/sulfate media. The foregoing observations demonstrate that enzymatic systems exist in both prokaryotes and eukaryotes for the utilization and conservation of the bond energy of pyrophosphate; however, we have not found any reports concerning either the utilization of PP_i as a source of energy by intact cells of prokaryotes or eukaryotes or the occurrence of PP_i in natural environments.

Growth of Desulfotomaculum on Pyrophosphate

Gram negative bacteria do not appear to utilize PP_i as such [40] and it is believed to be split to P_i by hydrolytic enzymes present in the periplasmic space. The observations concerning the utilization of PP_i in the sulfate reducing bacteria suggested the possibility that intact cells of Desulfotomaculum might be capable of utilizing PP_i in the presence of fixed carbon as a source of ATP for growth. The effect of PP_i on the growth of D. vulgaris and Dt. ruminis in a medium containing reduced levels of lactate and sulfate is compared in Table 1. In the presence of lactate, sulfate, and PP_i, a 2-3 fold stimulation of the growth of Dt. ruminis is observed over growth on lactate plus sulfate ($-PP_i$) and significant hydrolysis of PP_i is found. PP_i does not stimulate the growth of D. vulgaris but rather appeared to inhibit growth. Both microorganisms were dependent on the presence of sulfate for growth, but only Dt. ruminis exhibited good growth in the absence of lactate. Deletion of acetate decreased the growth of Dt. ruminis by 50% but appeared to stimulate the growth of D. vulgaris. The presence of yeast extract is required for the growth of Dt. ruminis. A medium has now been devised for the growth of Dt. orientis, Dt. ruminis, and Dt.

Table 1

The Effect of PP_i on the Growth of the Sulfate Reducing Bacteria, *D. vulgaris* and *Dt. ruminis*

	Dt. ruminis		*D. vulgaris*	
Medium	Growth (O.D. 580 nm)	% hydrolysis of PP_i	Growth (O.D. 580 nm)	% hydrolysis of PP_i
Complete	0.618	32	0.157	5
-sulfate	0.083	3	0.007	14
-lactate	0.372	23	0.101	11
-PP_i	0.262	--	0.324	--
-acetate	0.296	11	0.335	10
-yeast extract	0.021	3	0.170	4

nigrificans on PP_i in the absence of lactate and the optimal conditions for growth of *Dt. orientis* are presented in Table 2. In the absence of PP_i this basal medium containing acetate, yeast extract, sulfate, and salt does not support significant growth of *Dt. orientis*. The data in Figure 1 illustrate the growth response of *Dt. ruminis* to increasing concentrations of PP_i. The growth response is proportional to PP_i concentrations up to 0.04% PP_i and growth is accompanied by the hydrolysis of PP_i to P_i. In the absence of growth, there is little hydrolysis of the added PP_i and, above 0.05% PP_i, there appears to be inhibition of growth and lysis of cells. Growth is as good as that normally observed on lactate/ sulfate medium and orthophosphate equivalent to the added PP_i does not support the growth of these sulfate reducing bacteria. Neither *D. vulgaris* or *D. gigas* were capable of growth on this medium. Yeast extract probably meets the requirements of the bacteria for cell carbon and sulfate may provide the microroganism with an electron sink with which to adjust the oxidation level of the added fixed carbon. The requirement for acetate was unexpectedly high with little growth observed below a concentration of 0.2%; however, the physiological basis for the acetate requirement has not been investigated. The stimulatory effect of PP_i on growth does not appear to be due to the facilitation of anaerobic acetate oxidation

Table 2

The optimal Growth Conditions of Desulfotomaculum orientis in Acetate plus PP_i-sulfate medium.

1.	Acetate concentration	$CH_3COONa \cdot 3H_2O$	0.3%
2.	Sulfate concentration	Na_2SO_4	0.4%
		$MgSO_4 \cdot 7H_2O$	0.2%
3.	Mg^{+2} concentration	$MgCl_2 \cdot 6H_2O$	0.05%
4.	PP_i concentration	$Na_4P_2O_7 \cdot 10H_2O$	0.04%
5.	Yeast Extract concentration	Difco	0.25%
6.	pH range		5.8-6.2

*The other components of the medium are: Ferrous sulfate, 10 mg/l; K_2HPO_4, 0.5 g/l; $CaCl_2$, 0.2 g/l; Cysteine·HCl, 0.25 g/l; Na_2S, 0.125 g/l.

[43] by PP_i, as the ratio of acetate disappearance to sulfide production was 3:14 rather than the expected ratio of 1:1.

The specific activities of various enzymes involved in the energy metabolism of Dt. orientis have been determined in extracts of PP_i and lactate/sulfate grown cells [22]. The reductases of respiratory sulfate reduction, APS reducsae [6], thiosulfate reductase [27], bisulfite reductase [18], and ATP sulfurylase [45] have about the same levels of activity in each cell preparation. Fumarate reductase [27] is absent in both preparations and nitrite reductase [38], formate dehydrogenase [27], PP_i:acetate kinase [35], pyrophosphase [27] and pyruvate dehydrogenase [37], are present at similar specific activities. The specific activity of hydrogenase was five fold higher in PP_i than in lactate/sulfate grown cells. This may be due to the fact that growth with PP_i more closely approximates growth under sulfate limiting conditions or interspecies H_2 transfer which lead to an increase in hydrogenase activity [28].

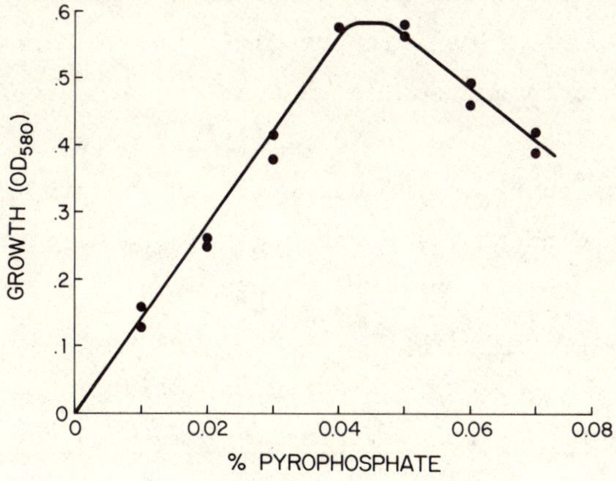

Fig. 1. The effect of pyrophosphate concentration on the growth of Desulfotomaculum ruminis. Growth conditions as in Table 2 except for varying concentrations of PP_i.

Because of the unique occurrence of these enzymes, the results indicate that the bacteria growing on PP_i and lactate/sulfate media are identical and that cells grown on PP_i exhibit no basic changes in their metabolic pattern as has been reported for D. vulgaris when grown on different media [14]. From these observations, it has been concluded that three species of Desulfotomaculum have the ability to utilize PP_i as a source of energy for growth and that a PP_i:acetate kinase activity is responsibile for this utilization of PP_i.

Studies with PP_i Enrichment Cultures

There is no reason to believe that the utilization of PP_i as a source of energy for growth is limited to Desulfotomaculum and in order to gain an idea of the generality of this phenomenon, we prepared PP_i enrichment cultures from anaerobic marine and fresh water environments. For the marine enrichments, mud samples were obtained from a spartina swamp and utilized to inoculate (5%) the basal medium employed for the growth of Desulfotomaculum supplemented with NaCl (2.5%) with and without PP_i under aerobic and anaerobic conditions. Within 24 h at 37°C, only the anaerobic media containing PP_i

showed extensive microbial growth and these enrichment cultures have been transferred ten times without diminution of growth. Photomicrographs of the microorganisms in the enrichment cultures are shown in Figure 2 which demonstrate the diversity of morphological types of bacteria growing on PP_i. The bacteria were both motile and non-motile and both Gram positive and negative. The diversity of cell-types strongly suggests that PP_i respiration is not restricted to the genus, Desulfotomaculum, which are characterized as spore-forming rods. Five new genera of sulfate reducing bacteria (Desulfobacter, Desulfobulbus, Desulfonema, Desulfococcus, and Desulfosarcina) have been recently described by Widdel and Pfennig [30,42] and it has been suggested on the basis of bioenergetic considerations that these bacteria may possess PP_i:acetate kinase activity [2]. Thus, the diversity of bacterial types found in these enrichment cultures may be due to growth of these new types of sulfate reducing bacteria and possibly other, yet to be described, genera and species of sulfate reducing bacteria; however, there is no direct evidence that these microorganisms are only sulfate reducing bacteria. The absence of a large precipitate of FeS in these enrichment cultures indeed suggests that the sulfate reducing bacteria do not constitute a significant fraction of the microorganisms in these cultures. As was observed with Desulfotomaculum, the composition of the media and the concentration of its components can be important for the growth of bacteria on PP_i. The composition of the media can select for the growth of different types of microorganisms and changes in the type of fixed carbon or electron acceptor may lead to the growth of completely different bacterial populations in enrichment cultures.

For the fresh water enrichments, mud samples were obtained from a local lake in an area where gas was being actively produced and used to inoculate the medium shown in Table 3 with and without PP_i. Tubes were incubated at 37°C under aerobic and anaerobic conditions. Visible growth was observed within 24 h only in tubes incubated

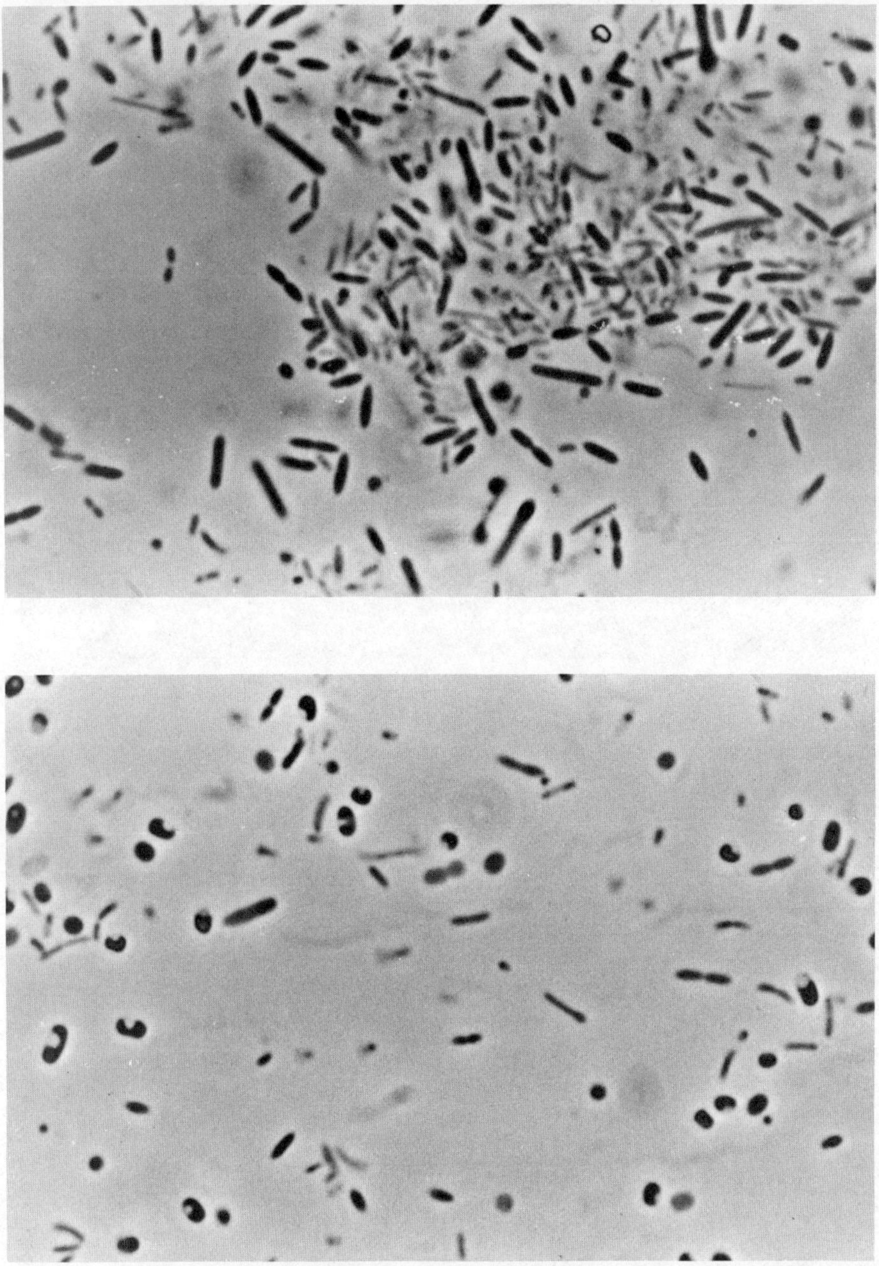

(a)

(b)

Fig. 2. Photomicrographs of microorganisms growing in a PPP_i enrichment of marine mud (a). Basal medium (see Table 3) supplemented with 2.5% NaCl (b).

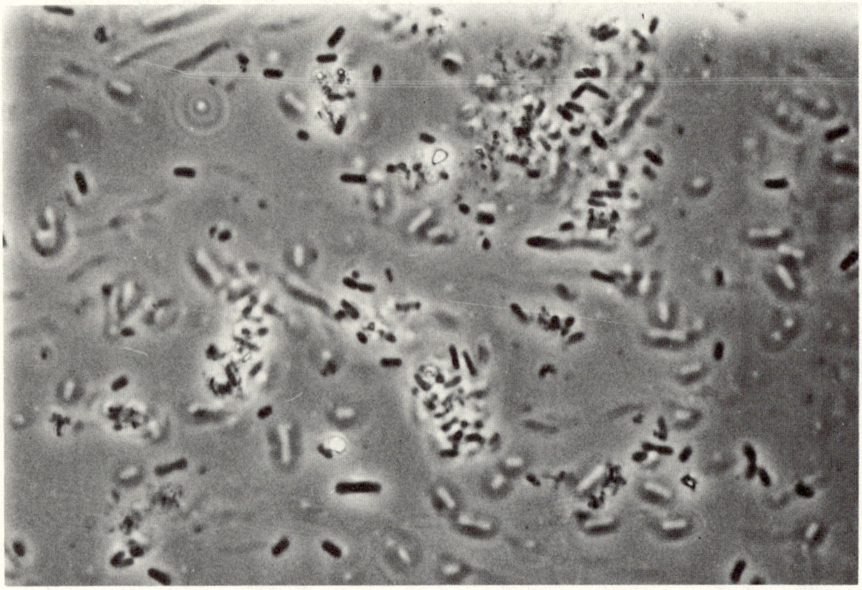

(b)

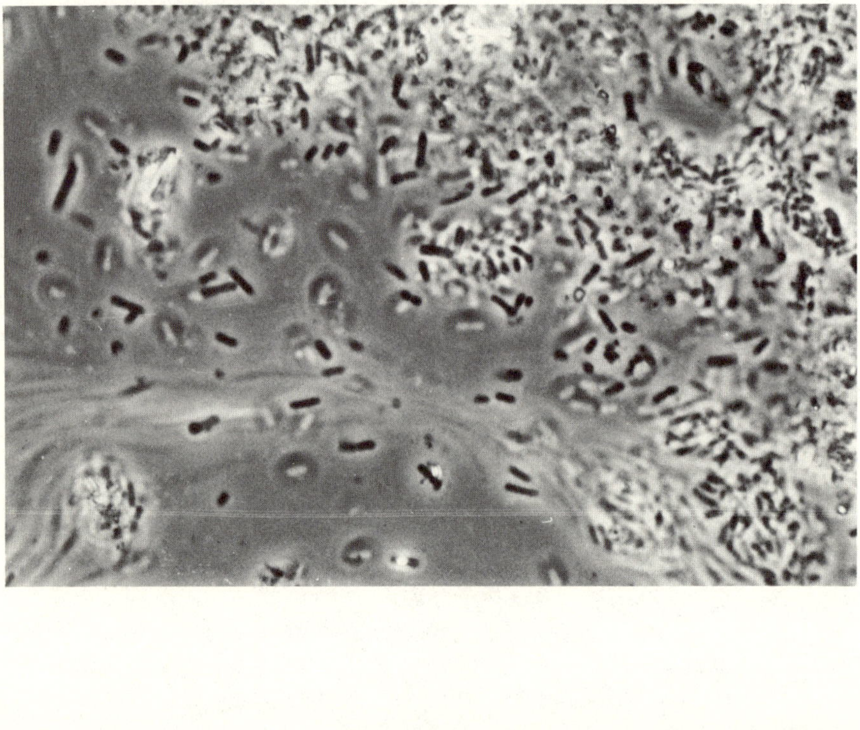

(a)

Fig. 3 Photomicrographs of microorganisms growing in tripolyphosphate (a) and tetrapolyphasphate enrichments (b) medium, see Table 3.

Table 3

Medium Utilized for Fresh Water PP_i Enrichments

	g/l
Na_2SO_4	3.0
KH_2PO_4	0.2
NH_4Cl	0.25
NaCl	1.0
$MgCl_2 \cdot 6H_2O$	0.4
KCl	0.5
$CaCl_2$	0.15
$CH_3COONa \cdot 3H_2O$	3.0
Yeast Extract (Difco)	5.0
Trace element solution*	(1.0 ml)
Cysteine·HCl	1.25
$Na_2S \cdot H_2O$	1.25
$Na_4P_2O_7 \cdot 10H_2O$ (filter sterilized)	5.0
Resazurin	1×10^{-3}

*pH 7.5 with N KOH or HCl.

anaerobically and containing PP_i. As with the marine enrichments, a diversity of morphological types were observed which were both motile and non motile and Gram negative and positive. Also, as with the marine enrichments, there was little formation of FeS. Direct colony counts of the numbers of PP_i utilizing bacteria in the mud samples ranged from 36-124 bacteria per ml. The results from these enrichment culture studies suggest that microorganisms capable of utilizing PP_i as a source of energy for growth are widely distributed in nature and are not limited to the sulfate reducing bacteria.

Studies with Tripolyphosphate (PPP_i) and Tetrapolyphosphate ($PPPP_i$) Enrichment Cultures

Our observations concerning the growth of microorganisms on PP_i suggested the possibility that microorganisms exist which can utilize higher polyphosphates as a source of energy for growth. A mud sample was obtained from the same lake as described above and used to inoculate (0.1 gm dry weight) the basal enrichment medium (200 ml) containing (mg/l) NH_4Cl, 200; $FeSO_4 \cdot 7H_2O$,10; $MgCl_2$, 400; Na_2SO_4, 200; K_2HPO_4, 13.6; NaCl, 100; $CaCl_2$, 10; yeast extract (Difco), 1000 peptone (Difco), 2000; trace elements [46] supplemented with selenium (Na_2SeO_3) and nickel($NiCl_2 \cdot 6H_2O$), 10^{-7}M, 5.0 ml; resazurin, 1; cysteine, 1250 and $Na_2S:H_2O$, 1250 and after sterilization each tube received 1% of a vitamin solution containing in mg/five liters: biotin, 2; folic acid, 2; pyridoxine-HCl, 10; riboflavin, 5; thiamine, 5; nicotinic acid, 5; pantothenic acid, 5; vitamin B_{12}, 0.1; p-amino benzoic acid, 5; and lipoic acid, 5. Individual tubes were then supplemented with filter sterilized orthophosphate, pyrophosphate, tripolyphosphate (penta sodium salt) and tetrapolyphosphate (hexa ammonium salt) and incubated aerobically and anerobically at 37^oC with shaking (100 rpm). Within 24 h visible growth was evident in all tubes incubated anaerobically except for the tubes containing P_i. The cultures containing $PPPP_i$ did not contain a precipitate of FeS; however, the culture containing $PPPP_i$ exhibited a large precipitate FeS suggesting that the different polyphosphates were selective for different microbial populations. Microscopically, the morphological types growing on PPP_i and $PPPP_i$ appeared to be as diverse as those growing on PP_i (Figure 3). Both enrichment cultures grew well when transferred to PP_i media, however; the PPP_i enrichments showed poor growth on $PPPP_i$ and the $PPPP_i$ enrichments showed poor growth on PPP_i. Isolates from the PPP_i and PPP_i are being studied with the goal of investigating the enzymology and physiology of polyphosphate utilization.

Characterization of PP_i Utilizing Bacteria from Fresh Water Environments

Four strains (I, II, III, and IV) of bacteria which are capable of rapid growth on PP_i have been isolated from the fresh water enrichment cultures. The bacteria exhibited a limited substrate specificity and, in addition to PP_i, were only capable of growth on purines and alanine but strain I and IV could grow on glucose. Growth on PP_i, uric acid, alanine, and hypoxanthine is shown in Table 4 and it should be noted that growth on each substrate is approximately equivalent. Growth on purines was not stimulated in the presence of PP_i; however, we have not yet determined whether PP_i effects the composition of the fermentation products. The parameters of growth on PP_i have been studied extensively with strains II and III which were morphologically distinct. The basal medium ($-PP_i$), which did not support growth was the same as that described in the previous section. Optimum growth of strain II as measured by optical density at 600 nm was obtained at a PP_i concentration of 0.14-0.15%; however, strain III exhibited optimal growth over a wide range of PP_i concentrations (0.1-.15%). With both strains, higher concentrations of PP_i resulted in an inhibition of growth as has been observed with *Desulfotomaculum*. The optimum requirement for yeast extract was between 0.1-0.15% for both strains of microorganisms. It is possible that PP_i stimulates growth on yeast extract by removing inhibitory metal ions; however, this possibility is considered as unlikely as other sources of fixed carbon such as peptone and casamino acids can successfully replace yeast extract. Interestingly, tryptone did not support growth. Growth as indicated by increase in optical density and protein is proportional to the concentration of added PP_i below the optimal concentration and the hydrolysis of PP_i as indicated P_i formation is proportional to growth.

Table 4

Utilization of Uric Acid, Hypoxanthine and Alanine on the Growth of the Fresh Water Isolates With and Without Pyrophosphate

Additions	Bacterial Strains I	II	III	IV
$+PP_i$	0.289	0.301	0.270	0.416
+Uric Acid	0.254	0.300	0.280	0.400
$+PP_i$ + Uric Acid	0.288	0.315	0.282	0.420
+ Alanine	0.260	0.272	0.288	0.292
$+PP_i$ + Alanine	0.270	0.289	0.290	0.400
+Hypoxanthine	0.290	0.310	0.300	0.322
$+PP_i$ + Hypoxanthine	0.288	0.312	0.274	0.398

Both strains exhibited a typical bacterial growth curve on PP_i and, at 36°C, generation times of 2.7 and 3.1 h for strains II and III respectively were calculated.

None of the four strains grew well on tetrapolyphosphate but strains II and IV grew well on tripolyphosphate. This observation again suggests that the utilization of polyphosphates involves different mechanisms. The nutritional situation as regards growth on pyrophosphate is much simpler than that found with Desulfotomaculum as only yeast extract and salts are required. It is curious that the faster growing bacteria from the fresh water PP_i enrichments are purine fermenting bacteria; however, the physiological significance of this observation has not been determined.

The Effect of PP_i on Methane Formation

Because of the role of the sulfate reducing bacteria as acetogenic bacteria in the microbial consortium responsible for the conversion of cellulose to methane and CO_2, the effect of PP_i on the

Table 5

The Effect of PP_i on the Establishment of Cellulose/Methane Enrichment Cultures

Days	Methane Production* (mmol)	
	$-PP_i$	$+PP_i$
7	0.03	0.06
9	0.04	0.15
11	0.07	0.64
13	0.15	2.04
15	0.24	2.97
17	0.38	3.63

*Medium was that of Dilworth et al. (9) containing 0.03% PP_i.

establishment of cellulose/methane enrichment cultures was investigated. Cellulose enrichment cultures were prepared using the medium of Dilworth et al. [9], inoculated from a fresh water mud sample, and methane production followed as a function of time. As shown in Table 5, there was ten times as much methane produced in the presence of PP_i as in its absence in the enrichment culture. On subsequent transfers of the PP_i cellulose enrichment cultures, the stimulation of methane formation by PP_i was only 2-3 fold. These observations suggested that the growth of the methane bacteria might be stimulated by the presence of PP_i. Thus far, we have observed the stimulation of methane formation by PP_i in cultures of *Methanobacterium formicium* grown on formate and *Methanosarcina barkeri* grown on methanol, H_2 plus CO_2, and acetate. In all cases, we have observed only marginal increases in cell mass; however, in cultures of *Ms. barkeri*, grown with H_2 plus CO_2, acetate now appears as a fermentation product in the presence of PP_i (Table 6). Similarly, when *Ms. barkeri* is grown on methanol in the presence of PP_i, there

Table 6

The Effect of PP_i on Methane Formation, Acetate Formation and Growth of *M. barkeri* on $H_2 + CO_2$

Days	CH_4 Formation (μmoles)		Cell Protein (mg/5ml)		Acetate Accumulation (mmole)	
	$-PP_i$	$+PP_i$	$-PP_i$	$+PP_i$	$-PP_i$	$+PP_i$
0	22.23	22.69	1.75	1.9	0	0.039
1	33.38	36.82	1.95	2.2	0	0.075
2	35.22	39.94	2.78	2.51	0	0.12
3	42.62	45.32	3.43	3.74	0	0.285
4	61.12	102.2	4.86	5.45	0	0.46
5	153.14	233.6	8.51	9.2	0	0.725
6	208.09	311.4	13.2	15.2	0	0.84
7	219.93	376.3	16.18	17.4	0	0.97

occurs a transient accumulation of acetate. The acetate is produced during the active phase of methane formation and itself appears to be converted to methane. We have not yet determined the origin of the acetate or its biochemical and physiological significance; however, these observations illustrate the potential of PP_i as a bioenergetic or metabolic probe for investigations of the physiology and biochemistry of the metabolic pathways of anaerobic bacteria.

The Effect of PP_i on the Growth and Metabolism of Other Microorganisms

Another approach for evaluating the generality of PP_i utilization as a source of energy for the growth of anaerobic bacteria has been to determine the effect of PP_i on the growth of laboratory strains of different microorganisms. These and the previously discussed results are summarized in Table 7. In these studies, it should be emphasized that negative results tend to be meaningless as an alteration of the growth conditions can result in growth of a bacterium on PP_i. Thus, in the absence of at least 0.3% acetate,

Table 7

The Effect of PP_i on the Growth and Metabolism of Various Microorganisms

Microorganism	Growth Supporting	Metabolic Effects
Dt. nigrificans, Dt. orientis and Dt. ruminis	+	
D. gigas, D. vulgaris	-	
E. coli	-	
Mb. formicium	?	stimulates methane formation from formate
Ms. barkeri	?	stimulates methane formation from acetate, methanol and H_2 plus CO_2; acetate accumulation from methanol and H_2 plus CO_2
Thermoanaerobacter ethanolicus	+	
Purine-fermenting isolates	+	
Clostridium thermocellum	+	
Icelandic isolate - RB-3	+	increases ethanol production from 20 to 40 mM.
Mb. thermoautotrophicum	-	
Micrococcus lactilyticus	-	
Desulfobacter postgatei	-	

Desulfotomaculum does not exhibit a growth response to added PP_i. We were unable to detect a stimulation of the growth of Escherichia coli by PP_i under aerobic conditions; however, the possible effect of PP_i under anaerobic conditions has not yet been investigated. Thermoanaerobacter ethanolicus, a thermophilic ethanol producing bacterium recently described by Wiegel and Ljungdahl [44] has been found to utilize PP_i (0.05%) as a growth substrate in the presence of yeast extract (0.2%) and salts. Clostridium thermocellum has also been observed to utilize PP_i as a source of energy for growth but it has not yet been established whether this is valid for all clostridia. A new isolate RB-3 from Iceland which grows at pH 8 from 45-90°C and ferments starch to several products including ethanol, lactate, acetate, and CO_2 also grows with yeast extract plus PP_i as the sole source of energy [23]. In the presence of starch and PP_i, the amount of ethanol is increased from 20 to 40 mM and suggests the possible utility of PP_i for altering fermentation patterns of anaerobic bacteria. No effect of PP_i on the growth of Mb. thermoautotrophicum, Micrococcus lactilyticus and Desulfobacter postgatei have as yet been observed.

The Enzymology of PP_i Utilization

PP_i:acetate kinase activity has been reported to be present in extracts of Dt. nigrificans, Dt. ruminis, and Dt. orientis [21] and proposed to be an essential enzyme for the reduction of sulfate by Desulfotomaculum, We have purified the PP_i:acetate kinase in good yield (50%) from extracts of T. ethanolicus grown at 50^oC on glucose. A molecular weight of 58,500 was obtained from gel filtration on a standardized Sephedex G-150 and the enzyme was judged to be pure based on the observation of a single band of protein by polyacrylamide disc gel electrophoresis. Electrophoresis on SDS polyacrylamide gels indicates a single protein subunit of molecular weight, 56,000. Interestingly the enzyme exhibited acetate kinase activity (Eq. 6) in addition to PP_i:acetate kinase (Eq. 5) in a ratio of about 2 and was free of adenylate kinase activity. Both activities had an absolute requirement for Mg^{+2} and several divalent cations, (Co^{+2}, Cd^{+2}, Ni^{+2}, Ca^{+2}) were found to replace Mg^{+2}.

$$6. \quad ATP + acetate \xrightleftharpoons{Mg^{+2}} acetyl\text{-}P + ADP$$

The acetate kinase activity was found to be reversible; however, we were unable to detect the formation of PP_i from acetyl phosphate plus P_i. Consistent with the presence of both PP_i acetate kinase and acetate kinase activities, the purified enzyme catalyzed the acetate dependent formation of ATP and P_i from PP_i and ADP (Eq. 7).

Table 8

PP_i Dependent Acetate Kinase Activity in Various Bacteria

Microorganism	Activity (μ mol/min./mg)
C. thermohydrosulfuricum	0.47
C. formicoaceticum (SMG 92)	0.30
C. tertium (NCTC 541)	0.19
C. thermoaceticum	0.34
E. coli (from Sigma)	0.11
D. desulfuricans (27774 strain MB)	0.26
C. thermoautotrophicum	+
D. gigas	+
C. thermocellum (27405 strain VP17372)	+
Methanosarcina barkerii	0.14
Dt. nigrificans (ATCC 19998)	0.22
T. ethanolicus (strain JW200)	0.40

PP_i dependent activity was determined with dialyzed crude extract. All assays were performed at 37°C or 40°C with 0.068 M PP_i, K Acetate 1.00 M, Tris/HCl pH 8.0 0.1 M, $MgCl_2$ 0.005 M, in the presence of about 35 μg of protein in a volume of 1 ml. The reaction was stopped with $HgCl_2$ and the presence of acetyl phosphate was determined by the procedure of Lipmann and Tuttle (19).

7. $$PP_i + ADP \longrightarrow ATP + P_i$$

The distribution of PP_i:acetate kinase in various bacteria has been investigated and the results are presented in Table 8. It is clear that this activity is widely distributed among bacteria as is acetate kinase; however, there is no positive correlation between the ability to utilize PP_i as a source of energy and the presence of PP_i: acetate kinase activity. Alternatively another PP_i:acetate kinase may be involved in the microbial utilization of PP_i and this possibility is being explored.

DISCUSSION OF DATA

The utilization of inorganic pyrophosphate and other polyphosphates as a source of energy for the growth of microorganisms is an entirely new observation and a unique concept regarding the energy metabolism of anaerobic bacteria and possibly aerobic microorganisms. It appears to have many important ramifications for basic biology, microbial ecology, and applied microbiology. As we now understand the system in the sulfate reducing bacteria belonging to the genus Desulfotomaculum, it represents, overall, the simplest ATP generating system in the biological world requiring only one specific enzyme, acetate kinase. Clearly, information regarding the basic biology of the microorganisms capable of utilizing PP_i plus the physiology and biochemistry of the phenomenon will add to our basic understanding of biology, specifically microbial bioenergetics and their ecological relationships.

The complex nutritional situation required for the growth of Desulfotomaculum on PP_i is not completely understood. The membranes of these and other bacteria must be permeable to PP_i; however, the factors involved in its transport by anaerobic bacteria have not been defined. Similarly, the physiological basis for the high acetate required for growth of Desulfotomaculum has not been examined but it may involve the bioenergetics of the permeation of acetate into the bacteria [13] and, thus far, this requirement appears to be unique to Desulfotomaculum. With other microorganisms the nutritional situation for the growth of PP_i appears to be quite simple, requiring only yeast extract and salts in addition to PP_i. From our studies with PP_i enrichment cultures, growth of existing strains of microorganisms and enzymological studies, the ability to utilize PP_i as a source of energy appears to be widely distributed among anaerobic bacteria. This utilization of PP_i can be indicated by growth with PP_i serving as the energy source or by alteration of metabolic activities without increase in growth such as the stimulation of methane formation and acetate accumulation by *Ms. barkeri* induced by the inclusion of PP_i in growth media. The growth of bacteria on PP_i has been demonstrated by increase in bacteria counts, increase in protein and the hydrolysis of PP_i occurring concomitantly with growth. The possibility that PP_i allows growth on yeast extract by removing inhibitors seems to be excluded by the fact that peptone or casamino acids can substitute for the yeast extract during growth on PP_i by the purine-fermenting isolates.

From our biochemical studies, it appears that PP_i can be converted to ATP by a single protein having PP_i:acetater kinase and acetate kinase activities. Thus a bacterium possessing this enzyme but unable to grow on PP_i should be able to generate excess ATP. This additional energy may be wasted or effect regulatory control by altering the adenylate pool. With *Ms. barkeri* and *T. ethanolicus* we have observed changes in fermentation patterns and suggest that PP_i may be useful as a metabolic probe for the investigation of unknown metabolic pathways and enzyme regulation in anaerobic microorganisms.

The utilization of tripolyphosphate and tetrapolyphosphate as growth substrates for anaerobic bacteria is a recent observation and the fact that it has been possible to carry enrichment cultures through ten successive transfers on both substrates demonstrates that such organisms do indeed exist. There appear to be different microbial populations involved in the utilization of these two polyphosphates and we are in the process of isolating pure cultures of these bacteria from each type of enrichment culture. Polyphosphates are known to be synthesized by a large number of microorganisms [12] and, from the standpoint of microbial ecology, a widespread occurrence of polyphosphate utilizing anaerobic bacteria may indicate that these organisms participate in a new type of energy cycle. The enzymatic mechanism of polyphosphate utilization has not been investigated; however the fact that all enrichment cultures grow rapidly on PP_i suggests that tripolyphosphate and tetrapolyphosphate are converted to PP_i by specific phosphatases prior to utilization. The failure of tripolyphosphate enrichment cultures to grow rapidly on tetrapolyphosphate and tetrapolyphosphate enrichment cultures to grow rapidly on tripolyphosphate implicates different enzyme systems in the utilization of these compounds.

PP_i:acetate kinase has only been found in extracts of *Entamoeba histolytica* by Reeves and Guthrie [35] but they did not extensively purify the enzyme because of the difficulty in obtaining sufficient amounts of amoeba. The enzyme did not exhibit acetate kinase activity with ATP and acetate or ATP formation in the reverse reaction with ADP and acetyl phophate. In the direction of acetyl phosphate formation, the rate of the reaction catalyzed by the enzyme is only 2% of the rate of the reaction in the direction of PP_i formation. Purification of the PP_i acetate kinase from *T. ethanolicus* yields an enzyme which has ATP:acetate kinase activity and does not catalyze the formation of PP_i from P_i and acetyl phosphate. At the present time it is not clear as to the relationship between these two kinase activities or whether there exists a second enzyme possessing only PP_i:acetate kinase activity, similar to that found in *E. histolytica*, in extracts of some of these anaerobic bacteria. The widespread distribution of acetate kinase in bacteria and its ability to utilize either ATP or PP_i as phosphoryl donor would [29] explain the utilization of PP_i as a source of energy in anaerobic bacteria.

The stimulation of microbial growth by PP_i has a number of potential applications in applied microbiology and it should be noted that PP_i is a common and inexpensive chemical. The growth on PP_i of *T. ethanolicus*, a thermophilic fermentative anaerobe, was unexpected but the fact that these types of organisms can metabolize PP_i suggests the possibility that PP_i can be used to modify or alter the pattern of fermentation products. Thus, *T.ethanolicus* forms, from a mole of glucose, 1.8 moles of ethanol, 0. 1 moles of acetate and 0.1 moles lactate. The accumulation of acetate and lactate limit the usefulness of the organism for the continuous production of ethanol but the addition of PP_i may remove, reduce, or eliminate the formation of acetate and lactate and thereby facilitate the continuous production of ethanol by this organism. *Desulfotomaculum* and *Methanosarcina* are intimately involved in the microbial conversion of cellulose or biomass to methane and carbon dioxide. As the conversion of acetate to methane and carbon dioxide (*Methanosarcina*) and the conversion of fermentation products (lactate, fatty acids, alcohols) to acetate, CO_2, and H_2 (*Desulfotomaculum*) are limiting steps in this important biological process, the stimulatory effects of PP_i on these bacteria suggest the possibility that PP_i may significantly stimulate the rate of methane formation and concomitant degradation of biomass. We now have preliminary evidence which indicates that this is indeed the case. If our results are substantiated by further investigation they will have significant impact on the production of methane from biomass for energy and the removal of organic wastes.

ACKNOWLEDGEMENTS

These studies were supported by a grant from the U.S. Department of Energy under contract No. DEAS-09-79-ER-10499 to Harry D. Peck and Lars G. Ljungdahl; the University of Georgia Research Foundation and the National Science Foundation, PCM 8205593 to Harry D. Peck.

REFERENCES

1. Akagi, J.M. and L.L. Campbell. 1962. Studies on thermophilic sulfate-reducing bacteria III Adenosine triphosphate sulfurylase of *Clostridium nigrificans* and *Desulfovibrio desulfuricans*. J. Bacteriol. 84:1194-1201.

2. Akagi, J.M. and L.L. Campbell. 1963. Inorganic pyrophosphatase of Desulfovibrio desulfuricans. J. Bacteriol. 86:563-568.

3. Badziong, W. and R.K. Thauer. 1978. Growth yields and growth rates of Desulfovibrio vulgaris (Marburg) growing on hydrogen and sulfate and hydrogen and thiosulfate as sole energy sources. Arch. Microbiol. 117:209-214.

4. Baltscheffsky, H. and L. von Stedingk. 1966. Bacterial photophosphorylation in the absence of added nucleotide. A second intermediate state of energy transfer of light-induced formation of ATP. Biochem. Biophys. Res. Commun. 22:722-725.

5. Baltscheffsky, M. 1969. Energy conversion-linked changes of carotenoid absorbance in Rhodospirillum rubrum chromatophores. Arch. Biochem. Biophys. 130:646-652.

6. Bramlett, R.N. and H.D. Peck, Jr.1975. Some physical and kinetic properties of adenylyl sufate reductase from Desulfovibrio vulgaris. J. Biol. Chem. 250:2979-2986.

7. Cagen, L.M. and H.C. Friedman. 1972. Enzymatic phosphorylation of serine. J. Biol. Chem. 247:3382-3392.

8. Carnal, N.W. and C.C. Black. 1979. Pyrophosphate-dependent 6-phosphofructokinase, a new glycolytic enzyme in pineapple leaves. Biochem. Biophys. Res. Commun. 86:20-26.

9. Dilworth, G., J. Wiegel, L.G. Ljungdahl, and H.D. Peck, Jr. 1980. Reconstitution of mesophilic microbial associations which ferment cellulose to various products. In "Colloque Cellulose Microbienne" Centre National de la Recerche Scientifique, Marseille pp. 111-126.

10. Evans, H.J. and H.G. Wood. 1968. The mechanism of the pyruvate phosphate dikinase reaction. Proc. Natl. Acad. Sci. (US) 61:1448-1453.

11. Hatch, M.D. and C.R. Slack. 1968. A new enzyme for the interconversion of pyruvate and phosphopyruvate and its role in the CH_4 dicarboxylic acid pathway of photosynthesis. Biochem. J. 106:141-146.

12. Harold, F.M., 1966. Inorganic polyphosphates in Biology:

structure, metabolism and function. Bacteriol Rev. 30:772-794.

13. Kell, D.B., M.W. Peck, G. Roger, and J.G. Morris. 1981. On the permeability to weak acids and bases of the cytoplasmic membrane of Clostridium pasteurianum. Biochem. Biophys. Res. Commun. 99:81-88.

14. Kobayashi, K., Y. Morisawa, T. Ishitoka, and M. Ishimoto. 1975. Biochemical studies on sulfate reducing bacteria. XIV. Enzyme levels of adenylyl sulfate reductase, inorganic pyrophosphatase, sulfite reductase, hydrogenase and adenosine triphosphatase in cells grown on sulfate, sulfite and thiosulfate. J. Biochem. (Tokyo) 78:1079-1085.

15. Kornberg, A. 1957. Pyrophosphorylases and phosphorylases in biosynthetic reactions. Adv. Enzymol. 18:191-240.

16. Kulaev, I.S., E.B. Mansurova, E.B. Borlakova, and V.F. Dukhovich. 1980. Why ATP instead of pyrophosphate? Interrelation between ATP and pyrophosphate production during evolution and in contemporary organisms. Bio. Systems. 12:177-180.

17. Lawson, J.W.R., R.W. Guynn, M. Cornell, and R.L. Veech. In: "Gluconeogenesis, its regulation in mammalian species (Ed. R.W. Hanson and M.A. Mehlman) pp. 48. Wiley, New York 1976.

18. Lee, J.P., J. LeGall, and H.D. Peck, Jr. 1973. Isolation of assimilatory and dissimilatory-type sulfite reductases from Desulfovibrio vulgaris. J. Bacteriol. 115:529-542.

19. Lipmann, F. and L.C. Tuttle. 1945. A specific micro-method for the determination of acylphosphates. J. Biol. Chem. 259:21-28.

20. Lipmann, F. 965. Projecting backward from the present stage of the evolution of biosynthesis. In (S.W. Fox, Ed) "The Origins of Prebiological Systems", pp. 259-280. Academic Press, N.Y.

21. Liu, C.-L. and H.D. Peck, Jr. 1981. Comparative bioenergetics of sulfate reduction in Desulfovibrio and Desulfotomaculum sp. J. Bacteriol. 145:966-973.

22. Liu, C.-L., N. Hart, and H.D. Peck, Jr. 1982. The utilization of inorganic pyrophosphate as a source of energy for the growth

of sulfate reducing bacteria, Desulfotomaculum sp. Science (in press).

23. Ljungdahl, L.G., F. Bryant, L. Carreira, T. Saiki, and J. Wiegel. 1981. Some aspects of thermophilic and extreme thermophilic anaerobic microorganisms. In Trends in the Biology of Fermentations for Fuels and Chemicals. (Hollaender, A. Ed.) Plenum Press, N.Y. Vol. 18. Basic Life Sciences, pp. 397-419.
24. Macy, J.M., L.G. Ljungdahl, and G. Gottschalk. 1978. Pathway of succinate and propionate formation in Bacteroides fragilis. J. Bacteriol. 134:84-91.
25. Mansurova, S.E., Yu. A. Schakhov, and I.S. Kolaev. 1977. Mitochondrial pyrophosphatase is a coupling factor of respiration and pyrophosphate synthesis. FEBS Lett. 74:31-34.
26. O'Brien, W.E., S. Bowien, and H.G. Wood. 1975. Isolation and characterization of a pyrophosphate-dependent phosphofructokinase from Propionibacterium shermanii. J. Biol. Chem. 250: 8690-8695.
27. Odom, J.M. and H.D. Peck, Jr. 1981. Localization of dehydrogenases, reductases and electron transfer components in the sulfate-reducing bacterium, Desulfovibrio gigas. J. Bacteriol. 147:161-169.
28. Odom, J.M. and H. D. Peck, Jr. 1981. Hydrogen cycling as a general mechanism for energy coupling in the sulfate reducing bacteria, Desulfovibrio sp. FEMS Lett. 12:47-50.
29. Peck, H.D., Jr. 1962. Comparative metabolism of inorganic sulfur compounds in microorganisms. Bacteriol. Rev. 26:67-94.
30. Pfennig, N. and F. Widdel. 1981. Ecology and physiology of some anaerobic bacteria from the microbial sulfur cycle in "Biology of Inorganic Nitrogen and Sulfur". (Ed. H. Bothe and A. Trebst). pp. 169-177. Springer-Verlag, Berlin.
31. Pfleiderer, C. and J.-H. Klemme. 1980. Pyrophosphate-abhangige D-fructose-6-phosphate phosphotransferase in Rhodospirillaceae. Z. Natur forsch. 35c:229-238.
32. Postgate, J.R. 1979. The sulphate-reducing bacteria. Cambridge

University Press, Cambridge, England.

33. Reeves, R.E. 1968. A new enzyme with the glycolytic function of pyruvate kinase. J. Biol. Chem. 243:3202-3204.
34. Reeves, R.E., D.J. South, H.J. Blytt, and L.G. Warren. 1974. Pyrophosphate: D-fructose 6-phosphate 1-phosphotransferase. A new enzyme with the glycolytic function of 6-phosphofructokinase. J. Biol. Chem. 249:7737-7741.
35. Reeves, R.E. and J.B. Guthrie. 1975. Acetate kinase (pyrophosphate). A fourth pyrophosphate-dependent kinase from *Entamoeba histolytica*. Biochem. Biophys. Res. Commun. 66:1389-1395.
36. Reeves, R.E. 1976. How useful is the energy in inorganic pyrophosphate? TIBS 1:53-55.
37. Rubtzov, P.M., N.V. Efremovich, and I.S. Kulaev. 1976. The light-dependent synthesis of pyrophosphate in chloroplasts. Dokl. AN USSR 230:1236-1237.
38. Searcy, R. L., N.M. Simms, J.A. Foreman, and L.M. Bergquist. 1965. A study of the specificity of the Berthelot reaction. Clin. Chim. Acta. 12:170-175.
39. Siu, P.M.L. and H.G. Wood. 1962. Phosphoenolpyruvic carboxytransphosphorylase, a CO_2 fixation enzyme from propionic acid bacteria. J. Biol. Chem. 237:3044-3501.
40. Stewart, G.J. and J.W. Fitzgerald. 1982. Metabolism of exogenous uridine 5'-triphosphate, adenosine 5'-triphosphate and pyrophosphate by alkyl-sulfatase-producing bacteria. Int. J. Biochem. 13:1019-1026.
41. Ware, D.A. and J.R. Postgate. 1971. Physiological and chemical properties of a reductant-activated inorganic pyrophosphatase from *Desulfovibrio desulfuricans*. J. Gen. Microbiol. 67:145-160.
42. Widdel, F. 1980 . Anaerober Abbau von Fettsauren und Benzioesaure durch neu isolierte Arten sulfalreduzierender Bakterien Dissertation, Univ. Gottingen.
43. Widdel, F. and N. Pfennig. 1977. A new anaerobic sporing

acetate oxidizing sulfate-reducing bacterium Desulfotomaculum (emend) acetoxidans. Arch. Microbiol. 112:119-122.

44. Wiegel, J., and L.G. Ljungdahl. 1981. Thermoanaerobacter ethanolicus gen. nov., spec. nov., a new extreme thermophilic anaerobic bacterium. Arch. Microbiol. 128:343-348.

45. Wilson, L.G. and R.S. Bandurski. 1958. Enzymatic reactions involving sulfate, sulfite, selenate and molybdate. J. Biol. chem. 233:975-981.

46. Wolin, E.A., M. J. Wolin, and R.S. Wolfe. 1963. Formation of methane by bacterial extracts. J. Biol. Chem. 238:2882

47. Wood, H.G. 1977. Some reactions in which inorganic pyrophosphate replaces ATP and serves as a source of energy. Fed. Proc. 36:2197-2205.

48. Wood, H.G., W.E. O'Brien, and G. Michaels. 1977. Properties of carboxytransphosphorylase; pyruvate phosphate dikinase; pyrophosphate phosphofructokinase and pyrophoshate-acetate kinase and their role in the metabolism of pyrophosphate. Adv. Enzymology 45:85-155.

DISCUSSION

Q. C. COONEY (MIT): Can you comment on the problems of synthesizing, inorganically, pyrophosphate or the pholyphosphates?

A. PECK: You can buy pyrophosphate for 37 cents a pound FOB Jolliet, Illinois, and its price is not out of reach for using it in some of these fermentations if its effect is catalytic. It is a common inorganic chemical and is used extensively in agriculture.

Q. P.STARLINGER (Universitat zu Köln): How long will it be before the prices of phosphate and phosphate derivatives go up as the price of oil had done recently, and will there be any bacteriological breakthrough to recover phosphate from wastewater?

A. PECK: You're quite right, increased use of PP_i could well at some time change its economics. One of the things that we're considering is that PP_i and polyphosphate are involved in cyclic energy metabolism possibly in microbial mats. In microbial mats there may be a polyphosphate transfer system because as you know, many of the algae and the bacteria that comprise the mat make polyphosphates. Perhaps we'll be actually recovering phosphate through some of these biological systems since they are really widespread in nature.

C. A. BULL (Univ. of Kent at Canterbury): If I may make a brief a comment on that very last point, a recent process development in the activated sludge process has led to exactly this situation and, in fact, by some rather interesting multistate systems going from anaerobic to anoxic to aerobic tanks, one can encourage this slude to over accumulate phosphate to a very large measure phosphate in this way.

Q. PECK: Do you know if it accumulate as orthophosphate or as polyphosphate.

A. BULL: I think it's polyphosphate.

C. PECK: That's really very exciting. We thought that possibly one of the reasons that people have not found PP_i in nature is that PP_i is an intermediate in energy transfer. In the rumen fermentation, hydrogen was for a long time difficult to identify as an intermediate because while it was indeed an intermediate, it never accumulated in large amounts and it was necessary to look at turn over rates to demonstrate that hydrogen is an intermediate in this fermentation. If pyrophosphate is an intermediate in a phosphate energy transfer system in nature,its concentration is bound to be very low and it will be necessary to look at turnover rates.

Q. J. E. TREND (3M Company): Would you speculate about the importance of inorganic phosphate energy systems in the evolution of microbes that predate ATP as an energy system?

A. PECK: Many years ago, Fritz Lipmann proposed that inorganic pyrophosphate is an evolutionary precursor of ATP. We've done some biochemical studies to look at the enzyme systems involved in PP_i utilization and we've found that acetate kinase which is universally distributed among bacteria is able to use inorganic pyrophosphate in addition to ATP. One can add inorganic pyrophosphate, plus ADP in the presence in a trace amount of acetate and make ATP and Pi. When you give pyrophosphate to these anaerobic bacteria they can very rapidly convert it to ATP. Now, as far as whether it is an intermediate in energy metabolism some of these fermentations that involve pyrophosphate may be really hangovers from other evolutionary times and are able to use pyrophosphate instead of ATP. But I would point that pyrophosphate metabolism goes in and out of vogue and I suspect that many of these reactions haven't really been extensively with tested with pyrophosphate as a phosphate donor.

GENETIC STRATEGIES IN STRAIN DESIGN FOR FERMENTATIONS

Graham C. Walker
Biology Department
Massachusetts Institute of Technology
Cambridge, Massachusetts 02139

INTRODUCTION

The impact of biotechnology on the production of fuels and chemicals will depend in part upon advances in our ability to genetically manipulate microorganisms of commercial interest. Many of the goals of successful fermentations such as high product yield, high rates of product formation, absence of undesired side products, reduced production of cell mass, and lack of end-product inhibition can be achieved, at least in principle, by the use of a combination of genetic and *in vitro* recombinant DNA approaches. However, many of the bacteria, particularly anaerobes, that are useful for producing fuels and chemicals have not yet been the object of detailed genetic or molecular biological study.

In this paper I will review some of the genetic strategies that my laboratory has found useful for strain design with *Escherichia coli*, an organism with a well developed system for genetic study. A number of these strategies can be employed with other bacteria after the investment of only a relatively modest amount of developmental work. I will focus particularly on applications of insertion mutagenesis and on the use of operon fusions, and will try to emphasize the power of combining genetic techniques with in vitro recombinant DNA techniques. I will then attempt to assess the possibility of implementing similar methods of strain construction in two groups of anaerobic bacteria that are of particular interest for the production of fuels and chemicals, the clostridia and the methanogens.

Transposable Elements as Tools for Strain Construction

Many of the recent advances in bacterial genetics have been based on the innovative application of transposable elements - segments of DNA that are capable of inserting more or less randomly into other DNA molecules. In bacteria, transposable elements include: (i) insertion sequences (IS), which are relatively short pieces of DNA (600-2000 bp) that encode only a function necessary for the IS to transpose; (ii) transposons, which are somewhat longer pieces of DNA (2500-40,000 bp) that encode not only a transposition function but also some other function such as a drug resistance, bacteriocin production, a particular metabolic capability etc.; and (iii) certain bacteriophage, such as Mu, that are capable of integrating into the host chromosome essentially at random. These elements appear to be ubiquitous in nature and have probably played significant roles in evolution.

Transposable elements possess a number of desirable properties that make them particularly valuable as tools in strain construction. Mutations generated by the insertion of a transposable genetic element tend to be null alleles resulting in complete loss of function; furthermore, since many such elements are polar, loss of function can result not only from insertion within the gene of interest but also from insertion upstream within the same transcriptional unit. The presence on transposons of positively-selectable markers, such as drug resistance, facilitates the mapping and genetic manipulation of mutations generated by the insertion of such elements. Furthermore, since the insertion of a transposable element into a gene results in the introduction of a new segment of DNA, the position of that insertion can be mapped by the use of physical techniques such as restriction endonuclease cleavage analysis, Southern blotting, and electron microscopic heteroduplex analysis. We have repeatedly taken advantage of these properties in our studies of gene function, regulation, and organization in *E. coli*.

Efficient Screening. Insertion mutagenesis is particularly helpful when the desired mutant cannot be selected for and must be identified by screening for a particular phenotype. Transposons are usually introduced into the bacterium on a vector such as a defective bacteriophage, temperature-sensitive plasmid, or "suicide" plasmid that cannot replicate or exist stably in that host.

Derivatives in which the element has transposed from the vector into the host's DNA can be obtained by selecting for the marker, such as a drug resistance, carried by the transposon. Screens of such derivatives are maximally efficient since each bacterium examined is a mutant and furthermore each bacterium is, in general, a single mutant.

Much of the work in my laboratory has been concerned with mutagenesis and DNA repair, and many of the mutations we have worked with have had to be identified by screening procedures.

For example, we have used insertion mutagenesis in order to obtain mutations in *umuC* (nonmutable with UV and many other mutagens, apparently defective in "error-prone repair" [4,16]) mutH, L, S, and uvrD (spontaneous mutators, apparently defective in methyl-instructed mismatch repair [49]), uvrA and uvrB (UV-sensitive, defective in excision repair [27]), and recB/C (sensitive to methyl methanesulfonate and recombination deficient, defective in exonuclease V [W.G. Shanabruch and G.C. Walker, unpublished results]). In addition, auxotrophs can be obtained at a frequency of approximately 1-2% and, as described below, we have used transposon mutagenesis in conjunction with operon fusions to isolate regulatory mutants.

Insertion mutagenesis is particularly useful when one is attempting to manipulate functions encoded on bacterial plasmids. Transposons are introduced into a bacterial cell carrying the plasmid of interest and derivatives are obtained as described above in which the transposon has inserted into either the bacterial or plasmid DNA. By then conjugating or transforming the plasmids to a new host and selecting for the marker carried by the transposon it is possible to obtain a set of derivatives of the plasmid, each of which carries a random insertion of the transposon. We have worked extensively with the mutagenesis-enhancing plasmid pKM101 which has played a critical role in the success of the Ames' test [34,35]. For example, mutagenesis by the transposon Tn5 has been used to obtain mutants of pKM101 (Fig. 1) that no longer increase the susceptibility of cells to mutagenesis (muc; ref. 48), cannot conjugally transfer (tra; ref. 30), lack β-lactamase activity (bla; ref. 30), exhibit a faster growth rate on minimal medium (slo; ref. 30), do not suppress the fertility of P-group plasmids (fip; S.C. Winans and G.C. Walker, unpublished observations), and are maintained with altered stability (S.C. Winans, P. Diamandis, and G.C. Walker, unpublished observations).

While it is useful to be able to carry out insertion mutagenesis directly in the bacterium of interest, it is still possible to exploit insertion mutagenesis to some extent even if no suitable transposable elements have yet been identified in that bacterium or no suitable vectors for introducing a transposon have been developed. This can be achieved by using a "shuttle" cloning vector that can replicate not only in the desired bacterium but also in some other bacterium such as *E. coli* that has a well developed genetic system. Insertions of transposons in cloned DNA of the organism can be obtained in *E. coli*, and the genes carrying insertion mutations can then subsequently be reintroduced into the original organism.

For example, Ruvkun and Ausubel [42] have used this strategy to obtain mutants of *Rhizobium meliloti* that are defective in nitrogen fixation.

Ease of Genetic Manipulation. Mutations generated by the insertion of a transposon are particularly easy to manipulate genetically since the mutations can be identified not only by the alteration in phenotype that they cause but also by the positively-selectable marker carried by the transposon. This makes them easy to map by whatever method of genetic exchange is employed - conjugation [26,27], transduction [16,26,36,49], or transformation - and aids in such strain constructions as making double mutants [49].

A transposon insertion does not even have to be within a gene of interest in order to be useful in strain constructions but only needs to be genetically linked to a desired mutation. For example, we routinely use a *srl*::Tn*10* mutation to introduce a *recA* mutation (which abolishes homologous recombination) into desired strains [54] and also use a Tn*5* insertion, which is not in a known gene but is genetically linked to the *umuC* locus, to move *umuC* mutations from one strain to another (C.J. Kenyon and G.C. Walker, unpublished results). Furthermore, once a transposon insertion has been obtained that is genetically linked to a gene of interest it is

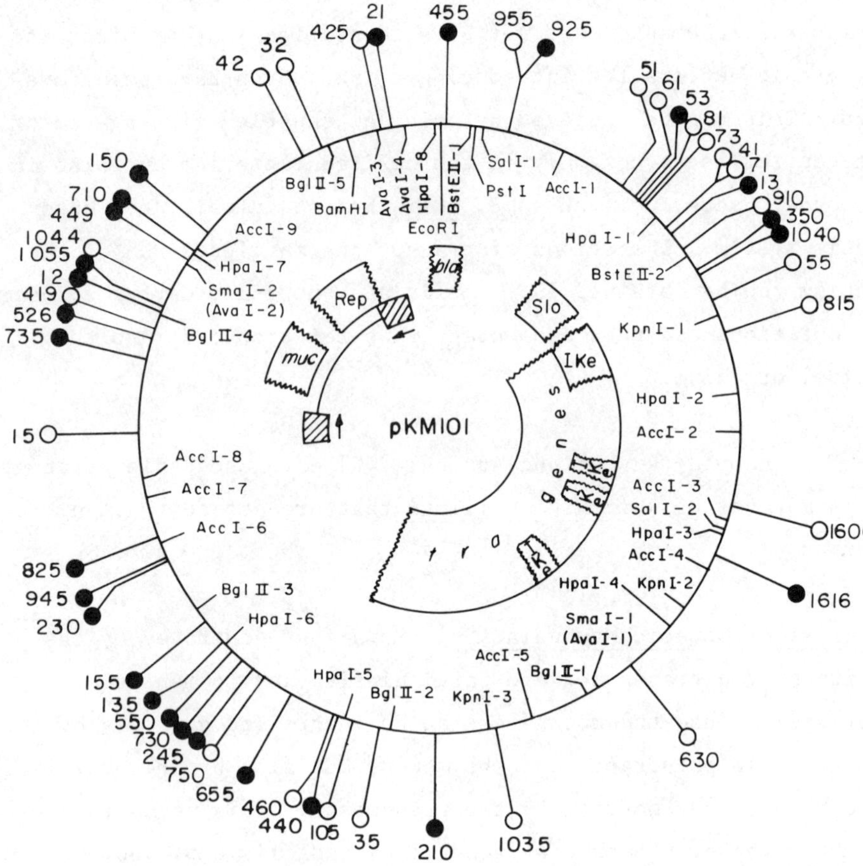

Fig. 1. pKM101 restriction map showing the position of 49 Tn5 insertions and regions of pKM101 DNA essential for pKM101 phenotypes. Restriction enzyme cleavage sites are numbered according to their clockwise order from the EcoRI site. Symbols: 0, Tn5 DNA in the minus orientation; 0, Tn5 in the plus orientation. The isolation numbers of Tn5 insertions are shown next to the symbols. The regions of DNA essential for pKM101 phenotypes are as follows: bla, ampicillin, resistance; Slo, slow growth; IKe, sensitivity to phage IKe; tra, conjugal transfer; muc, enhancement of UV and chemical mutagenesis; Rep, region essential for plasmid replication. The pKM101 inverted repeat and loop region is indicated by the two cross-hatched boxes connected with a line. Arrows indicate inverted repeats [30].

possible to then use techniques of "localized mutagenesis" to efficiently obtain base substitution mutations in that gene [29].

Physical Mapping of Insertion Mutations. Mutations resulting from the insertion of a transposable element into a cell's DNA can be mapped and manipulated by a variety of physical techniques. For example, mutants (*muc*) of the plasmid pKM101 were obtained after N-methyl-N'-nitro-N-nitrosoguanidine treatment that were unable to increase the susceptibility of cells to UV and chemical mutagenesis [53], however these mutants could not easily be mapped genetically because of their difficult phenotype and because of problems caused by the phenomenon of plasmid incompatibility. We therefore generated equivalent mutations by the insertion of the transposon Tn*5* into pKM101 and mapped them with relative ease by restriction endonuclease cleavage analysis [48]. The positions of the *muc* locus and other genetic loci on the pKM101 map are shown in Fig. 1 [30]. These same mutations were also mapped by electron microscopic procedures that took advantage of the fact that the ends of Tn*5* are inverted repeats; these experiments led to the additional interesting observation that the *muc* genes of pKM101 are themselves surrounded by inverted repeats and thus might be part of a transposon [30]. In another example, we recently used Tn*5* insertion mutagenesis to obtain regulatory mutations affecting the expression of genes induced by DNA damage (J.H. Krueger and G.C. Walker, unpublished observations). Certain of these mutations were in *lexA*, a gene which encodes a repressor for many of these damage-inducible genes. We were able to establish the exact position of these Tn*5* insertions in the *E. coli* chromosome by carrying out Southern blotter experiments using a probe [8] to the *lexA* gene (J.H. Krueger and G.C. Walker, unpublished results).

Transposable Elements as Mobile Restriction Sites. Once a series of insertion mutants have been obtained they are often useful for *in vitro* recombinant DNA experiments since the insertion of a transposable element into a DNA molecule results in the introduction of a set of restriction endonuclease sites at that position. It was relatively easy to delete the small SalI fragment (Fig. 1) from pKM101 by digesting pKM101 DNA with SalI, diluting and religating. Since Tn*5* has a SalI site, it was then possible to use Tn*5* derivatives of pKM101 to generate a series of deletion mutants that had lost increasingly larger amounts of plasmid DNA. For example, repeating the experiment with the pKM101 derivative carrying the Tn*5* insertion numbered 630 resulted in the deletion of DNA from the SalI-1 site to the positions of insertion 630 [30]. We have also used insertions to provide convenient sites for subcloning. For example, the *muc* genes were subcloned on a fragment that extended from the HpaI-7 site to the HpaI site in the Tn*5* insertion number 735 [38].

Identification of Gene Products. Proteins coded for by recombinant plasmids and other small plasmids can be visualized by the use of minicells [32] or "maxicells" [43]. However, since such plasmids may often code for several proteins, further work is usually necessary to identify the region of DNA coding for the protein of interest. Besides subcloning, an extremely useful approach is to obtain insertion mutations in the plasmid that disable the gene of interest and to then examine the protein products of that mutated plasmid. For example, Sancar *et al*. [30] used this approach to identify the *uvrA* gene product and we have used it to identify the *muc* and *umuC* gene products [16,38]. Since the truncated polypeptides can often be visualized, the direction of transcription of the gene of interest can also be established by this procedure.

Generating Probes to Genes of Interest. Some genes can be particularly difficult to clone, and transposable elements can sometimes be used to help identify the desired gene in a recombinant DNA library. For example, we were unsuccessful in identifying the umuC gene, whose product is required for UV and chemical mutagenesis, by screening recombinant plasmids for the ability to complement the nonmutability of a umuC mutant. We then employed the alternative strategy of using a umuC::Tn5 insertion mutant to generate a probe to the umuC gene. This was obtained by cloning the kanamycin resistance gene of Tn5 along with a piece of the adjacent DNA (Fig. 2). This probe was then used to screen a recombinant DNA library and the umuC gene was successfully identified and subsequently subcloned [16]. We are also using the same strategy to clone the mutH, L, S, and uvrD genes that are required for methyl-instructed mismatch repair [49; P. Pang and G.C. Walker, unpublished results.]

An interesting sidelight concerns the requirement for umuC function for UV and much chemical mutagenesis. E. coli is normally mutable by UV, methyl methanesulfonate, 4-nitroquinoline-1-oxide and many other mutagens, but a umuC mutation renders it nonmutable by these agents [25]. This fact argues strongly that the mutagenesis caused by UV and many agents requires the intervention of an active cellular process often termed "error-prone repair". In contrast, mutagens such as ethyl methanesulfonate and N-methyl-N'-nitro-N-nitrosoguanidine can introduce directly mispairing lesions (for example 0^6-alkylguanine) that do not require the participation of error-prone repair to be mutagenic. Interestingly a number of types of bacteria, for example methylotrophs, Proteus, and Haemophilus are nonmutable by UV [9] and thus may lack umuC function. In fact, the introduction of the umuC genes or analogs of these genes into Proteus mirabilis [20] and Salmonella typhimurium [12, G.C. Walker, unpublished results] greatly increases the susceptibility of these strains to mutagenesis by UV, arguing that they are nonmutable or poorly mutable because they are deficient in umuC function. Thus, in choosing mutagens for a new organism, it is useful to consider not only the possibility that the cells might have a very efficient

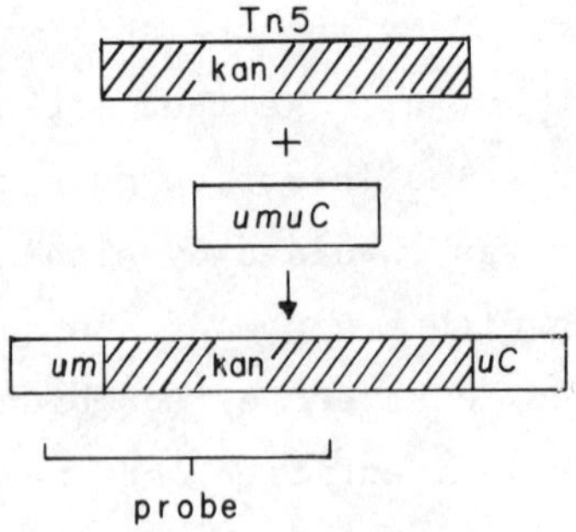

Fig. 2. Use of a Tn5 insertion mutation to generate a probe to the umuC gene of E. coli.

efficient accurate repair system for certain classes of DNA lesions but also the possibility that they may lack the ability to process certain types of lesions in such a way that mutations result.

Genetic Strategies Involving Operon Fusions

Another factor contributing to the power of modern bacterial genetics has been the development of facile methods for the construction of operon and gene fusions. By substituting a gene with an easily assayable product for the gene of interest, it is possible to analyze gene regulation in a relatively straightforward manner no matter what the function of the original gene. The gene most frequently used to date in constructing fusions is lacZ which codes for β-galactosidase but, in principle, any convenient gene could be used.

Two basic methods have been developed for the construction of lac operon fusions. The first is to use in vitro recombinant DNA technology to join a piece of DNA that contains the structural information for β-galactosidase but lacks the lac promoter/regulatory region to the promoter/regulatory region of the gene of interest [11]. This approach can be used in any organism for which cloning vectors are available. For *E. coli* and related bacteria, an *in vivo* method for creating *lac* operon fusions has been developed [10]. These operon fusion techniques give strains in which normal β-galactosidase molecules are produced. Analogous *in vitro* and *in vivo* methods have been developed for the construction of gene fusions in which hybrid β-galactosidase molecules are produced [11, 46].

Operon fusions allow studies of the regulation of any gene to be carried out conveniently and greatly facilitate the construction of strains that overproduce desired gene products. For example, we have used *lac* operon fusions in *E. coli* to investigate both the regulation of genes induced by DNA damage [28] and the regulation of genes involved in methionine biosynthesis [36]. In each case we have used the Mud(Ap, *lac*) bacteriophage constructed by Casadaban and Cohen [10] that allows operon fusions to be constructed *in vivo* in a single step. Mud(Ap, *lac*) is a derivative of bacteriophage Mu that is capable of integrating randomly into the bacterial chromosome. In Mud(Ap, *lac*), some of the phage genes have been removed and a β-lactamase gene has been introduced; thus Mud(Ap, *lac*) resembles a transposon in that it can insert randomly into DNA, and cells in which an insertion has occurred acquire a drug resistance. Mud(Ap, *lac*) also carries the structural genes for the *lac* operon but no promoter for those genes. Thus, when Mud(Ap, *lac*) inserts into the chromosome or a plasmid, no β-galactosidase is synthesized unless the insertion occurred downstream from a promoter and in the correct orientation, in which case an operon fusion results.

We used the Mud(Ap, *lac*) phage to search for genes that could be induced by DNA damage [26] and to obtain operon fusions to genes we suspected of being turned on in response to DNA damage. Once such fusions had been obtained, we were able to analyze the regulation of these din (damage-inducible) genes even though the functions of the din gene products are difficult to study physiologically or biochemically [4,26,28]. Similarly, we were able to use Mud(Ap, lac)-generated operon fusions in a study of the regulation of methionine biosynthesis [36]. We made random Tn5 insertions into metB::Mud(Ap, lac) and metE::Mud(Ap, lac) strains and screened for derivatives that expressed β-galactosidase at high levels even in the presence of high methionine. In addition to obtaining a number of mutants that caused increased production of methionine biosynthetic enzymes, we also obtained mutants affecting the transport of vitamin B12. Since these regulatory mutations had been generated by the insertion of the transposon Tn5, they were easy to study and manipulate genetically.

Anaerobic Fermentations

Anaerobic fermentations are of particular interest for the production of fuels and chemicals for a number of reasons including: (i) the wide range of substrates fermented and products formed; (ii) the high yields and rates with which substrates can be converted to products; (iii) the ability of a number of anaerobes to grow under unusual conditions such as high temperature, low pH, or high concentration of a solvent; and (iv) the technological advantages of anaerobic fermentations. Since there is not a need to constantly supply O_2, anaerobic fermentations can be carried out in reactors of simpler design and of larger volume. With thermophiles, the process heat can help reduce the energy cost of recovering volatile products.

There has been a particular interest in the possibilities of using anaerobic bacteria to ferment biomass, or substrates derived from biomass, to produce useful chemicals or fuels. The clostridia have attracted a considerable amount of attention because of their abilities to degrade biomass and their abilities to produce industrially useful organic molecules. Another interesting group of bacteria are the methanogens which are the organisms responsible for the production of the gaseous fuel methane. I will briefly review the possibilities of developing more powerful tools for strain construction with these two types of organisms.

Clostridia

A number of clostridia have properties which are useful in industrial applications. For example, *C. acetobutylicium* can be used to produce acetone-butanol [47] from a variety of low cost substrates including pentose sugars derived from biomass residues [57]. The homoacetic species, *C. formicoaceticum* [3] and *C. thermoaceticum* [17], are useful for the production of acetic acid. *C. thermosaccharolyticum* produces butyric acid as the major fermentation product during exponential growth [22]. Two thermophilic species are particularly promising for the production of ethanol from biomass: *C. thermocellum* [37], because of its ability to degrade cellulose, and *C. thermohydrosulfuricum*, [58] because of the high yields of ethanol that it produces.

In most cases, processes that utilize clostridia for the production of chemicals and fuels could be greatly improved if these bacteria could be readily manipulated by genetic and *in vitro* recombinant DNA technologies. For example, the production of known fermentation products could be optimized or metabolic pathways could be altered so that different products accumulate. In some cases, altering the side products that are produced might make the fermentation more economically attractive. These goals can be achieved by the isolation of regulatory mutations, by overproduction of particular enzymes, by blocking certain pathways, by isolating mutants resistant to end-product inhibition, etc.

Prospects for Genetic Manipulation. Clostridia have been the object of relatively few genetic studies. A simple defined medium has been developed for *C. thermocellum* [24] and a few auxotrophs were isolated after penicillin enrichment [33]. Mutagenesis by UV is apparently only modestly effective and it is possible that *C. thermocellum* carries out relatively little "error-prone repair". Other mutagens such as ethyl methanesulfonate (EMS) that do not require error-prone repair processing might be more effective. EMS has been used to mutagenize *C. acetobutylicum* during the isolation of an autolysis-deficient mutant [1]. Some clostridia mutants that have been described, such as a derivative of *C. thermoacetium* capable of growth and acid production at pH 4.5, probably contain multiple mutations [45].

An insertion sequence has been identified in *C. thermocellum* that is capable of transposition in *E. coli* as well as in its original host [19]. The IS sequence is 1.4 kb in length and seems to have similar properties to insertion sequences found in *E. coli*. The identification of this transposable element opens up the possibilities for using insertion mutagenesis techniques similar to those described above for *E. coli*.

Many transposons in *E. coli* such as Tn*9* and Tn*5* consist of a gene for a selectable marker flanked by two copies of an IS sequence. Thus, even if naturally-occurring transposons are not identified in *Clostridia* species it should be possible to use *in vitro* recombinant techniques to construct useful transposons. Interestingly, studies of the *C. perfringens* plasmid, pIP401, revealed that the plasmid frequently lost a 6 kb segment of DNA that carried chloramphenicol resistance [7]; this phenomenon might possibly indicate the presence of a chloramphenicol-resistance transposon or at least an insertion sequence on this plasmid.

In addition to improving methods for making mutations, it will be necessary to develop methods for the transfer of genetic information so that constructions of desired strains can be carried out. Once again, relatively little work has been done on this problem, but a few results are quite encouraging. For example, during their studies of _C. perfringens_ plasmids, Brefort _et al_. [7] were able to obtain a derivative that was capable of promoting the exchange of chromosomal genes apparently by a conjugational process. Eklund and Poysky [15] reported an apparent instance of transduction in _C. botulinum_, an observation that suggests it may be possible to isolate transducing phage for various clostridial strains. A recent paper by Allcock _et al_. [2] has described the production and regeneration of stable _C. acetobutylicum_ protoplasts, and preliminary experiments with bacteriophage DNA indicated that these protoplasts could be used for transformation. The availability of a method for producing protoplasts opens the possibility of using protoplast fusion techniques [21] in clostridia.

Prospects for In Vitro Recombinant DNA Approaches. A bank of _C. thermocellum_ DNA has been prepared in _E. coli_ [19] but no direct cloning of clostridia DNA in clostridia has yet been reported.

However, the prospects for the development of clostridial host/vector system seems quite good. A number of plasmids have been reported in _C. perfringens_ such as pIP401 (54 kb, Tc^R and Cm^R, conjugally transferable) [7], pIP402 (63 kb, Em^R and Cl^R) [7], pCW3 (30.6 megadaltons, Tc^R, conjugally transferable)[42], pCW 4 (36.4 megadaltons, cryptic) [42] and pHB101 (2.1 megadaltons, caseinase activity)[6]. In addition a series of toxinogenic plasmids have been described in _C. perfringens_ [13]. Some of the smaller plasmids such as pHB101 might be relatively easily manipulated *in vitro* to produce a suitable cloning vector for, at least, *C. perfringens*. Whether such a vector would replicate in other species of *Clostridium* would need to be established empirically. In the case of the conjugally proficient plasmids, it may be possible to test their ability to replicate in a particular species by introducing them by a conjugal transfer. For other industrially important species of clostridia, systematic efforts should be made to screen for drug resistance plasmids that could be used as cloning vectors.

Besides the need for a vector, the other requirement for a host vector system is a means of introducing the recombinant DNA back into the host. The preliminary results referred to above concerning transformation of *C. acetobutylicum* protoplasts are certainly encouraging in this regard [2]. Once a suitable vector and transformation system is available, a number of the strategies I have discussed for strain construction could begin to be used in *Clostridium*.

Methanogens

The methanogens are a specialized group of microorganisms, operating at the terminus of an anaerobic food chain, that produce methane mostly from acetate and hydrogen/carbon dioxide. They are strict anaerobes and a number of thermophilic strains have been isolated [56,58]. Methanogens are of interest not only because they produce the gaseous fuel methane but because of their importance in the anaerobic digestion of biomass. By removing H_2, methanogens provide a thermodynamically more favorable environment for other organisms to ferment more complex organic molecules [31] and by utilizing acetate they prevent short chain organic acids from building up to inhibitory levels [58].

A recent treatment of the taxonomy of the methanogens based on a comparative analysis of their 16S ribosomal RNAs has led to the methanogens being classified as archaebacteria, a group which also includes the extreme halophiles and the thermoacidophiles [5,18]. The archaebacteria have a number of characteristics that set them apart from other bacteria (eubacteria), and the suggestion has been made that the archaebacteria constitute a third "primary kingdom" separate from the eubacteria and the eukaryotes.

Regardless of the evolutionary significance of the classification of methanogens as archaebacteria, the fact remains that the methanogens differ in a number of significant respects from most of the microorganisms that have been the object of genetic and microbiological study, and these differences will have to be considered in the development of tools for strain construction.

For example, the cell walls of the archaebacteria contain no muramic acid and so do not contain the rigid cell wall polymer, peptidoglycan, which is a universal constituent of the cell walls of true bacteria [18]. Furthermore, they do not contain D-amino acids, diaminopimellic acid, or teichoic acid [5,55]. Practical consequences of these differences are that methanogens are sensitive to neither penicillin nor cycloserine, drugs commonly used for mutant enrichment, nor are they susceptible to lysozyme, an enzyme widely used in plasmid isolations and in protoplast formation. In another example, the RNA polymerases of the archaebacteria seem to have radically different subunit structures from the $\beta\beta'\alpha_2{}^{o}$ structure of eubacterial RNA polymerase [59], and it is still unclear to what extent our knowledge of the properties of eubacterial polymerases can be extrapolated to archaebacterial polymerases.

Prospects for Genetic Manipulation. There have been to date no genetic studies of methanogens. However, the nutritional requirements of most of the methanogens are known. For example, *Methanobacterium thermoautotrophicum* can grow at 65°C using H_2/CO_2 as its sole energy and carbon source [56]. It should be possible to initiate genetic studies by isolating auxotrophs although, as noted above, penicillin enrichments could not be used.

Since so little work has been done with methanogens, the prospects for genetic manipulation can probably best be judged by consideration of the properties of the extreme halophiles, organisns apparently closely related to the methanogens [18]. Spontaneous mutants of *Halobacterium halobium* arise at very high frequency [44] and mutants defective in pigment synthesis arise at a frequency of approximately 10^{-3} (R. Dunn, personal communication). Sapienza and Doolittle [44] have shown that two strains of *H. halobium* contain 400 dispersed repetitive sequence families, at least some of which are insertion sequences or transposons. Many of the mutants of *H. halobium* which have been isolated apparently result from the insertion of these mobile elements (U.L. RajBhandary, personal communication). These observations suggest that methanogens will probably contain transposable elements but also raise the possibility that they would be relatively genetically unstable and difficult to work with. However, even if that were the case, individual strains might be found which contained fewer native mobile elements and were more stable. There have been several reports of bacteriophage growing on *Halobacterium* [51,52], so it seems likely that phage could also be found for methanogens and a transductional system of genetic exchange possibly developed. Similarly, the discovery of plasmids in *Halobacterium* strains makes it seem likely that plasmids will also be present in methanogens so that a conjugational system of genetic exchange would also be a possibility.

Prospects for In Vitro Recombinant DNA Approaches. To date very little work has been done in the molecular biology of methanogens. It would be relatively straighforward to clone methanogen DNA into *E. coli* or some other eubacteria, however the chances of an archaebacterial promoter being recognized by eubacterial polymerase seems fairly small so that appropriate promoters and ribosomal binding sites might well have to be provided in order to obtain gene expression. The bacteriorhodopsin gene from *H. halobium* has been cloned and sequencing of the upstream region of the gene suggests that the promoter may be quite different and that there is not a ribosome binding site of the type found in eubacterial mRNAs [14]. A substantial amount of work remains to be done before recombinant DNA approaches can be used in methanogens themselves. The discovery of plasmids in the archaebacterium, *H. halobium* [39,40], suggests that plasmids will also be found in methanogens so that vectors could be developed. The development of suitable vectors will be somewhat more difficult than for some systems, since there have been no genetic studies of methanogens and drug resistance genes active in archaebacteria yet described; as noted above, archaebacteria are naturally resistant to some of the drugs that kill eubacteria. In addition, a suitable procedure will need to be developed for transformation. As discussed above, methanogens are resistant to lysozyme because of the unusual composition of their cell walls, however, two instances of protoplast formation by methanogens have been reported [23,50]. Whether such spontaneously arising protoplasts are suitable for transformation and can be regenerated remains to be determined.

ACKNOWLEDGEMENTS

I thank T. Sinskey, R. Gomez, and J. Krueger for their helpful discussions and L. Withers for help in preparing the manuscript. This work was supported by Grant R01-CA21615 from the National Cancer Institute and Grant R01-GM28988 from the National Institute of General Medical Sciences. G.C.W. was a Rita Allen Scholar.

REFERENCES

1. Allcock, E.R., S.J. Reid, D.T. Jones, and D.R. Woods. 1981. Autolytic activity and an autolysis-defective mutant of Clostridium acetobutylicum. Appl. Environ. Microbiol. 42: 929-935.
2, Allcock, E.R., S.Reid, D.T. Jones, and D.R. Woods. 1982. Clostridium acetobutylicum protoplast formation and regeneration. Appl. Environ. Microbiol. 43:719-721.
3. Andreesen, J.R., G. Gottschalk, and H. Schlegel. 1970. Clostridium formicoaceticum nov. spec. Isolation, description, and distinction from C. aceticum and C. thermoaceticum. Arch. Microbiol. 72:154-174.
4. Bagg, A., C.J. Kenyon, and G.C. Walker. 1981. Inducibility of a gene product required for UV and chemical mutagenesis in Escherichia coli. Proc. Natl. Acad. Sci. USA 78:5749-5753.
5. Balch, W.E., G.E. Fox, L.J. Magrum, C.R. Woese, and R.S. Wolfe. 1979. Methanogens: reevaluation of a unique biological group. Microbiol. Rev. 43:260-296.
6. Blaschek, H.P. and M. Solberg. 1981. Isolation of a plasmid responsible for caseinase activity in Clostridium perfringens ATCC 3626B. J. Bacteriol. 147:262-266.
7. Brefort, G., M. Magot, H. Ionesco, and M. Sebald. 1977. Characterization and transferability of Clostridium perfringens plasmids. Plasmid 1:52-66.
8. Brent, R., and M. Ptashne. 1980. The lexA gene product represses its own promoter. Proc. Natl. Acad. Sci. USA 77:1932-1936.
9. Bridges, B.A. 1976. Mutation induction, pp. 7-14. In K.D. MacDonald (ed.), Second international symposium on the genetics of industrial microorganisms. Academic Press, Inc., New York.
10. Casadaban, M.J., and S.N. Cohen. 1979. Lactose genes fused to exogeneous promoters in one step using a Mu-lac bacteriophage: In vivo probe for transcriptional control. Proc. Natl. Acad. Sci. USA. 76:4530-4533.

11. Casadaban, M.J., J. Chou, and S.N. Cohen. 1979. In vitro gene fusions that join an enzymatically active β-galactosidase segment to the amino-terminal fragments of exogenous proteins: Escherichia coli plasmids vectors for the detection of cloning of translational initiation signals. J. Bacteriol. 143:971-980.

12. Dobson, P.P., and G.C. Walker. 1980. Plasmid (pKM101)-mediated Weigle-reactivation in Escherichia coli K-12 and Salmonella typhimurium LT2: genetic dependence, kinetics of induction, and effect of chloramphenicol. Mutat. Res. 71:25-41.

13. Duncan, C.L., E.A. Rokos, C.M. Christenson, and J.I. Rood. 1978. Multiple plasmids in different toxigenic types of Clostridium perfringens: possible control of β-toxin production, pp 246-248. In D. Schlessinger (ed.), Microbiology 1978. American Society for Microbiology, Washington, D.C.

14. Dunn, R., J. McCoy, M. Simsek, A. Majumdar, S.H. Chang, U.L. RajBhandary, and H.G. Khorana. 1981. The bacteriorhodopsin gene. Proc. Natl. Acad. Sci. USA 78:6744-6748.

15. Eklund, M.W., and F.T. Poysky. 1974. Interconversion of type C and D strains of Clostridium botulinum by specific bacteriophages. Appl. Microbiol. 27:251-258.

16. Elledge, S.J., and G.C. Walker. Proteins required for UV and chemical mutagenesis: identification of the products of the umuC locus of Escherichia coli. (Submitted for publication).

17. Fontaine, F.E., W.H. Peterson, E. McCoy, M.J. Johnson, and G.J. Ritter. 1942. A new type of glucose fermentation by Clostridium thermoaceticum n. sp. J. Bacteriol. 43:701-715.

18. Fox, G.E., E. Stackebrandt, R.B. Hespell, J. Gibson, J. Maniloff, T.A. Dyer, R.S. Wolfe, W.E. Balch, R.S. Tanner, L.J. Magrum, L.B. Zablen, R. Blakemore, R. Gupta, L. Boene, B.J. Lewis, D.A. Stahl, K.R. Luehrsen, K.N. Chen, C.R. Woese. 2980. The phylogeny of prokaryotes. Science 209:457-463.

19. Gomez, R.F., B. Snedecor, and B. Mendez. 1981. Development of genetic principles in Clostridium thermocellum. Developments in Industrial Microbiol. 22:87-95.

20. Hofmeister, J., H. Kohler, and V.D. Fillipov. 1979. DNA repair in Proteus mirabilis: plasmid-mediated recovery and mutagenesis. Molec. Gen. Genet. 176:265-273.

21. Hopwood, D.A. 1981. Genetic studies with bacterial protoplasts. Ann. Rev. Microbiol. 35:237-272.

22. Hsu, E., and E.J. Ordal. 1970. Comparative metabolism of vegetative and sporulating cultures of Clostridium thermosaccharolyticum. J. Bacteriol. 102:369-376.

23. Jarrell, K.F., J. R. Colvin, and G.D. Sprott. 1982. Spontaneous protoplast formation in Methanobacterium bryantii, J. Bacteriol. 149:346-353.

24. Johnson, E.A., A. Madia, and A.L. Demain. 1981. Chemically defined minimal medium for growth of the anaerobic cellulolytic thermophilic Clostridium thermocellum. Appl. Environ. Microbiol. 41:1060-1062.

25. Kato, T., and Y. Shinoura. 1977. Isolation and characterization of mutants of Escherichia coli deficient in induction of mutations by ultraviolet light. Molec. Gen. Genet. 156:1212-131.

26. Kenyon, C.J., and G.C. Walker. 1980. DNA-damaging agents stimulate gene expression at specific loci in Escherichia coli. Proc. Natl. Acad. Sci. USA 77:2819-2823.

27. Kenyon, C.J., and G.C. Walker. 1981. Expression of the uvrA gene of Escherichia coli is inducible. Nature 289:810-812.

28. Kenyon, C.J., R.Brent, P. Ptashne, and G.C. Walker. The regulation of damage-inducible genes in Escherichia coli. J. Molec. Biol. (In Press).

29. Kleckner, N., J. Roth, and D. Botstein. 1977. Genetic engineering in vivo using translocatable drug-resistance elements. J. Molec. Biol. 116:125-159.

30. Langer, P.J., W.G. Shanabruch, and G.C. Walker. 1981. Functional organization of the plasmid pKM101. J. Bacteriol. 145:1310-1316.

31. Mah, R.A., D.A. Ward, L. Baresi, and T.L. Glass. 1977. Biogenesis of methane. Ann. Rev. Microbiol. 31:309-341.

32. Meagher, R.B., R.,C. Tait, M.B. Betlock, and H.B. Boyer. 1977. Protein Expression in *E. coli* minicells by recombinant plasmids. Cell 10:521-536.

33. Mendez, B.S., and R.F. Gomez. 1982. Isolation of *Clostridium thermocellum* auxotrophs. Appl. Environ. Microbiol. 43:495-496.

34. McCann, J., E. Choi, E. Yamasaki, and B.N. Ames. 1975. Detection of carcinogens as mutagens in the *Salmonella*/microsome test: assay of 300 chemicals. Proc. Natl. Acad. Sci. USA 72:5135-5139.

35. McCann, J., and B.N. Ames. 1976. Detection of carcinogens as mutagens in the *Salmonella*/microsome test: assay of 300 chemicals: discussion. Proc. Natl. Acad. Sci. USA. 73:950-954.

36. Mulligan, J.T., W. Margolin, J.H. Krueger, and G.C. Walker. 1982. Mutations affecting the regulation of methionine biosynthetic genes isolated by the use of *met-lac* fusions. J. Bacteriol. (In Press).

37. Ng, T.K., P.J. Weimer, and J.G. Zeikus. 1977. Cellulolytic and physiological properties of *Clostridium thermocellum*. Arch. Microbiol. 114:1-7.

38. Perry, K.L. and G.C. Walker, Identification of Plasmid (pKM101)-Coded Proteins Involved in Mutagenesis and UV-Resistance, (Submitted for publication).

39. Pfeifer, F., G. Weidinger, and W. Goebel. 1981. Characterization of plasmids in halobacteria. J. Bacteriol. 145:369-374.

40. Pfeifer, F., G. Weidinger, and W. Goebel. 1981. Genetic variability in *Halobacterium halobium*. J. Bacteriol. 145:375-382.

41. Rood, J.I., V.N. Scott, and C.L. Duncan. 2978. Identification of a transferable tetracycline resistance plasmid (pCW3) from *Clostridium perfringens*. Plasmid 1:563-570.

42. Ruvkun, G.B. and Ausubel, F.M. 1981. A general method for site-directed mutagenesis in prokaryotes. Nature 289:85-88.

43. Sancar, A., R.P. Wharton, S. Seltzer, B.M. Kacinski, N.D. Clarke, and W.D. Rupp. 1981. Identification of the uvrA Gene Product. J. Molec. Biol. 148:45-62.

44. Sapienza, C., and W.F. Doolittle. 1982. Unusual physical organization of the Halobacterium genome. Nature 295:384-389.

45. Schwartz, R.D., and F.A. Keller, Jr. 1982. Isolation of a strain of Clostridium thermocellum capable of growth and acetic acid production at pH 4.5 Appl. Environ. Microbiol. 43:117-123.

46. Silhavy, T.J., and J. Beckwith. Isolation and characterization of Escherichia coli mutants affected in protein localization. In Biomembanes: membrane biogenesis, sorting, and transport of membrane constitutents. Academic Press, Inc., New York, in press.

47. Spivey, M.J. 1978. The acetone/butanol/ethanol fermentation. Process Biochem. 13(11):2-25.

48. Shanabruch, W.G., and Walker. G.C. 1980. Localization of the plasmid (pKM101) gene(s) involved in recA+lexA+-dependent mutagenesis. Molec. Gen. Genet. 179:289-297.

49. Shanabruch, W.G., I. Behlau, and G.C. Walker. 1981. Spontaneous mutators of Salmonella typhimurium LT2 generated by the insertion of transposable elements. J. Bacteriol. 147:827-835.

50. Sprott, G.D., J.R. Colvin, R.C. McKellar. 1979. Spheroplasts of Methanospirillum hungatii formed upon treatment with dithiothreitol. Can. J. Microbiol. 25:730-738.

51. Torsvik, T., and I.D. Dundas. 1974. Bacteriophage of Halobacterium salinarium. Nature 248:680-682.

52. Wais, A.C., M. Kon, R.E. MacDonald, and B.D. Stollar. 1975. Salt-dependent bacteriophage infecting Halobacterium cutirubrum and H. halobium. Nature 256:314-315.

53. Walker, G.C. 1978. Isolation and characterization of mutants of the plasmid pKM101 deficient in their ability to enhance mutagenesis and repair. J. Bacteriol. 133:1203-1211.

54. Walker, G.C. and P.P. Dobson. 1979. Mutagenesis and repair

deficiencies of Escherichia coli umuC mutants are suppressed by the plasmid pKM101. Molec. Gen. Genet. 172:17-24.

55. Woese, C.R., L.J. Magum, and G.E. Fox. 1978. Archaebacteria. J. Molec. Evol. 11:245-252.

56. Zeikus, J.G., and R.S. Wolfe. 1972. Methanobacterium thermo-moautotrophicus sp. n., anaerobic, autotrophic, extreme thermophile. J. Bacteriol. 109:707-713.

57. Zeikus, J.G. 1980. Chemical and fuel production by anaerobic bacteria. Ann. Rev. Microbiol. 34:423-464.

58. Zeikus, J.G., A. Ben-Bassat, and P. Hegge. 1980. Microbiology of methanogenesis in thermal, volcanic, environments. J. Bacteriol. 143:432-440.

59. Zillig, W., K.O. Stetter, W. Schulz, and D. Janekovic. 1980. In P. Moldner and B. Ries (eds.) Trends in enzymology: enzyme regulation and mechanism of action. pp 159-178. Pergamon Press.

DISCUSSION

Q. C. COONEY (MIT): I have a brief question on the work you do with the umuC gene. Are umuC mutations likely to be useful in increasing the stability of desirable strains of certain bacteria?

A. WALKER: Loss of umuC and thus loss of error-prove repair has very little effect on the spontaneous mutation rate and therefore would be of little use in stabilizing strains. In contrast, umuC function is required to process damaged DNA in such a way that you get mutations. I think that one way umuC genes might be useful, at least in the case of gram negatives, would be to change a strain that is non-mutable by UV to one that is mutable. UV is a particularly useful mutagen because it gives you all kinds of different base changes. In fact, that's been done with Proteus which is normally non-mutable by

UV. If you introduce a plasmid that carries an analogue of the umuC gene, that organism that was previously non-mutable becomes highly mutable and I think that that may be the sort of application that one might make. However, these bacteria could be mutated in any case by chosing a mutagen that does not require the participation of error-prone repair in order to cause mutations.

Q. P. STARLINGER (Universitat Zu Kohn): I have a question with regard to the umuC. Have you, or has anybody else, looked whether a umuC+ strain has a growth advantage over an umuC$^-$ strain using a chemostat? I mean a complicated function like that should bring some evolutionary advantage to the cell besides just the mutations that are being brought about by this gene. Can one show that having a higher mutation rate in a changing environmental condition brings an advantage to the cell?

A. WALKER: I'll stress again that a umuC$^-$ mutation has a minimal impact on the spontaneous mutation rate. However, a fundamental teleological question that often comes up at this point in the discussion is does the cell really want to have a higher mutation rate? Does it say "I'm getting in trouble I'd better mutate." The alternative interpretation is that there is a small but important increase in UV resistance if a cell has umuC function. In that way of thinking about it a cell would like to live and it doesn't mind if it pays a price in terms of a modest loss of genetic fidelity. I don't know the answer to that. If we get some insight into the biochemistry I think that may be a considerable help.

Q. P. STARLINGER (Universitat Zu Kohn): I was not thinking about teleology but I was thinking for instance of a very old experiment reported in 1950 by Ryan and his associates who grew a mixture of wild type and his$^-$ cells in the chemostat. They showed that mutants would accumulate steadily and then they would abruptly go away. The idea was that there is once in a while a mutation in the cell which conveys an unknown growth advantage if this occurs in the majority of faction and this was going on and on and was looking like a see-saw, this picture of the chemostat. I don't know whether anybody has ever tried to repeat this, but it would be nice to know which kinds of mutations there are that convey growth advantage and accumulated at a rather high rate within days within a chemostat.

A. WALKER: We haven't done any chemostat experiments. However, there haven't been any obvious differences in growth rate between $umuC^+$ and $umuC^-$ cells that we have noticed while doing ordinary growth curves.

Q. M. BARTER (Economics Lab.) I was very curious about your operon fusion. Have you, or do you know of anyone, who has made operon fusions to let's say extracellular enzymes that are normally inducible and then used those to make constituitive mutants? I ask, because I was wondering if there were any operons that are susceptible to being modified so that they become, in effect, hyperproducers of extracellular enzymes.

A. WALKER: Jon Beckwith has done a lot of studies on proteins that get transported and in particular has made gene fusions. However the fusion proteins cannot be transported and get jammed in the membrane and this has been used to select for mutants involved in the transport of proteins. I'm not aware of any studies of where the fusion protein actually gets transported. If you wanted to do such studies, you might well want choose something beside lacZ to make the fusion. For example, you might be able to modify β-lactamase or something that you know can get transported and use that to monitor the gene that you're interested in.

Q. S. HAYES (Univ. of Saskatchewan): Could you comment a bit more on your mention about the possible umuC type mutation in Clostridium or its insensitivity to radiation mutagenesis.

A. WALKER: Clostridium thermacellum seems to be very ineffectively mutated by UV even though it is mutated quite well by ethyl methanesulfonate. That is a characteristic that one would associate with the *umuC*$^-$ mutants of *E. coli* that are deficient in this basically still unknown process that is referred to as error-prone repair. I'm suggesting that, on the basis of this phenotype, maybe clostridia are somewhat deficient in error-prone repair, nothing more profound than that. Although, it's certainly the kind of thing that could be tested if someone wanted to look into it.

Q. S. HAYES (Univ. of Saskatchewan): In looking at the UV effects on Clostridium, we find that there's very little UV killing so this may be related to that.

A. WALKER: Certainly one thing to stress is that *umuC*$^-$ mutations have very small effects on resistance to UV-killing. Their effects are not nearly as striking as mutations that knock out excision repair or disable *recA* functions.

C. C. COONEY (MIT): I would like to thank Dr. Walker again.

ANAEROBIC PRODUCTION OF CHEMICALS

James C. Linden and Antonio Moreira*
Colorado State University
Department of Agricultural and Chemical Engineering
Fort Collins, Colorado 80523

INTRODUCTION

Anaerobic fermentations are among the oldest industrially practiced fermentation processes. The production of acetone and butanol, for example, by the well-known Weizmann process, dates as far back as 1916 [1]. In spite of such a long record, anaerobic processes are not, at the present time, among the most important fermentation-based industries. This has resulted from the tremendous development of the petrochemical industries starting in the 1950s and the consequent displacement of the fermentation routes by the more economically attractive petrochemical processes.

In recent years, the dramatic increase in the price of petroleum derivatives, especially after the 1973 oil embargo, has

---

* Present address: International Flavors and Fragrances, Inc. 1515 Highway 36, Union Beach, NJ 07735

Table 1

Main Features of Anaerobic Fermentations

Advantages

- Broad spectrum of end products
- A variety of substrates can often be metabolized
- Low mixing requirements
- Aeration not required
- Cooling requirements lower than for aerobic fermentations
- Low substrate consumption for cell mass production

Disadvantages

- Anaerobes are difficult to handle
- Low product concentrations
- Low productivities
- High sterility required
- Large quantities of undesirable by-products typically formed

generated a renewed interest in the production of key organic chemicals via fermentation-based technology. Due to their wide spectrum of end products, anaerobic processes occupy a central position in future biochemical industries and are thus being extensively investigated by a large number of researchers all over the world. Two basic approaches are being pursued in such studies. While some researchers are looking carefully at older fermentation processes (such as the acetone-butanol fermentation) in an effort to improve such processes by "modernizing" the corresponding technology, totally new fermentations (utilizing either newly discovered or genetically engineered microorganisms) are in the process of being developed and becoming technically feasible.

In this paper an overview is presented of those anaerobic processes which show a strong potential of becoming economically attractive for the production of key organic chemicals in a short-to-medium term. The acetone-butanol fermentation is then discussed as a typical example of the problems facing most anaerobic processes before commercialization and to show how research programs such as the one at Colorado State University can contribute to the solution of such problems.

General Characteristics of Anaerobic Processes

Anaerobic processes are characterized by their ability to proceed in the absence of air. As a consequence of this basic feature, these processes are endowed with a number of characteristics strikingly different from aerobic fermentations as summarized in Table 1.

Metabolic pathways are usually rather complex in anaerobic microorganisms, as these organisms accomplish only partial substrate decomposition and devise ingenious alternatives to oxidative phosphorylation in order to generate energy (ATP) and rebuild their reducing power (NADH, NADPH). Such complex metabolism allows anaerobic microorganisms to typically produce a large spectrum of end-products. Although this could be envisioned as a disadvantage for anaerobes since it does represent a decrease in the yield of a specifically desired final product, the possibility of deriving many important chemicals (as will be seen later) makes anaerobic processes very often more attractive than aerated fermentations.

Along with the multitude of fermentation products, a large variety of substrates can often be metabolized by anaerobic microorganisms. These substrates can be classified into three major categories: (1) sugar-based materials, to include molasses and crops such as sugar cane, sugar beets, fodder beets, and sweet sorghum; [2] starch-based materials, primarily crops such as corn, wheat, milo, rye and barley, as well as cassava; and (3) cellulose-based substrates, such as agricultural and forest residues and municipal solid waste. While the fermentation of sugar and starch-based crops is a well-established technology, the fermentation of cellulosic materials is primarily still at the research stage and it will be some time before large-scale production of chemicals from cellulose will become a commercial reality. Since lignocellulose, the substrate of the future, is intrinsically heterogeneous in composition, microorganisms which are able to convert cellulose directly to chemicals, or which can metabolize a mixture of sugars as opposed to utilizing glucose only, will have a direct advantage in future processes. As will be seen later, some of the anaerobic microorganisms currently under investigation do have such characteristics (e.g., *Clostridium thermocellum*).

Power requirements for anaerobic processes are typically rather low when compared with aerated systems. This results not only from the fact that large air compressors are not required, but also because mechanical mixing requirements are quite low since mass transfer from gas to liquid is nonexistent. In addition, due to the lower cell yield in anaerobic systems, less energy is dissipated into the environment and consequently, cooling requirements are usually much lower than those observed in aerated fermentations.

Although the above characteristics can be taken as possible advantages for anaerobic systems, other considerations indicate difficulties associated with these processes. Among them, the primary requirement for an anaerobic sterile environment is probably one of the most critical. Special handling techniques must be adopted in order to prevent oxygen from leaking into the system and consequently fermentation media usually become expensive, as special reducing compounds must be present in order to maintain anaerobiosis.

Another very important drawback is the low product concentrations and low productivities typically observed in these fermentations. These result in large capital expenditures for the fermentation plant as well as in large energy costs associated, for instance, with media sterilization and end-product recovery.

Finally, and as mentioned earlier, anaerobic fermentations tend

Table 2

Potentially Important Anaerobic Fermentation Systems

Microorganism	Carbon Source(s)	Major Fermentation Product(s)
S. cerevisiae	glucose, sucrose	ethanol
Z. mobilis	glucose, sucrose	ethanol
Cl. thermocellum	glucose, sucrose	ethanol, acetic acid, lactic acid
Cl. thermosaccharolyticum	glucose, xylose, cellobiose	ethanol, acetic acid, lactic acid
Cl. thermohydrosulfuricum	glucose, xylose, cellobiose	ethanol, acetic acid, lactic acid
Schizosaccharomyces pombe	xylulose	ethanol
Kluyveromyces lactis	xylulose	ethanol
Pachysolen tannophilus	glucose, xylose	ethanol
Thermobacteroides saccharolyticum	xylose, xylan, glucose, cellobiose, starch	ethanol
Thermoanaerobacter ethanolicus	glucose, cellobiose, xylose, starch	ethanol, acetic acid, lactic acid
Cl. acetobutylicum	glucose, xylose, arabinose	acetone, butanol
Cl. thermoaceticum	glucose, fructose, xylose	acetic acid
Cl. propionicum	α-alanine, β-alanine	propionic acid, acetic acid, acrylic acid
Aeromonas hydrophilia	xylose	ethanol, 2,3-butanediol

to produce an array of end products instead of a single final product. Although this might be advantageous, the presence of large quantities of undesirable by products can represent significant losses in process yields. Means must then be devised to minimize such losses, or alternatively, to find potential uses for such by-products. Thus, the CO_2 and H_2 gases evolved in the acetone-butanol fermentation were recently converted to methanol [2] as in earlier days [3] using an improved methanol synthesis technology.

Production of Chemicals by Anaerobic Fermentation

In this section, a summary will be presented of those anaerobic processes which have been reported as having potential for large-scale development in the future.

Ethanol has received by far the most attention to date as a fuel and chemical to be obtained by fermentation. Yeast (*Saccharomyces cerevisiae*) has traditionally been utilized as the organism to achieve such a conversion. However, in recent years, the bacterium *Zymomonas mobilis* has attracted increased interest as an ethanol producer [4]. *Zymomonas* uses the Entner-Doudoroff pathway for ethanol production. This pathway results in a lower ATP yield than the EMP pathway utilized by the yeast and thus a lower cell mass is observed with the *Zymomonas* fermentation with a consequent increase in the ethanol yield and fermentor productivity.

As mentioned earlier, it is anticipated that cellulose will be the ultimate substrate for modern age fermentation processes, and thus improved cellulose fermentation processes must be devised in the future. An interesting approach has been developed by Emert and collaborators [5] where a simultaneous cellulose saccharification and yeast ethanol fermentation (SSF) is performed in the same vessel. An extension of this concept, supplementing *Z. mobilis* with cellulases from *Trichoderma reesei*, has also been reported [6].

Another alternative process for converting cellulose into ethanol involves mixed cultivation of cellulolytic and non-cellulolytic microorganisms. Processes involving *Clostridium thermocellum* [7,8] and *Clostridium thermosaccharolyticum* [9] or *Clostridium thermohydrosulfuricum* [10] have been proposed. In these processes, *Cl. thermosaccharolyticum* and *Cl. thermohydrosulfuricum* have the potential of fermenting pentoses (xylose) to ethanol. Although *S. cerevisiae* will not ferment xylose to ethanol, it has been recently shown that some yeasts (*Schizosaccharomyces pombe* and *Kluyveromyces lactis*) can ferment xylulose obtained by isomerization of xylose [11]. Yet another interesting possibility is the fermentation of xylose directly to ethanol by the yeast *Pachysolen tannophilus* [12]. Lastly, a new thermophilic anaerobic bacterium tentatively named *Thermobacteroides saccharolyticum* has been reported [13] to produce ethanol at temperatures as high as 70°C. These high temperatures have also been reported for *Thermoanaerobacter ethanolicus* [14].

The production of acetone and butanol by fermentation is also of great industrial significance. Although several anaerobic bacteria belonging to the genus *Clostridium* can be used, *Clostridium acetobutylicum* is probably the most widely known producer [1]. The ratio of acetone to butanol produced is strongly dependent on the microorganism and type of substrate used. A more detailed description of this fermentation will be presented in the next section of this paper.

Clostridium thermoaceticum is another thermophilic anaerobe of great interest for the production of acetic acid [14]. In this fermentation, one mole of glucose is fermented to three moles of acetate via a complex reaction scheme from which many details are still missing.

The formation of acrylic acid as an intermediate in the metabolic pathway of *Clostridium propionicum* has been recently demonstrated by Sinskey *et al*. [15]. Acrylic acid and its ester derivatives have considerable value as chemical feedstocks and are used primarily in the form of polymers. Although acrylic acid is not a metabolic end product during the anaerobic fermentation of *Clostridium propionicum* (as in propionic acid), its estabishment as an intermediate for propionate formation raises the possibility of converting biomass to acrylate under suitable fermentation conditions.

Table 3

U.S. Annual Production of Chemicals

Chemical	10^6 lbs
Acetic acid	2,706
Acetone	2,167
Acrylonitrile	2,006
1,3-Butadiene	3,046
n-Butanol	823
Ethanol (synthetic)	1,157
Ethylene	28,867
Isopropyl alcohol	1,644
Methyl ethyl ketone	626
Vinyl acetate	1,934
Vinyl chloride	6,720

* Source: Ref. 17.

Finally, the production of 2,3-butanediol has also received some attention from the research community. The facultative anaerobe Aeromonas hydrophilia has been shown to produce a mixture of the diol plus ethanol when grown anaerobically on xylose [16]. Methyl ethyl ketone can then be obtained from the diol by an acid-catalyzed dehydration.

In summary, ethanol, butanol, acetone, acetic acid, 2,3-butanediol, and acrylic acid are some of the most important chemicals currently under strong consideration for production via anaerobic fermentation. These chemicals and potential derivatives are among the major organic chemicals produced annually in the United States (as shown in Table 3) and could very well serve as the basis for establishment of a fermentation industry for the production of chemicals in the United States if economic viability can be assured.

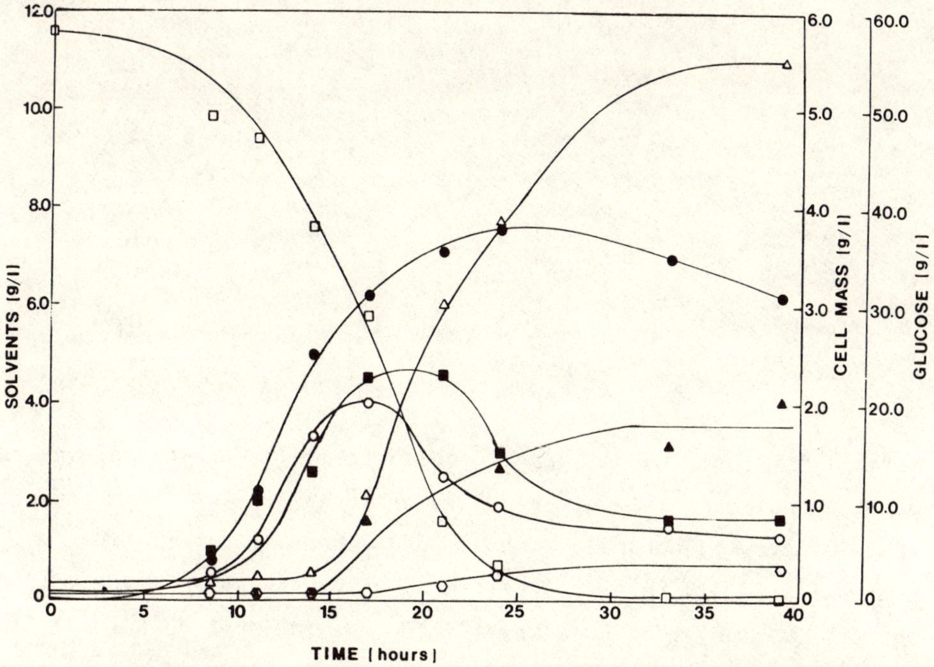

Fig. 1. Production of solvents by Clostridium acetobutylicum grown on soluble medium with pH controlled at 5.0 in batch culture.

Acetone-Butanol Fermentation

As stated above, dilute product concentrations are one of the major drawbacks of the anaerobic fermentations. In order to overcome this problem, two options exist: improve the fermentation so as to continually remove product, as by *in situ* extraction; or improve the microorganisms so as to produce higher concentrations of the desired product. The following discussion describes the rationale and results for the second option.

A. Alcohol Effect on Fermentation. The production of acetone and butanol by *Clostridium acetobutylicum* was inhibited at 2% solvents by weight [18]. The results of a 39-hour batch fermentation are shown in Figure 1. During the exponential phase of growth

Table 4

Summary of Growth Inhibition Data

Product	Threshold Conc.	Conc. at which growth was inhibited by 50%	
	M	M	g/1
Butyric Acid	0.02	0.07	6.0
Butanol	0.05	0.15	11.0
Acetic Acid	0.04	0.13	8.0
Ethanol	0.25	1.10	51.0
Acetone	0.36	0.88	43.5

a small increase in the butanol concentration was observed, whereas acetone and ethanol levels remained constant. After the exponential phase of growth, butanol, acetone, and ethanol concentrations increased rapidly to near their final values in approximately 10 hours. To study the inhibitory factors of the acetone-butanol fermentation, the growth rates of C. acetobutylicum in the presence of each fermentation product were determined. The end products used in this study included ethanol, butanol, acetone, acetic acid, and butyric acid. From the slopes of the least squares regression lines of optical density vs. time data, the maximum specific growth rates in the presence of varying concentrations of each inhibitor (μ^i_m) were determined. There appeared to be a threshold concentration which must be reached before growth inhibition occurred. This concentration was found to vary with each inhibitor studied. Concentrations causing a 50% reduction in growth rate were also determined. A summary of the inhibition data obtained is given in Table 4.

The inhibitory effects of the solvents on the growth rate of C. acetobutylicum were evaluated in comparison with concentrations obtained as fermentation products. The levels of acetone and ethanol typically observed during fermentation (5 g/1 and 1.5 g/1 respectively) were found to be noninhibitory to cell growth. The highest concentrations of butyric acid and acetic acid which we have observed during fermentation are in the range of 3.5 to 4.0 g/l. These levels of acids approach those causing 50% inhibition of growth. Typical butanol concentrations observed during a fermentation are 11-12 g/l. Butanol is the only product that reaches levels actually causing 50% inhibition of growth. The inhibitory effects of all of the solvents contribute additively to shut down the fermentation.

B. Alcohol Effect on Membrane Composition. Changes in the lipid composition of bacterial membranes have been described which result from exposure of growing cells to an environment containing aliphatic alcohols. Adaptation of *Escherichia coli* to ethanol has been reported by Ingram [19] to result in decreased saturated to unsaturated fatty acid (S/U) ratios, whereas alcohols of chain length greater than four produced the opposite effect, i.e., increased the S/U ratio. Buttke and Ingram [20] proposed a mechanism for alcohol-induced compositional changes, based upon the observation that ethanol inhibited the synthesis of saturated fatty acid *in vivo*. Similar modification of membrane composition, following a reduction in temperature, has been shown to occur so rapidly as to indicate that the enzymes involved in adaptation reactions must exist *in situ* as integral membrane proteins [21]. Higher growth temperatures result in bacterial cell membranes containing saturated and branched fatty acids.

Butanol increases membrane fluidity, an effect opposite to that observed for ethanol. The literature contains reports of spin label [22] and fluoresence probe [23,24] work which show the membrane-fluidizing effects of butanol. In an effort to maintain constant membrane fluidity, the physiological response of cell adaptation to butanol and higher growth temperature would be the same, i.e., an increased ratio of saturated to unsaturated fatty acids in

Table 5

Fatty Acyl Compositions of Membranes from Mesophilic and Thermophilic Species of Bacillus and Clostridium [27]

% of Total Fatty Acids

	Saturated			Unsaturated			Branched			
	14	16	18	14	16	18	15	16	17	19
B. subtilis	1	10					51	10	25	
B. stearo-	2.9	3.1	1.2	4.2	23.5	1.2	30.7		33.2	
thermophilis	2.3	42.1			10.9		32.8	3.1	8.5	
B. species PS3		5.7					35.3	10.8	49.9	
C. butyri- (acyl)	6.5	52.0	2.0	0.9	19.0	2.2			9.4*	4.5*
cum (ether)	2.4	49.0	6.2		17.0	7.9	1.5*		9.0*	5.2*
C. thermo-saccharolyticum	19.6	15.7	6.7	16.7	16.6	6.2			10.9+	

* cyclopropane formed only by this species of Clostridium by formation of methyl bridge across double bond

+ fatty alcohol

membranes. Hence, the membrane properties of thermophilic microorganisms, in such a case, would be desirable for butanol tolerance. This notion is supported in the report by Yoshida et al. [25] where extracted ATPase complexes of the thermophilic PS3 Bacillus sp. microorganism remained active in 10 M ethanol and 12 M acetone. These concentrations were several-fold greater than those tolerated by similar preparations of the F1-ATPase complex from Bacillus stearothermophilus (3 M ethanol and 2 M acetone). Optimal growth temperature of the thermophile PS3 was reported to be 75°C; that of the mesothermophile B. stearothermophilus was 50°C. Interestingly, the fatty acyl groups were almost completely saturated in the membranes of PS3 [26]. By comparison, the fatty acyl groups of the mesophiles were relatively more unsaturated as shown in Table 5. Branched fatty acid membrane components were also a property of thermophiles.

Published membrane compositions for a mesophilic Clostridium butyricum and a thermophilic Cl. thermosacchrolyticum, also

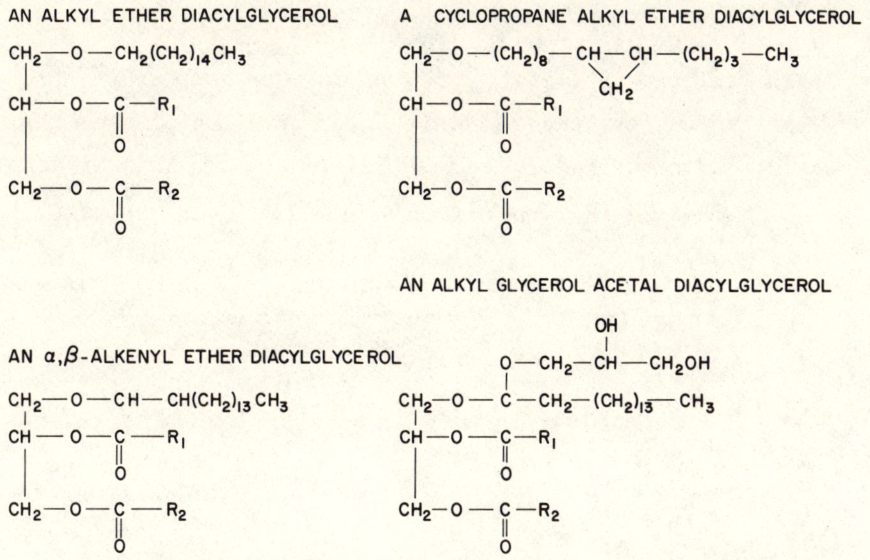

Fig. 2. Structural formulas of plasmologen molecules containing ether-linked fatty acid glycerides isolated from anaerobic bacteria [42].

tabulated in Table 5, did not exhibit the same thermotropic relationship between saturated and unsaturated fatty acids exhibited by the Bacillus species. The difference may be accounted for by the large percentage of plasmalogen linkages in Clostridium species membranes. Plasmalogens are glycerolipids containing ether-linked fatty acid residues on the C-1 of glycerol as shown in Figure 2. The C-2 is linked by the usual ester to a fatty acid and a phosphate ester occurs at C-3. The long-chain composition of the fatty acids and fatty aldehydes derived from esters and ethers respectively were similar [27] (Table 5). C. acetobutylicum phospholipids contained a molar ratio of the ether linkage to phosphorus of 0.72-0.92, which was greater than that of 0.40 from C. butyricum [19].

Brain tissue membranes share similarities with C. acetobutylicum membranes in that approximately 75% of the total lipid content of both are plasmalogens. Long-term exposure in vivo of brain cells to ethanol (as in cases of alcoholism) elicits the necessity for

Table 6

Correlation Between the Log of the Octanol/Water Partition Coefficient and the Reciprocal Log of the Concentration to Produce a Given Relative Biological Effect

	Dupperay(33) log P[a]	Paterson (24) 50% change in spin label enthalpy	Grisham (22) 50% of (Na+ - K+) ATPase activity	Lenaz (23) 50% fluoresence intensity	Linden (31) 50% rate cellular functions
Ethanol	-0.16		-0.66		-0.02
n-Propranol	0.34	0.04			
t-Butanol	0.37		0.11		0.47
n-Butanol	0.88	0.22	0.40	0.74	0.93
n Pentanol	1.40	1.00	0.96	1.00	
n-Hexanol	2.03	1.10			2.00
n-Heptanol	2.53	2.00	2.10		

[a] P is the octanol/water partition coefficient.

greater concentrations of ethanol in order to maintain normal functionality. The brains of mice adapted to ethanol exhibited responses from electrophysiological studies showing rapid detoxification of localized mouse cerebellar and hippocanysal neurons, which may point to appropriate changes in membrane composition within seconds of challenging with ethanol [28]. In addition, relative doses of n-butanol, t-butanol, and ethanol required to induce alcoholic stupor in mice [29] were proportional to the relative concentrations of the same alcohols required to inhibit C. acetobutylicum cell growth [30] and cell membrane functionality [31].

C. Alcohol Effect on Membrane Structure. The ability of aliphatic alcohols to increase the fluidity of cell membranes is proportional to the chain length of the alcohol. This is thought to be related to greater solubility of longer chain alcohols in the core of phospholipid bilayers. Hydrophobicity, as measured by the octanol-water partition coefficient, has been correlated with a number of biological membrane properties [22,23,24,32,33]. Table 6 shows the log of the partition coefficients of various alcohols. In numerous cases, the partition coefficient would correlate with the ability of an alcohol to generate a given effect, especially when the effect involves biological membranes. Also in Table 6 are the reciprocal logarithms of aliphatic alcohol concentrations which have been found to cause the listed biological effects [33]. The correlations between the C. acetobutylicum growth, nutrient uptake and membrane ATPase inhibitions with the partition coefficients are also remarkably similar. Longer chain lengths were effective at correspondingly lower concentrations in increasing fatty acyl mobility within the membrane and in disrupting interactions between the phospholipids and proteins embedded in the membrane. In cases where enzymatic activities or protein-affected processes were involved, the disruption of aliphatic-chain packing may have caused lower activity or process rates to occur.

The importance of the membrane interface may provide explanations for the fact that butyric acid was more toxic than butanol and that acetic acid was more toxic than ethanol [34]. Emerging in the literature is spectroscopic evidence that fundamental differences exist in the effects of local and general anaesthetics on membranes [29,35]. The class of general anaesthetics, into which aliphatic alcohols would fall, appears to cause membrane expansion by occupation of volume in the hydrophobic core of the membrane. The local anaesthetic effect can be attributed to the approach of a position charge to the phosphate of the phospholipid, which resides at the membrane interface with the environment [36]. In the case of butyric acid, strengthening of a weak interaction of divalent cations with the negative-charged phospholipids, such as phosphatidylcholine and phosphatidylethanolanine, may be hypothesized. The amphiphatic character of butyric acid could localize its interaction at the membrane surface where a combination of membrane expansion and interface effects may be acting.

D. Alcohol Effect on Membrane Function. Hydrophobicity has been correlated with a number of biological membrane properties. The hydrophobic properties of aliphatic alcohols have been shown to increase with the number of carbon atoms in the alcohol [22]. The molar concentrations of the alcohols which caused 50% inhibition of membrane-bound adenosine triphosphatase (ATPase) were given in Table 6. The same concentrations also effected the maximum change in the enthalpy required to orient a spin label compound in the membrane lipid bilayer [22].

Lenaz *et al*. [37] determined that the activation energy of membrane-bound ATPase was increased three-fold by 0.35 *M* butanol. The enzyme was not extracted from the membrane, but changes in the conformation of the enzyme proteins could be correlated to butanol induced mobility changes in the lipid environment. The Arrhenius plot was found to break at 18°C in the absence of butanol but not in its presence, in which case the higher activation energy was observed at both high and low temperatures. In another study, Lenaz *et al*. [23] concluded that there was more constriction of spin label orientation in biological membranes than in phospholipid vesicles because of protein interaction with the lipids. Increased mobility of the spin label at low butanol concentrations was more striking in biological membranes than in the vesicles because butanol removed some of the protein induced restraints on surrounding lipids in the membrane. This emphasized the importance of interactions between membrane-bound proteins and annular lipids which surround the proteins [38]. The association of a discrete number and type of lipid molecules with the ATPase molecules embedded in the membrane has been shown to be an important factor determining the activity of the enzyme [39].

Our findings have shown the dependence of the uptake of sugars [30] and amino acids [31] in *C. acetobutylicum* on an energy generaing source, i.e., on ATP hydrolysis (Table 7). The inhibition of

Table 7

Concentrations of Aliphatic Alcohols which Limit Various *C. acetobutylicum* Cellular Functions to Half-maximal Rates

Half Maximal Rates	Concentration (M)		
	EtOH	BuOH	HxOH
Cell Growth	1.10	0.15	0.015
Alanine Uptake	0.91	0.13	0.006
3-0-Me Glucose Uptake	1.00	0.10	0.007
ATPase Activity	0.82	0.09	0.015

the membrane-bound ATPase activity occurs instantaneously upon addition of aliphatic alcohols to the reaction mixture. The data plotted in Figure 3 show the hydrolysis of ATP by *C. acetobutylicum* membrane preparations as a function of time in the presence of 1.10 *M* ethanol, 0.15 *M* n-butanol and 0.01 *M* n-hexanol. The respective rates of inorganic phosphate release from ATP were 38, 25, and 20 percent of controls; where controls yielded 0.113, ethanol-inhibited membranes yielded 0.043, n-butanol treatment yielded 0.028, and n-hexanol, 0.023 μmole Pi/min/mg protein. These data also show the inhibition of membrane functionality at concentrations similar to those which inhibited growth and nutrient uptake. The inhibition of the various cellular functions by the three aliphatic alcohols has been summarized in Table 7. Descriptions of experiments for obtaining these data have been presented elsewhere [30,31].

The hydrophobic correlation of the aliphatic alcohol inhibition of cellular growth and nutrient uptake points strongly to the membrane as the site of inhibitory interaction. The ATPase enzyme components which are associated with active transport processes not only must be incorporated in the phospholipid bilayer to be active, but must have the proper phospholipid species present in the bilayer for full activity [39]. Inhibition of the ATPase by butanol supports the model of Ingram [19] for insertion of short chain

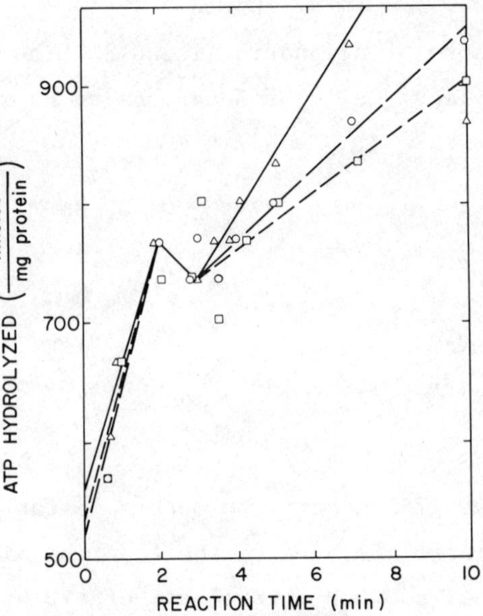

Fig. 3. Membrane-bound ATPase activity as a function of time with addition of challenge alcohols after 2.5 minutes: 1.10 M ethanol, Δ; 0.15 M n-butanol, 0; and 0.01 M n-hexanol, X. ATP hydrolysis was measured by release of inorganic phosphate as described in text. Cytoplasmic membranes prepared from log phase *C. acetobutylicum* cells as described previously [31].

aliphatic alcohols into the lipid bilayer. Insertion of the short chain alcohols into the hydrophobic interior of the membrane would restrict movement of the fatty acids making the membrane less fluid. Longer chain alcohols would introduce gaps in the phospholipid packing and increase the freedom of fatty acyl chains. Lenaz *et al.* have presented evidence based on fluorescence measurements for the binding of butanol to membrane proteins [23]. However, the long-range lipid-protein interaction rather than annulus of strongly bound phospholipids around the proteins appeared to be affected by butanol. The maintenance of membrane fluidity is important in normal lipid-protein interactions and in maintenance of the activity of membrane-bound enzymes.

E. Alcohol Effect on Modified Cells. Broquist and Snell [40] found that biotin became completely non-essential for cell growth of *C. butyricum* in media supplemented with oleic, linoleic, and linolenic acids. Goldfine and Johnston [41] defined the auxotrophic relationship of biotin to fatty acid incorporation. In completely biotin-free media, the incorporation of oleate and elaidate into both acyl (glycerol ester linkage) and alkyl-enyl (glycerol ether linkage) chains of *C butyricum* was enriched more than 90 percent in the fed fatty acids. Also, Goldfine *et al*. [42], working with *C. butyricum*, showed that oleic acid (cis 18:1) and elaidic acid (trans 18:1) could be incorporated into the cell membrane to effect, respectively, greater and lesser fluid characteristics to the membrane.

Growth of *C. acetobutylicum* under similar conditions in medium supplemented with oleic acid and with elaidic acid have been conducted in our laboratory. Experiments designed to establish the tolerance of cells with modified membranes ot butanol have included growth rate and ATPase activity measurements. Cell growth experiments have been conducted in which the normal, oleate, and elaidate cells were exposed to various concentrations of butanol during logarithmic growth. Significant differences were observed in the responses to butanol challenge, when maximum specific growth rates of the three cell populations were analyzed as a function of butanol concentration (Table 8). The oleate-adapted cells exhibited half-maximal growth at 0.30 *M* (22 g/l); half-maximal growth rate for elaidate-adapted cells was 0.22 *M* butanol (16 g/l); whereas comparable values for control cells were 0.15 *M* (11 g/l). Tolerance to butanol had been extended up to two-fold.

Table 8

Concentrations of Butanol which Limit to Half-Maximal Rates, the Growth and Membrane ATPase Activity of C. acetobutylicum when Grown on Normal Soluble Media, on Media Supplemented with Avidin and Oleic Acid and on Media Supplemented with Avidin and Elaidic Acid

Half Maximal Rates	Butanol (M)		
	Normal	Oleate	Elaidate
Cell Growth	0.15	0.30	0.22
Membrane ATPase Activity	0.06	0.09	0.16

Membranes were prepared from C. acetobutylicum cells grown in normal medium, from cells grown in medium supplemented with avidin and oleic acid, and from cells grown in medium supplemented with avidin and elaidic acid. Depending on the medium used, adenosine triphosphatase (ATPase) activity associated with the particulate membranes exhibited different responses to inhibition of butanol added to the assay mixture. Hydrolysis of ATPase was determined by analyzing for release of inorganic phosphate following short periods (minutes) of incubation at 37°C. Such inhibition experiments, conducted in butanol concentrations varied from 0 to 0.16 M and were analyzed based on Folin-Lowry protein content of the membrane preparations. The nanomoles of ATP hydrolyzed per minute per mg protein as a function of butanol concentration yielded linear relationships representing the butanol inhibition of ATPase activity in membranes prepared from normal, oleate, and elaidate grown cells. The data clearly showed that the membrane-associated activity from modified fermentations exhibited lower inhibition by to butanol than did that from normal cells (Table 8). Half-maximal reaction velocities were noted at butanol concentrations as follows: normal cell membranes at 0.06 M (4.4 g/l), oleate cell membranes at 0.09 M (6.7 g/l), and elaidate cell membranes at 0.15 M (11.1 g/l). According to these parameters, tolerance to butanol had been extended 150 percent by growth in oleate and by 250 percent by growth in elaidate.

These data would indicate that substitution of unsaturated fatty acids into the cell membrane of C. acetobutylicum may diminish the inhibition of growth and related membrane functionality by butanol. To understand the improvement in tolerance by both oleate and elaidate will require further investigation of the membrane composition and enzymology. Whether the modification of the cell membrane will allow the cell to actually produce greater levels of solvents during fermentation is another question under investigation.

CONCLUSION

The incorporation of unsaturated fatty acids was effective in making yeast tolerant to ethanol. Thomas and Rose [42] reported that populations of yeast with membranes enriched with linoleic [18:2] residues exhibited greater viability and a lower extent of nutrient uptake inhibition in 1.0 M ethanol than did yeast enriched in oleate [18:1]. However, Brown et al. [43] have shown that ethanol was less inhibitory toward fermentation than toward growth of yeast.

Wang et al. [44] have studied alcohol inhibition of C. thermocellum, which is a thermophilic anaerobe that produces ethanol and acetic acid. Whereas acetic acid may have inhibited membrane processes, their results showed that ethanol may have inhibited glycolysis. Generally, hydrophobic effects need not necessarily involve membrane interaction, but because the effects of butanol on fermentation and growth are consistent with those on membrane enzymology, we predict that modification of the membrane environment will enhance solvent productivity.

Because of their simplicity, such biochemical approaches may be practiced before the potential of genetic engineering can be realized for improvement of alcohol tolerance. Indeed, the mechanism of alcohol toxicity must be understood through fundamental work in order to know whether a specific gene product could be the target of the genetic approaches.

ACKNOWLEDGEMENT

The authors wish to acknowledge the technical abilities of M.J. Moreira and S.M. Costa and for support of the Solar Energy Research Institute under contract XK-1-1315-1.

REFERENCES

1. Walton, M.J. and J.L. Martin. 1979. Production of Butanol-Acetone by Fermentation. In Microbial Technology, H.J. Peppler and D. Perlman (Eds.), Vol. I, Academic Press, New York, pp. 187-209.
2. Moreira, A.R., B.E. Dale, and M.G. Doremus. 1982. Utilization of the Fermentor Off-Gases from an Acetone-Butanol Fermentation. Paper presented at the Fourth Symposium on Biotechnology in Energy Production and Conservation, Gatlinburg, Tennessee, May 10-14.
3. Gabriel, C.L. 1928. Butanol Fermentation Process, Ind. Eng. Chem., 20, No. 10, p. 1063-1083.
4. Rogers, P.L, K.J. Lee, and D.E. Tribe. 1979. Kinetics of alcohol production by *Zymomonas mobilis* at high sugar concentrations. Biotechnol. Letters, 1, No. 4:165-170.
5. Becker, D.K., P.J. Blotkamp, and G.H. Emert. 1981. Pilot-Scale Conversion of Cellulose to Ethanol. In Fuels from Biomass and Wastes, D.L. Klass and G.H. Emert (Eds.), Ann Arbor Science, Ann Arbor, Michigan, pp. 375-392.

6. Vijkari, L., P. Nybergh, and M. Linko. 1981. Hydrolysis of Cellulose by T. reesei Enzymes and Simultaneous Production of Ethanol by Zymomonas sp. In Advances in Biotechnology, M. Moo-Young (Ed.), Vol. II, Pergamon Press, Toronto, pp. 137-142.

7. McGree, R.H. 1950. Anaerobic thermophilic cellulolytic bacteria. Bacteriol. Review, 14:51-63.

8. Ng, T.K., P.J. Weimer, and J.G. Zeikus. 1977. Cellulolytic and physiological properties of Clostridium thermocellum. Arch. Microbiol., 114:1-8.

9. Wang, D.I.C., C.L. Cooney, S.D. Wang, J. Gordon, and G.Y. Wang. 1978. Anaerobic biomass degradation to produce sugars, fuels, and chemicals. Proceedings of the 2nd Annual Biomass Energy Systems Conference. (Rensselaer Polytechnic Institute, Troy, NY), pp. 537-570.

10. Zeikus, J.G., A. Ben-Bassat and P.W. Hegge. 1980. Microbiology of methanogenesis in thermal, volcanic environments. J. Bacteriol., 143:432-440.

11. Wang, P.Y., B.F. Johnson, and H. Schneider, 1980. Fermentation of D-xylose by using glucose isomerase in the medium to convert xylose to D-xylulose. Biotechnol. Letters, 3:273-278.

12. Slininger, P.S., R.J. Bothast, J.E. Cauwenberg, and C.P. Kurtzman. 1982. Conversion of D-xylose to ethanol by the yeast Pachysolen tannophilus. Biotechnol. Bioeng. 24:371-384.

13. Anon. 1982. Gene looks, but doesn't leap, at thermophilic fermentation process. Biomass Digest, 4, No. 5:2-3.

14. Ljungdahl, L.G., F. Bryant, L. Carreira, T. Saiki, and J. Wiegle. 1981. Some Aspects of Thermophilic and Extreme Thermophilic Anaerobic Microorganisms. In Trends in the Biology of Fermentations for Fuels and Chemicals, A. Hollaender (Ed.), Plenum Press, New York, pp. 397-419.

15. Sinskey, A.J., M. Akedo, and C.L. Cooney. 1981. Acrylate Fermentations. In Trends in the Biology of Fermentations for Fuels and Chemicals, A. Hollaender (Ed.), Plenum Press, New York, pp. 473-492.

16. Flickinger, M. C. 1980. Current biological research in conversion of cellulosic carbohydrates into liquid fuels: How far have we come? Biotechnol. Bioeng., 22, Suppl. 1:27-48.

17. Heylin, M. (ed.). 1982. Facts and figures for the chemical industry. Chem. and Eng. News, 60 (24):31-81.

18. Wang, D.I.C., C.L. Cooney, A.L. Demain, R.F. Gomez, and A.J. Sinskey. 1979. Degradation of cellulosic biomass and its subsequent utilization for the production of chemical feedstocks. Quarterly Report to the U.S. Dept. of Energy, COG-4198-9:141-149.

19. Ingram, L.O. 1976. Adaptation of membrane lipids to alcohols. J. Bacteriol. 125:670-678.

20. Buttke, T.M. and L.O. Ingram. 1978. Mechanism of ethanol-induced changes in lipid composition of Escherichia coli: inhibition of saturated fatty acids synthesis in vivo. Biochem. 17:637-644.

21. Garwin, J.L. and J.E. Cronan, Jr. 1980. Thermal modulation of fatty acid synthesis in Escherichia coli does not involve de novo enzyme synthesis. J. Bacteriol. 141:1457-1459.

22. Grisham, C.M. and R.E. Barnett. 1973. The effects of long-chain alcohols on membrane lipids and the (Na^+ - K^+) - ATPase. Biochim. Biophys. Acta. 311:417-422.

23. Lenaz, G., E. Bertoli, G. Curatola, L. Mazzanti, and A. Bigi. 1976. Lipid protein interactions in mitochondria: spin and fluoresence probe studies on the effect of n-alkanols on phospholipid vesicles and mitochondrial membranes. Arch. Biochem. Biophys. 172:278-288.

24. Paterson, S.J., K.W. Butler, P. Huang, J. La Belle, I.C.P. Smith, and H. Schneider. 1972. The effects of alcohols on lipid bilayes: A spin label study. Biochim. Biophys. Acta. 266:597-602.

25. Yoshida, M., N. Sone, H. Hirata, and Y. Kagawa. 1975. A highly stable adenosine triphosphatase from a thermophilic bacterium: purification, properties, and reconstitution. J. Biol. Chem. 250:7910-7916.

26. Hirata, H., N. Sone, M. Yoshida, Y. Kakawa. 1976. Active transport of alanine of thermo-stable membrane vesicles isolated from PS3. J. Biochem. (Tokyo). 76:1157-1166.

27. Laskin, A.I. and H. Lechevalier (eds). 1971. Lipoidal contents of specific microorganisms. CRC Handbook of Microbiology. Vol. 3: 297-298.

28. Sorensen, S., T. Dunwiddie, G. McClearn, R. Freedman, and B. Hoffer. 1981. Ethanol-induced depressions in cerebellar and lippocampal neurons of mice selectively bred for differences in ethanol sensitivity: an electro-physiological study. Pharmacol. Biochem. Behavior. 14:227-234.

29. Baker. R., C. Melchior and R. Deitrich. 1980. The effect of halothane on mice selectively bred for differential sensitivity to alcohol. Pharmacol. Biochem. Behavior. 12:691-695.

30. Moreira, A.R., D.C. Ulmer, and J.C. Linden. 1981. Butanol toxicity in the butylic fermentation. Biotechnol. Bioeng., Symp. No. 11:567-579.

31. Linden, J.C., D.C. Ulmer, and A.R. Moreira. 1981. A mechanism for aliphatic alochol-induced toxicity in Clostridium acetobutylicum. Presented at 182nd Natl. ACS Meetings, New York City.

32. Sullivan, K.H., M.K. Jain, and A.L. Koch. 1974. Activation of the β-galactoside transport system in E. coli ML-308 by n-alkanols. Biochim. Biophys. Acta. 352:287-297.

33. Duperray, B., M. Chastrette, M.C. Makabeh, and H. Pacheco. 1976. Analyse de l'activite bactercide de populations d'alcools alphatiques et de β-naphtols suivanto les methodes de Hansch et Darc-Pelco: effet d'allongement de chaine. Eur. J. Med. Chem-Chimica Therapeutica. 11:433-437.

34. Costa, J.M. and A.R. Moreira. 1982. Kinetics of the acetone-butanol fermentation. Presented at the Winter Symposium on the Fundamentals of Biochemical Engineering, Boulder, CO. January 17-20.

35. Boulanger, Y., S. Schreier, and I.C.P. Smith. 1981. Molecular details of anesthetic-lipid interaction as seen by deuterium

and phosphorus-31 nuclear magnetic resonance. Biochem. 20:6824-6830.

36. Browning, J.L. and H. Akutsu. 1982. Local anesthetics and divalent cations have the same effect on the headgroups of phosphatidylcholine and phosphatidylethanolamine. Biochim. Biophys. Acta. 684:172-178.

37. Lenaz, G., G. Parenti-Castelli, and A.M. Sechi. 1975. Changes in mitochondrial adenosine triphosphatase activity induced by n-butanol. Arch. Biochem. Biophys. 167:72-79.

38. Hesketh, T.R., G.A. Smith, M.D. Houslay, K.A. McGill, N.J.M. Birdsall, J.C. Metcalfe, and G.B. Warren. 1976. Annular lipids determine the ATPase activity of a calcium transport protein complexed with dipalmitoyllecithin. Biochem. 15:4145-4151.

39. Meissner, G. 1981. Effect of lipid membrane structure on adenosine triphosphate hydrolyzing activity of the calcium-stimulated adenosinetriphosphatase of sacroplasmic reticulum. Biochem. 20:6810-6817.

40. Broquist, H.P. and E.E. Snell. 1951. Biotin and bacterial growth. J. Biol. Chem. 188:432-444.

41. Goldfine, H. and N.C. Johnston. 1980. Regulation of membrane fluidity in anaerobic bacteria. In Membrane Fluidity: Biophysical Techniques and Cellular Recognition. M. Kates and A. Kuksis (Eds.). The Human Press, Clifton, NJ. pp 365-380.

42. Thomas, D.S. and A.H. Rose. 1979. Inhibitory effect of ethanol on growth and solvent accumulation by Saccharomyces cerevisiae as affected by plasma-membrane lipid composition. Arch. Microbiol. 122:49-55.

43. Brown, S. W., S.G. Oliver, D.E.F. Harrison, and R.C. Righelato. 1981. Ethanol inhibition of yeast growth and fermentation: differences in the magnitude and complexity of the effect. Eur. J. Appl. Microbiol. Biotechnol. 11:151-155.

44. Wang, D.I.C., C.L. Cooney, A.L. Demain, R.F. Gomez, and A.J. Sinskey. 1981. Degradation of cellulosic biomass and its subsequent utilization for the production of chemical feedstocks.

Report to U.S. DOE under contract no. EG-77-S-02-4198, subcontract no. XR-9-8109-1.

DISCUSSION

Q. P. ROGERS (University of Minnesota): You mentioned an extractant on the surface of the butanol-acetone fermentation. What is the extractant you put on top of your culture, and when you add your butyric and acetic acid and got inhibition, is it pH adjusted or have you just added free acid?

A. LINDEN: In answer to the first question, in this case, I'm not at liberty to say what that extractant is, but MIT work with corn oil produced just about the same increase in productivity as we observed. Secondly, the pH of the media was controlled in the cases of butyric acid and acetic acid challenges with 2-(N-morpholino)ethane-sulfonic acid (MES) buffer. These were batch fermentations but the pH stayed between 5.5 and 6.

CONTINUOUS CULTURE FOR PRODUCTION

Alan T. Bull
Biological Laboratory
University of Kent at Canterbury
Canterbury, Kent CT2 7NJ, England

INTRODUCTION

First I would like to make a personal comment on the general development of biotechnology from the viewpoint of a microbial physiologist. The study of microbial physiology has suffered considerable neglect in recent years and this has implications for the overall pace and direction of biotechnological innovation. In contrast, the effort to understand and manipulate the genomes of microorganisms has attracted massive investment. One of the most remarkable features of microorganisms is their capacity for phenotypic variation, variation which can be manifest in metabolic, chemical, and structural terms. Such variation is a double-edged sword as far as the fermentation microbiologist is concerned: it provides an abundant scope for the development of novel processes but it may pose problems during process scale-up if the fermentation conditions are not sufficiently well reproduced. If one is considering the development of a continuous fermentation process, the difficulties - especially where genetically engineered strains are to be used - may be compounded; the strong selection pressures characteristic of continuous cultures can lead to the competitive displacement of the production strain. The dilemma has been put clearly by Tempest [40] as a basic incompatability between organism improvement by genetic manipulation and process improvement by utilizing continuous culture techniques. Consequently there is a pressing need to extend our understanding of the behavior of organisms under conditions of continuous culture so that strains, improved by whatever means, can be deployed in continuous processes without the problem of reversion or other forms of degeneration.

The fermentation industry has been based very largely on batch operations using stirred tank reactors. Of course, there are circumstances under which batch cultures are and will remain the process option of choice, but among the disadvantages of batch systems are:

(1) very limited capacity to manipulate organism specific growth rate (μ) without major alterations to the culture environment; μ is close to a maximum throughout most of the culture period;

(2) environment and organism change continuously as a function of time of culture: steady states cannot be attained;

(3) diseconomies of a non-continuous process.

Continuous culture appears to have been discovered several times this century. Empirical continuous processes for baker's yeast and ethanol were described in the 1920s while systematic studies of continous cultivation were made by Czech and Soviet microbiologists in the following decade [see Humphrey, 21; Malek and Fencl, 26]. The theoretical basis of continuous culture was laid in the 1950s with the studies of Monod [27], Novick and Szilard [28] and Herbert *et al.* [19]. But only in the following two decades were the possibilities of the technique widely appreciated and applications made to biochemical, physiological, genetic, and ecological research on microorganisms. The final phase of discovery is concerned with the impact of continuous culture theory on biotechnology and this paper examines some properties of continuous culture which recommend their adoption by fermentation technologists. My personal bias is to regard continuous culture not as a mere technique but as the catalyst of a basic change in approach to the study of microbial behavior. Such studies have provided a new dimension to the understanding of microbial physiology and have revealed novel properties not suspected from batch culture experiments. Most importantly it also offers the opportunity for a genuinely scientific approach to process design and optimization.

DISTINCTIVE PROPERTIES OF CONTINUOUS CULTURES

A large body of literature exists on the theory, practice, and range of continuous culture studies [see Malek and Fencl, 26; Pirt, 30 for comprehensive reviews] and on their application in microbiology research [Bull and Brown, 6; Tempest, 39]. It is not my intention to repeat such discussions, rather I wish to draw attention to those distinctive properties of continuous cultures that are germane to industrial exploitation. It is worth keeping in mind that the boundaries between different types of culture systems have become increasingly blurred and acceptance of the term "bioreactors" is a measure of the integration of ideas from fermentation technology, enzyme engineering, and chemical engineering.

The basic types of continuous culture are the chemostat, turbidostat, and plug-flow systems (Fig. 1) described as follows:

(1) Chemostat (Fig. 1a). The specific growth rate (μ) at steady state is determined by the rate of supply of

the growth-limiting substrate (F). The ratio F/V, where V is the constant culture volume, gives the dilution rate (D) and the latter equals μ in the steady state. Any component of the culture medium can be made the growth-limiting substrate and μ can be varied from very low values to values approaching a maximum simply by manipulating F.

(2) Turbidostat (Fig. 1b). The organism concentration of the culture is sensed by a photoelectric cell which activates the medium supply pump when the concentration exceeds a preset value. Thus, in the chemostat, D is preset and the organism concentration is self-adjusting to a steady state value while in the turbidostat organism concentration is fixed and the dilution rate is self-adjusting. Specific growth rate in a turbidostat is maximized due to the excess of all substrates. Control can be achieved by any parameter, ranging from CO_2 production to bioluminescense, which is directly linked to growth.

(3) Plug-flow (Fig. 1c). This system can be visualized as simulating in spatial terms the temporal changes characteristic of batch culture. The assumption is made that nutrient medium flows through the fermenter as a plug at constant rate, without forward or backward mixing, and that organisms contained in it grow as a batch culture. True plug-flow culture has not been realized at laboratory scale but has found application in the waste treatment and dairy industries (see 5 below).

The chief advantages of simple continuous cultures are summarized in Table 1. These systems can be elaborated in a variety of ways and two such modifications of the simple, single stage chemostat are of industrial concern.

1. Experimental manipulation of specific growth rate is possible over a full range and does not necessitate varying medium composition or environmental conditions.

2. Effects of physico-chemical environment can be evaluated systematically while maintaining constant specific growth rate.

3. Steady state and defined transient states can be analysed.

4. Establishment of unique culture conditions is possible by changing the nature of the growth-limiting substrate.

5. Maintenance of growth over long periods.

Fig. 1. Basic continuous culture systems. (a) chemostate, (b) turbidostate, (c) plug flow.

Table 1

Some Advantages of Simple Continuous Cultures

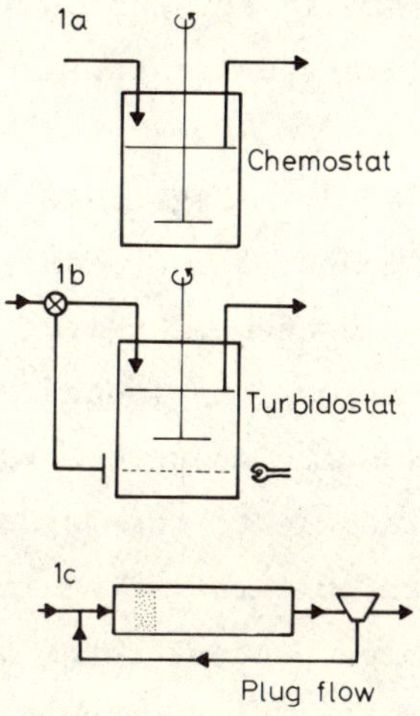

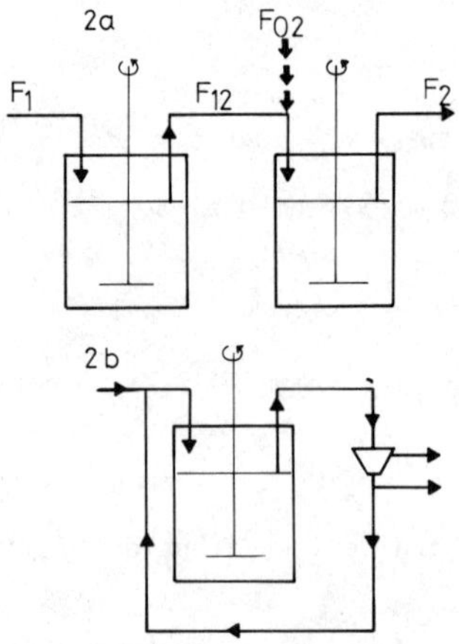

Fig. 2. Complex continuous culture systems. (a) multi-stage; $F_1 = F_{12} = F_2$. F_{02} indicates a subsidiary feed of materials into the second stage vessel. (b) feedback.

(4) Multi-stage (Fig. 2a). Here, two or more chemostats are linked in series. The environmental conditions may be varied in the different stages and supplementary feeds of medium or other materials may be made to the 2nd to the nth stages (flow F_{02} in Fig. 2a). There is no critical dilution rate in the 2nd or nth stages as long as the 1st stage is in steady state.

(5) Biomass Feedback (Fig. 2b). Continuous cultures which have some means of increasing the biomass concentrations of the simple chemostat are termed feedback systems. In practical terms centrifugation, sedimentation, and filtration provide the means of producing a concentrated suspension for recycle to the fermenter. The essential feature of feedback culture is the increased biomass concentration which enables process rates to be increased above those obtainable in a simple chemostat.

Table 2

Some Advantages of Complex Continuous Cultures

1. Growth or metabolism in presence of high excess of substrate (such conditions may be inhibitory in simple chemostat or batch culture.

2. Behaviour at very low or zero growth rates.

3. Utilization of mixed substrates at high overall rates.

4. Transformation of, or in the presence of, growth-inhibitory materials.

5. Synthesis on non-growth associated products.

6. High rates of processing of dilute substrates.

The chief advantages of multistage and feedback continuous cultures are summarized in Table 2. Two other elaborations of continuous culture relate to fluidized bed and fixed bed systems. These systems also increase significantly the operational versatility and control of continuous-flow bioreactors and among the advantages conferred are increased stability to shock loading and environmental perturbation and increased processing rates [Bull, 5].

There is one final feature of continuous cultures that has overriding signficance for biotechnological industries. Chemostat theory predicts that higher productivities of biomass and growth-related metabolites are possible compared with batch cultures operating with similar growth yields, final biomass concentrations, and inoculum sizes. The ratio of continuous to batch productivities is largely determined by the specific growth rate and the "down-time" incurred in batch operation. Figure 3 indicates that the advantage

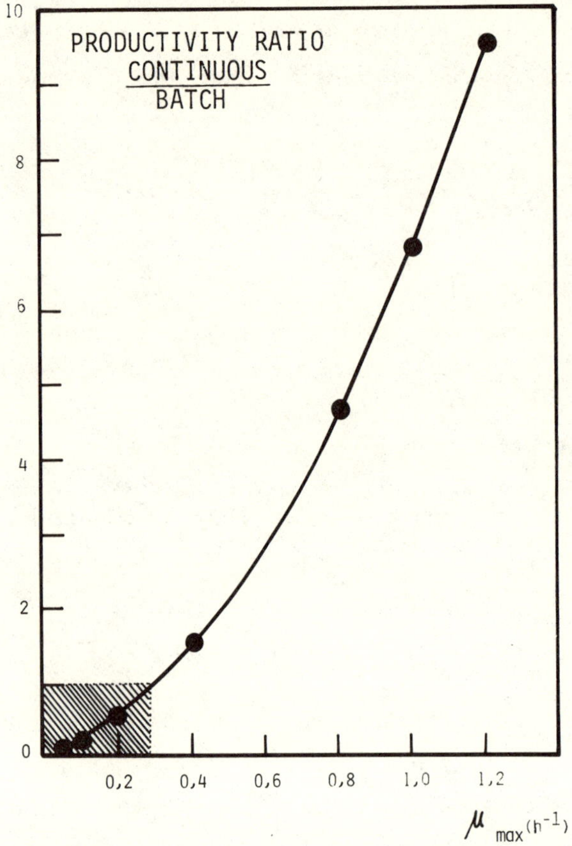

Fig. 3. Comparative biomass productivities of continuous and batch cultures. The productivity ratio is calculated as

$$\frac{(\ln(X_m/X_o + \mu_{max}\, t_L)\ \ D_{crit}\ Y}{(X_m - X_o)\ /\ X_m}$$

with $X_m/X_o = 0.95$, $X_m = 30\,g\,l^{-1}$, down time, $t_L = 10h$, $Y = 0.5g$ biomass g^{-1} substrate.

The hatched area indicates the operational range over which continuous culture offers no advantage.

of continuous culture increases as a function of μ, while Fig. 4 demonstrates the further impact that biomass feedback has on the relationship.

It would be sanguine to suggest that adoption of continuous culture methods is without problems. Some of the commonly voiced disadvantages of continuous culture are listed in Table 3. Of these, organism stability is of special concern to the fermentation microbiologist, a concern which is heightened by the advent of genetically manipulated strains. These problems will be addressed later in this paper.

THE IMPACT OF CONTINUOUS CULTURE ON THE BIOTECHNOLOGY-BASED INDUSTRIES

The potential and realized applications of continuous culture methodology in industry have been assessed with familiar regularity [Dawson, 11; Evans, 14; Herbert, 18; Hospodka, 20; Righelato and Elsworth, 33] and one might anticipate a progressive increase in its acceptance and diversity of application over the last three decades. This is patently not the situation. The waste treatment, baker's yeast, and brewing industries have deployed continuous culture but the impact on the production of pharmaceutical and other chemicals has been negligible. The reasons for such reticence are severalfold:

(1) an anticipation that continuous fermentations would prove to be less trouble-free in operation than batch equivalents, particularly regarding contamination;

(2) the capital investment required to install a new plant or to convert existing batch equipment even when a superior process is promised;

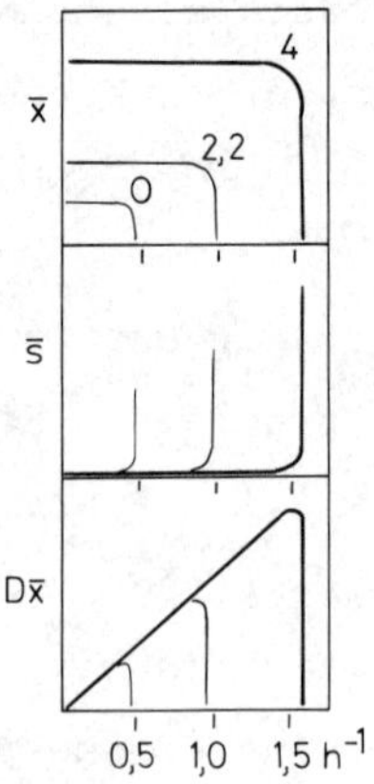

Fig. 4. The effect of biomass recycle on chemostat productivity $D\bar{x}$.

Table 3

Some Disadvantages (Real and Imagined) of Continuous Cultures

1. Organism stability; selection of spontaneous mutants; reversion of production strains to wild-types; loss of plasmids.

2. Prevention of contamination over long periods.

3. Equipment unreliability.

(3) the possibility that introduction of a new process will change product quality;

(4) uncertainty of demand for extra production over existing supply;

(5) some early failures or qualified successes inhibited development and prolonged the invention-innovation lag.

However, with three decades of experience behind us, changing economic trends especially with regard to organic feedstocks, and increased confidence in biotechnology-based industry, interest in continuous culture is certain to grow. In my view this interest will focus on continuous culture (a) as a potent tool in biotechnology research and development, and (b) as the means of achieving the large-scale, lowcost biotechnology necessary for bulk productions. A measure of the usefulness of the chemostat under the first heading can be judged from studies of nitrogen metabolism. Ammonia assimilation in bacteria can occur via the glutamate dehydrogenase (GDH) or the glutamine synthetase (GS) - glutamate synthase (GOGAT) pathways. The discovery of glutamate synthase came from analysis of ammonia-limited chemostat populations of *Klebsiella aerogenes*; it has a higher affinity for ammonia than glutamate dehydrogenase but requires an extra mol of ATP per mol NH_3 assimilated. Of considerable interest is the fact that the bacterium used by I.C.I. Ltd. (*Methylophilus methylotropus*) in their single cell protein process possesses the GS-GOGAT only. Windass *et al*. [41] have cloned the GDH gene from *Escherichia coli* into *M. methylotrophus* and the consequent energy-sparing in ammonia assimilation resulted in a 5% increase in protein yield from methanol. To date no reports have appeared on the performance of this manipulated strain in large-scale continuous fermenters.

Regarding very large-scale production, there is no question that continuous processes are essential. The I.C.I. pressure cycle fermenter with a capacity of 1500 m^3 is thought to be the largest production fermenter. The next generation of fermenters may be at least 10,000 m^3 capacity [Spinks, 38] and, as King [22] has pointed out: "If biotechnology is to play a part in replacing oil-based chemical products, then our ability to build and operate large-scale plants will be as important as it is currently for polyethylene, nylon, salt, or ammonia." The operation of such large continuous fermenters poses many problems for the biochemical engineer - the following two will serve to illustrate their magnitude. First, the rate of response of microorganisms to a changing environment is such that catabolism can be selectively accelerated by transient fluctuations in substrate supply under circumstances of carbon-limited growth. It is important to prevent the occurrence of such transients in very large-scale chemostats, but imperfect mixing and periodic adjustments to fermenter conditions may cause them. The consequences of discontinuous additions of substrate are shown dramatically in model experiments with methanol-limited *Pseudomonas methylotropha* [Brooks and Meers, 3] and glucose-limited *Klebsiella aerogenes* [Leegwater *et al.*, 25] (Figs. 5a and 5b). Thus, the growth yield of *P. methylotropha* was reduced by 21% when the interval between methanol additions was 100s and even much smaller intervals (20s) caused significant impairment of operational efficiency (yield reduced by 7%). Under the second heading we may consider the recycling, not of the biomass but of the spent fermentation broth consisting of water, mineral nutrients. As the scale of continuous fermentation increases, broth recycling becomes economically attractive and has been considered necessary in

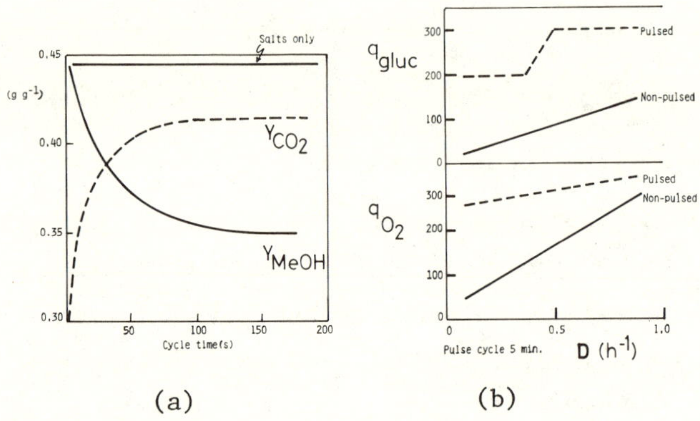

Fig. 5. The effects of discontinuous substrate additions on bacterial growth. (a) *Pseudomonas methylotropha*-methanol; (b) *Klebsiella aerogenes*-glucose.

large-scale SCP processes. Harrison [17] claims that considerable economies occur if greater than 90% water recycle can be achieved. The accumulation of metabolites in the recycled broth may cause problems; with 90% recycle of broth the amino acid content of SCP-methanol fermentations can increase 10-fold and have a deleterious effect on productivity. Carbon dioxide recycle in carbon-limited chemostat cultures of *Aspergillus nidulans* has been investigated by Bushell and Bull [9]. By optimizing the activities of anaplerotic carboxylases the biomass yield was increased by more than 20%.

R AND D IMPLICATIONS

The position of continuous culture in research and development, alluded to in the previous section, merits further attention. The continuous culture approach is an enormously powerful one and in this context it will be instructive to examine three areas of activity: organism selection for biotechnological processes, process optimization, and the development of novel bioreactors.

A crucial stage of exploratory research is the selection of organisms having desired properties, and in contrast to the usual requirements of academic research, organism selection has to be based on a spectrum of criteria relevant to optimizing the process [Bull, 5]. The traditional means of organism selection is via batch enrichment techniques and, useful as such techniques are, they are inherently inadequate. For example, batch enrichments select for organisms on the basis of maximum specific growth rate (because of the substrate excess), a characteristic which might not be of primary importance; sampling of enrichment cultures at a stage when the required organisms are dominant may be missed because conditions (and thereby populations) change as a function of time; and because of the complex succession of changes which occur during batch enrichments, the system is not well controlled and reproducibility tends to be restricted to enrichments made under extreme conditions. In contrast, continuous-flow enrichment techniques offer much improved control, reproducibility, and versatility. Turbidostats are advantageous when selecting for organisms having high maximum specific growth rates (a desirable property in SCP organisms) while enrichment under chemostat conditions enables selection to be based on different specific growth rates, substrate concentration or nutrient limitations. Continuous-flow enrichment invariably selects stable multispecies communities, a point which will be touched upon later.

Some varied examples of chemostat enrichment from my own laboratory illustrate its potential. The technique is particularly suited to the isolation of biodegradative organisms and selection of extracellular enzymes. A novel exopectin lyase specific for highly methylated substrates was isolated in this way [Almengor-Hecht and Bull, 1] and a two-stage enrichment chemostat was used for the isolation of potent yeast cell wall hydrolyzing bacteria (Stage 1, growth of yeast; Stage 2, enrichment on living yeast cells as substrate) [Rowley and Bull, 35]. Continuous-flow systems are ideal for the isolation of organisms resistant to toxic materials. Bryson's "turbidostatic selector" [Bryson, 4] was an early application of this sort and was used for the enrichment of neomycin resistant *Escherichia coli* and at the same time avoiding bacteriostasis. In our hands enrichment chemostats have been deployed for the selection of silver and copper resistant and bioaccumulative bacteria [Charley and Bull, 10; G.M. Dunn, P. Goddard and A.T. Bull, unpublished experiments]. Organisms can be "trained" to resist high concentrations of such metals by gradually increasing the concentration in the feed supply, while two-stage or biomass recycle modifications can prevent washout of populations under highly toxic conditions. All our experiments of this type have produced stable communities of organisms and frequently the bioaccumulative capacity of the

Table 4

Silver Bioaccumulation by a Chemostat-Enriched Community and its Dominant Component, Pseudomonas maltophilia

Population	Rate of Accumulation (mg silver g^{-1} biomass h^{-1})	Accumulation (mg silver g^{-1} (biomass)	K_i silver (nM)
Community[a)]	21.0	316	0.78
Ps.maltophilia	3.8	182	0.55

a) *Ps.maltophilia*, *Staphylococcus aureus*, coryneform organism.

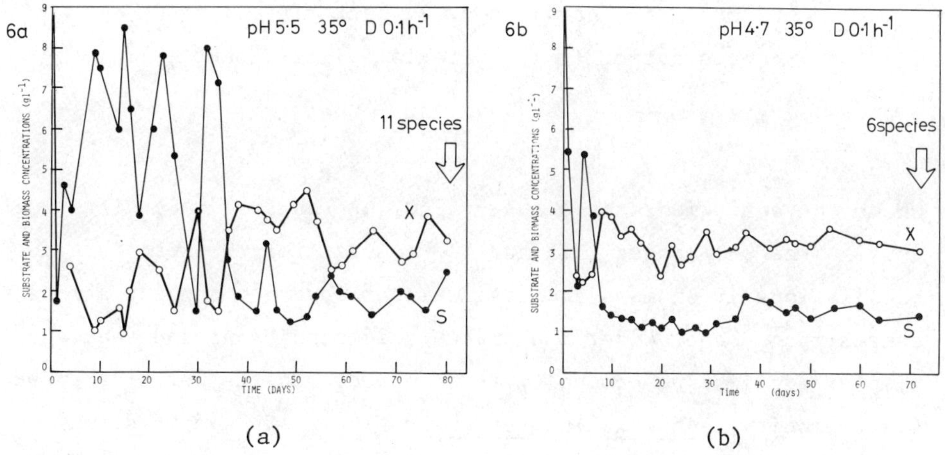

Fig. 6. Progress of chemostat enrichment isolations; starch was the growth-limiting substrate. (a) enrichment at pH 5.5; (b) enrichment at pH 4.7.

community is superior to that of any of the component species. Table 4 presents results from one silver bioaccumulation enrichment experiment. The final enrichment study relates to the selection of organisms for a starch-SCP process (J.R. Rodriquez and A.T. Bull, unpublished experiments). Figs. 6a and 6b show the results of two

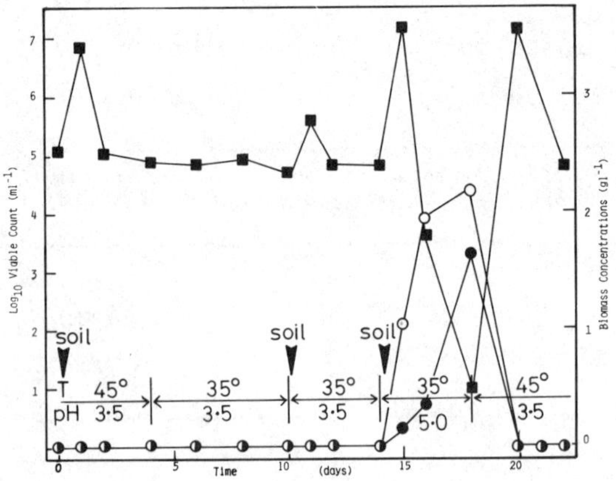

Fig. 7. Response of a starch=limited chemostat culture of <u>Aspergillus terreus</u> to deliberate contamination by soil heterotrophs (as shown by the vertical arrows) <u>A. terreus</u> biomass concentration (■), bacterial biomass concentration (●), bacterial viable count (O).

chemostat enrichments (D $0.10h^{-1}$,35°C, starch 10 g 1^{-1}) differing only in the pH imposed (5.5 and 4.7 respectively). Note that the oscillations in biomass and residual carbohydrate concentrations dampen much sooner under the higher acid conditions and that a simpler equilibrium community is selected. One member of the "pH 4.7 community", <u>Aspergillus terreus</u> has been studied in detail. This fungus is able to grow with maximum productivity at extremes of temperature and pH (45°C and pH 3.5) and, as illustrated in Fig. 7, is totally resistant to contamination by soil heterotrophs under these conditions. The implications will be obvious for long term, contamination-free production runs, or the development of septic "protected fermentations" in which no attempt is made to prevent access of contaminating organisms, but instead their establishment is prevented due to the selective conditions of culture.

Table 5

Optimization of Xanthan Gum Production:

The Influence of Nutrient Limitation

Nutrition Limitation	D (h^{-1})	Xanthan yield from glucose (%)	Culture Viscosity (cps)	Strain variation (weeks) a)
K	0.03	36	360	1
Mg	0.03	36	270	3
C	0.045	45	500	1
P	0.03	49	5000	3
S	0.035	61	18000	None
N	0.03	62	15000	None

a) Time on stream before the appearance of non-productive variations.

From Evans *et al.*, (15).

The utility of continuous cultures in process optimization studies is limited only by the perception of the investigator. Work on xanthan gum production, for example, has shown that product yield, product quality, and strain variation in continuous culture are simultaneously influenced by the nature of the nutrient limitation. In this case all three variables were optimized by the same nutrient limitation (Table 5).

The considerable benefit of partial biomass feedback on fermenter productivity was indicated in the earlier section on "Distinctive Properties of Continuous Culture". Recent work by D.N. Bull and Young [8] extends this principle to product formation and these authors incorporated a novel cross-flow filtration device to produce various recycle ratios (ratio of flow rate of cell-free stream to

Table 6

Effect of Partial Cell Recycle on the Fermentation of D-Sorbitol to L-Sorbose

D (h^{-1})	Recycle Ratio	S_R Sorbitol (gl^{-1})	Sorbose Concn. (gl^{-1})	Sorbose Productivity ($gl^{-1}h^{-1}$)	Enhancement %
0.28	0	199	160	45	
0.36	0	199	134	48	7
0.34	0.49	210	222	76	69
0.32	0.32	311	201	65	44
0.34	0.48	307	272	91	102
0.45	0.49	307	250	111	147

From Bull and Young (8).

total effluent flow-rate). Bull and Young [8] tested their system for the conversion of D-sorbitol to L-sorbose and glucose to 2-keto-gluconic acid and found that partial biomass recycle increased production rates decisively (Tables 6 and 7). These results are of great interest and greatly enhanced productivity of any substance for which the rate of synthesis is a positive function of biomass concentration, or μ, or both parameters.

My final comment in this section is reserved for the application of continuous culture strategy in the development of novel reactor designs. Several commentators have argued that the exploitation of microbial photosynthesis is the only feasible route to primary carbon production sufficient to replace fossil sources. Thus, in the last few years several groups have sought to maximize photosynthetic efficiency (biomass produced/light absorbed) and

Table 7

Effect of Partial Cell Recycle on the Fermentation of Glucose to 2-Ketogluconic Acid

D (h^{-1})	Recycle Ratio	S_R Glucose (gl^{-1})	2-KGA Concn. (gl^{-1})	2-KGA Productivity (gl^{-1} h^{-1})	Enhancement (%)
0.096	0	198	55	5.3	
0.097	0.50	198	79	7.7	45
0.102	0.76	198	111	11.3	113

From Bull and Young (8).

light-limited growth has been shown to be essential for this [Pirt et al. 31) and for maximum photoheterotrophic productivity [Kreuzberg and Hempfling, 23]. Pirt and his colleagues have used a continuous-flow loop reactor in their studies and have demonstrated that light-limited *Chlorella* has a maximum practical storage of total solar energy of 18%, a value about three times the maximum predicted for higher plants. More recently, Lee and Pirt [24] have assessed the effect of intermittent, short cycle illumination on biomass production. Populations exposed to dark periods greater than about 9s showed reduced specific growth rates and a loss of biomass through endogenous metabolism at a rate of 13.6% h^{-1}. The implication of this finding for the design of large-scale photobioreactors is considerable.

INDUSTRIAL PROCESSES

Continuous-flow processes exist at the industrial scale for

waste and water treatment, for biomass (SCP) production, and for certain foods and beverages. The next major sector of biotechnology to develop continuous production processes will be that of bulk chemicals, and there will be increased interest in processes as metal winning, biochemicals (e.g. amino acids), biopolymers, and agrochemicals (e.g., microbial pesticides, soil inoculants). Equally predictable is the large array of microbial products that will not be suitable for continuous production, either because the absolute market size is small (e.g., some vaccines, toxins, hormones, enzymes) or because the present understanding of biosynthetic pathways and their regulation is inadequate for the rational design of a continuous process (e.g., many secondary metabolic products). However, the sophisticated nature of continuous culture will prove attractive for the production of low volume material when precisely defined quality is at a premium. It is not my intention to take an itinerative view of existing industrial process but rather to focus on a few processes or products and illustrate the impact of continuous culture thereon.

Waste Treatment

A very thorough review of activated sludge technology was made recently by Humphrey [21]. The process basically operates as a multistage system with partial sludge recycle, usually the recycle ratio is about 0.25, and BOD removal greater than 90%. One of the most interesting developments in this field is the optimization of activated sludge processes for the removal of BOD, phosphorus, and nitrates [Osborn and Nicholls, 29; Figure 8]. The sequential removal of the influent sludge constituents is achieved by controlling the relative residence times in anaerobic, anoxic, and aerobic treatment tanks and the internal and external sludge recycle ratios. Polyphosphate kinase is induced in phosphate accumulating bacteria under anaerobic conditions and concomitantly large quantities of BOD are taken up. Nitrates inhibit kinase synthesis and are removed in

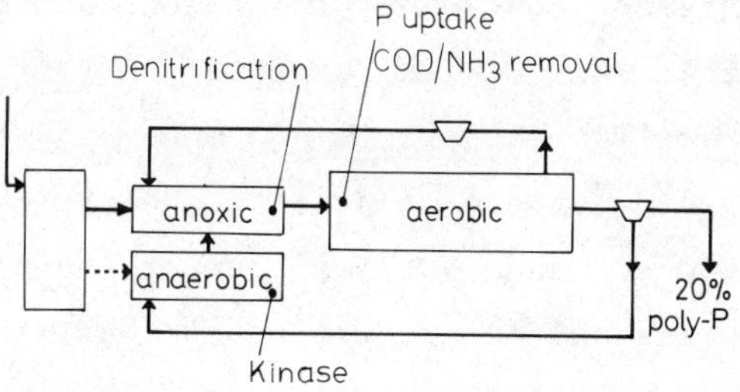

Fig. 8. Activated sludge process for the removal of BOD, phosphorus and nitrates.

the anoxic stage. Thus bacteria entering the aerobic, plug-flow stage oxidize the BOD and synthesize polymetaphosphate; the latter may comprise 20% of the biomass. Sludge from such a process would provide a useful slow-release P-fertilizer when applied to land.

Biomass

A vast literature exists on experimental, pilot- and production-scale activities in the biomass field [Rose, 34]. However, one problem common to all large-scale continuous culture operations, viz. maintenance of sterility (see 3 earlier section), has been tackled strenuously by SCP manufacturers and their protocols will be of interest to a broad audience of fermentation technologists. Smith [37] discusses this problem in detail with respect to the I.C.I. process and identifies three points of contamination risk: sterilization of feed streams, sterilization of the plant at start-up, and operation of the plant. The advent of the "sterile audit" means regular inspection of plant operations by independent auditors who have complete freedom of investigation.

Food

The manufacture of yoghurt illustrates a number of features of modern, sophisticated continuous fermented food production. Traditionally yoghurt, a mixed milk fermentation (*Streptococcus thermophilus*, *Lactobacillus bulgaricus*) is made by a batch process. Consumption of yoghurt during the past decade or so has lead to increased production demands but scale-up of the batch process caused problems of souring and deterioration of consistency. Consequently attention turned to continuous manufacture and the process developed at the Netherlands Institute for Dairy Research has proved very successful [Driessen, 12]. The basic unit stages in continuous yoghurt production are shown in Fig. 9. Prefermentation of the milk (D $2.0h^{-1}$) occurs with the two bacteria and the pH is maintained at 5.7 by continuous neutralization with fresh milk. The fermented milk is pumped to the coagulation tank where it is layered onto the surface of the acidifying milk via a centrifugal distributor. The acidifying milk passes through the coagulation tank in plug-flow fashion and a gradient of acidity and texture becomes established. At the bottom of the tank the yoghurt is stirred by a rotating plate which does not disturb the plug-flow character of the operation. Total residence time in a 4000 $\mu\ h^{-1}$ plant is about 3 hr. The continuous process results in an 80% saving in fermenter volume and yields a product having good organoleptic properties.

Beverages

Continuous fermentation has been exploited by the brewing industry for many years and both stirred tank and tower fermenters have been designed for ale and lager beers. Very high brewing rates can be achieved in continuous tower fermenters (residence time 4 to 5h) once the plug of flocculent yeast has built up at the base of the tower (up to 400 g l^{-1}). Unfortunately, unlike the experience with yoghurt, continuously brewed beer has suffered a number of problems - impaired flavor, difficulty in switching production from one beer to another, and increased expense of wort storage and pasteurization. Because of such problems brewers in various

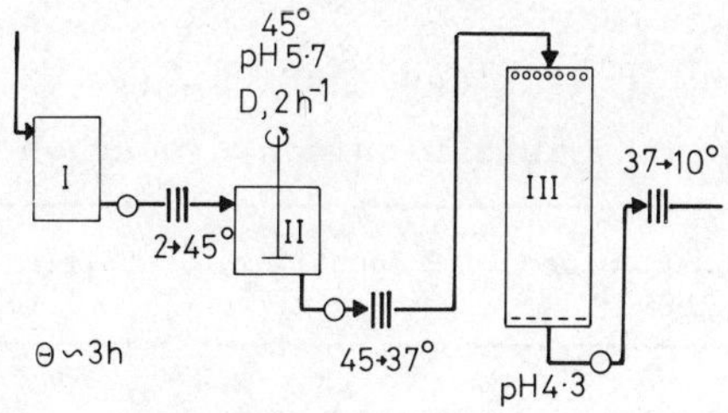

Fig. 9. Continuous yoghurt production. I, fresh milk holding tank; II, prefermentation tank; III, coagulation tank.

countries, particularly in the U.K., have reverted to batch brewing with cylindroconical vessels receiving considerable favor.

REFLECTIONS

The following are some final thoughts relating to large-scale continuous culture operations.

Trends in Reactor Design and Operation

The stirred tank fermenter is still the most popular industrial reactor and culture volumes of about $300m^3$ and power inputs of about $4kWm^{-3}$ appear to be maximum scale figures [Sittig, 36]. The new generation of fermenters will be at least one order of magnitude larger in size, and alternatives to stirred tanks will be imperative; continuous-flow air-life loop reactors of the I.C.I. SCP and Deep-shaft waste treatment types are indicative of current thinking. The selection of a reactor system for a designated process will be influenced not only by the scale required but also by the interaction between the organism and the physical environment within which it grows. One such situation has been reviewed by Bailey and

Table 8

Effect of Power Input per Unit Volume on Biomass Productivity in a Liquid Hydrocarbon Fermentation

Power Input (HPm^{-3})	Productivity ($gl^{-1}\ h^{-1}$)	Critical Dilution Rate (h^{-1})
0.10	0.17	0.090
0.25	0.29	0.130
0.50	0.38	0.150
1.00	0.49	0.168
1.50	0.54	0.172
2.00	0.59	0.177
2.50	0.63	0.180

Computed data from Bailey and Ollis (2).

Ollis [2], that of fluid mechanics in relation to biomass productivity in a liquid hydrocarbon fermentation (Table 8). For a 25-fold increase in power input, the productivity increased nearly 4-fold due to a doubling of the critical dilution rate, and the latter was a consequence of the effect of increased shear on hydrocarbon droplet size.

Downstream Implications

The attraction of biomass feedback has been emphasized in this discussion: the means of generating a concentrated feed-back stream for recycle can have implications for down-stream processing or product formulation. Thus, Gold *et al*. [16] have increased biomass productivity from sulphite waste liquor 150% by sedimenting cells with bentonite as part of the recycle step. In this particular case the sedimenting agent was present in low concentration and unlikely to affect subsequent processing. However, the consequence could be nocuous if this recycle tactic was to be used in other processes.

Biotechnology per se is the source of serious effluent problems. The adoption of large-scale continuous fermentation will exacerbate the problem and generate effluents of large volume and BOD (up to 7000 mg l^{-1} for whole cultures and 4000 mg l^{-1} for extracted spent broths; [Dunnill, 13], e.g., a 10,000 m^3/day brewery can produce effluent with a domestic sewage equivalent of 200,000 persons. Such facts will influence the siting of large scale plants and, in turn, continue to stimulate the development of high efficiency treatment plants.

Strain Stability

Many industrially useful strains have been heavily mutated over long time scales and their stability has been an ever-present problem for the fermentation industry. These problems are magnified when genes encoding for desirable properties are carried on plasmids and stability of these strains can be influenced by (a) growth conditions, (b) the copy number of the plasmids, (c) the nature of the gene(s) encoded on the plasmid, (d) the genetic characteristics of the host organism. Instability of manipulated strains may be manifest as total loss of a plasmid, change in the copy number or segregation leading to the loss of necessary DNA segments. There is an urgent need to study plasmid stability under a wide range of continuous culture conditions because results of studies made to date make it hazardous to draw general conclusions.

Mixed Cultures

The stability of mixed microbial populations in continuous cultures is now well established [Bull and Slater, 7] and, whereas many traditional food fermentations are based on spontaneous mixtures, the modern fermentation industry is becoming increasingly interested in the utility of defined mixed cultures. One incentive to the development of mixed culture processes has been the alleviation of substrate or metabolite inhibition of growth, e.g., methanol inhibition of methane- or methanol-based SCP processes. Secondary organisms present in such cultures frequently scavenge the inhibitory compounds so that they do not obtain inhibitory concentration. Scavenging activities of this type also are important in removing metabolic products from fermentation broths which otherwise could accumulate during water recycle and have deleterious effects on the fermentation (see "The Impact of Continuous Culture" above).

Alternative Production Strategies

Conventional continuous culture systems of the type highlighted in this paper are not or will not be suitable for all biotechnological objectives. Immobilized cell reactors, for example, will be deployed for many continuous product syntheses, while fed-batch and fill-and-draw systems have widespread use for secondary metabolite productions.

REFERENCES

1. Almengor-Hecht, M.L. and A.T. Bull (1978). Continuous-flow enrich ment of a strain of *Erwinia carotovora* having specificity for highly methylated pectin. Archives of Microbiology 119:163-166.
2. Bailey, J.E. and D.F. Ollis (1977). Biochemical Engineering Fundamentals. New York. McGraw-Hill Book Co.
3. Brooks, J.D. and J.L. Meers, (1973). The effect of discontinuous methanol addition on the growth of a carbon-limited culture

of Pseudomonas. Journal of General Microbiology 77:513-519.

4. Bryson, V. (1952). Microbial Selection II. The turbidostatic selector - a device for automatic isolation of bacterial variants. Science, N.Y. 116:48-51.

5. Bull, A.T. (1981). Strategies in microbial process optimization. In Global Impacts of Applied Microbiology Sixth International Conference, pp. 623-645. Edited by S.O. Emejuaiwe, O. Ogunbi and S.O. Sanni. London: Academic Press.

6. Bull, A.T. and C.M. Brown (1979). Continuous culture applications to microbial biochemistry. In International Review of Biochemistry, Vol. 21, Microbial Biochemistry pp.177-226. Edited by J.R. Quayle. Baltimore: University Park Press.

7. Bull, A.T. and J.H. Slater, (Eds.) (1982). Microbial Interactions and Communities, Volume 1. London: Academic Press.

8. Bull, D.N. and M.D. Young (1982). Enhanced product formation in continuous fermentations with microbial cell recycle. Biotechnology & Bioengineering 23:373-389.

9. Bushell, M.E. and A.T. Bull (1981). Anaplerotic metabolism of Aspergillus nidulans and its effect on biomass synthesis in carbon-limited chemostat. Archives of Microbiology 128:282-287.

10. Charley, R.C. and A.T. Bull (1979). Bioaccumulation of Silver by a multispecies community of bacteria. Archives of Microbiology 123:239-244.

11. Dawson, P.S.S. (1977). Continuous fermentations. Annual Reports of Fermentation Processes, Vol. 1, pp. 73-93. Edited by D. Perlman. New York: Academic Press.

12. Driessen, F.M. (1981). Protocooperation of yoghurt bacteria in continuous culture. In Mixed Culture Fermentation, pp. 99-120. Edited by M.E. Bushell & J.H. Slater. London: Academic Press.

13. Dunnill, P. (1981). Biotechnology and industry. Chemistry and Industry 4 April, 204-217.

14. Evans, C.G.T. (1965). The industrial application of continuous culture. Laboratory Practice, October, 1168-1174.

15. Evans, C.G.T., R.G. Yeo, and D.C. Ellwood (1979). Continuous culture studies of the production of extracellular polysaccharides by Xanthomonas juglandis. In Microbial Polysaccharides and Polysaccharases, pp. 51-68. Edited by R.C.W. Berkeley, G. W. Gooday & D.C. Ellwood. London: Academic Press.

16. Gold, D., A. Mohagheghi, C.L. Cooney, and D.I.C. Wang. (1981). Single-cell protein production from spent sulfite liquor utilizing cell-recycle and computer. Biotechnology and Bioengineering 23:2105-2116.

17. Harrison, D.E.F. (1978). Mixed cultures in industrial fermentation processes. Advances in Applied Microbiology 24:129-162.

18. Herbert, D. (1976). Stoicheiometry of microbial growth. In Continuous Culture 6. Applications and New Fields pp. 1-30. Edited by A.C.R. Dean, D.C. Ellwood, C.G.T. Evans & J. Melling. Chichester:Ellis Horwood.

19. Herbert, D., R. Elsworth, and R.C. Telling, (1956). The continuous culture of bacteria: A theoretical and experimental study. Journal of General Microbiology 14:601-622.

20. Hospodka, J. (1966). Industrial application of continuous fermentation. In Theoretical and Methodological Basis of Continuous Culture of Microorganisms, pp. 495-645. Edited by I. Malek & Z. Fencl. Prague: Publishing House of the Czechoslovak Academy of Sciences.

21. Humphrey, A.E. (1981). Continuous culture - its influence on engineering practice. In Advances in Biotechnology, Volume 1, pp. 203-210. Edited by M. Moo-Young, C.W. Robinson & C. Vezina Toronto: Pergamon Press.

22. King, P.P. (1982). Biotechnology. An industrial view. Journal of Chemical Technology & Biotechnology 32:2-8.

23. Kreuzberg, K. and W. Hempfling (1981). Properties of the green alga Chlorogonium elongatum during light-limited continuous culture in the phauxostat. In Advances in Biotechnology, Volume 1, pp. 287-293. Edited by M. Moo-Young, C.W. Robinson and C. Vezina. Toronto: Pergamon Press.

24. Lee, Y-K and S.J. Pirt (1981). Energetics of photosynthetic algae growth: Influence of intermittent illumination in short (40s) cycles. Journal of General Microbiology 124:43-52.

25. Leegwater, M.P.M., O.M. Neijssel, and D.W. Tempest (1982). Aspects of microbial physiology in relation to process control. Journal of Chemical Technology & Biotechnology 32:92-99.

26. Malek, I. and Z. Fencl (1966). Theoretical and Methodological Basis of Continuous Culture of Microorganisms. Prague: Publishing House of the Czechoslovak Academy of Sciences.

27. Monod, J. (1950). La technique de culture continuée. Theorie et application. Annales Institute Pasteur, Paris 79:390-410.

28. Novick, A. and L. Szilard, (1950). Experiments with the chemostat on spontaneous mutations of bacteria. Proceedings of the National Academy of Sciences, Washington 36:708-719.

29. Osborn, D.W. and H.A. Nicholls (1977). Optimization of the activated sludge process for the biological removal of phosphorus. International Conference Advanced Treatment and Redamation of Wastewater, pp. 23. Johannesburg: City Health Department.

30. Pirt, S.J. (1975). Principles of Microbe and Cell Culture. Oxford: Blackwell Scientific Publications.

31. Pirt, S.J., Y-K Lee, A. Richmond, and M. Watts Pirt, (1980). The photosynthetic efficiency of *Chlorella* biomass growth with reference to solar energy utilization. Journal of Chemical Technology and Biotechnology 30:25-34.

32. Righelato, R.C. (1980). Anaerobic fermentation: alcohol production. Philosophical Transactions of the Royal Society of London **B290**. 303-312.

33. Righelato, R.C. and R. Elsworth (1970). Industrial application of continuous culture: Pharmaceutical products, other products, and other processes. Adv. in Appl. Microb., 13:399-417.

34. Rose, A.H. (1979). Economic Microbiology, Volume 4. Microbial Biomass. London: Academic Press.

35. Rowley, B.I. and A.T. Bull (1977). Isolation of a yeast-lysing

Arthrobacter species and the production of the lytic enzyme complex in batch and continuous-flow fermenters. Biotechnology and Bioengineering 19:1260-1278.

36. Sittig, W. (1982). The present state of fermentation reactors. Journal of Chemical Technology and Biotechnology 32:47-58.
37. Smith, S.R.L. (1980). Single cell protein. Philosophical Transactions of the Royal Society of London B290, 341-354.
38. Spinks, A. (1982). The Philips Lecture, 1981. Targets in biotechnology. Proceedings of the Royal Society of London B214, 289-303.
39. Tempest, D.W. (1970). The place of continuous culture in microbiological research. Advances in Microbial Physiology 4:223-250.
40. Tempest, D.W. (1981). Microbiology, microbial physiology and biotechnology. European Federation of Biotechnology Workshop on "A Community Strategy for European Biotechnology", Working papers, pp. II 1 - II 9.
41. Windass, J.D., M.J. Worsey, E.M. Pioli, D. Pioli, P.T. Barth, K.T. Atherton, E.C. Dart, D. Byron, K. Powell, and P.J. Senior. (1980). Improved conversion of methanol to single-cell protein by *Methylophilus methylotrophus*. Nature, London 287:396-401.

DISCUSSION

Q. O. ZABORSKY (NSF): Could you tell us a little bit more about those microorganisms that accumulate copper and silver? Is that an internal or external accumulation?

A. BULL: It's hazardous to generalize. On the one hand, one can isolate organisms that produce a lot of slime in the presence of toxic heavy metals, and the heavy metal doesn't actually get into the cell; it's caught up, entrapped, or absorbed on the polysaccharide. We do have some silver accumulating organisms in which silver passes directly into the cell and initially it's an active process. However, there's a limit to the accumulation and ultimately, the internal concentration of silver leads to the death of the cell.

Q. R. SUBDEN (Univ. of Guelph): I know that you were talking about continuous fermentation, but you did compare it to batch fermentation with respect to the loss of plasmids. Have you any idea why the batch fermentations, especially with yeast, seem to accumulate plasmids, and other things such as double stranded RNA?

A. BULL: I can't comment on the last point that you made; I'm not familiar with the yeast area, unfortunately. The one thing that does impress me is the range of results people are getting on the stability of plasmids in bacterial systems. It seems to me that, although there isn't a vast literature yet the literature is very confusing. Some people claim that plasmid stability is a function of the type of nutrient limitation, or is dependent on the type of plasmid. In addition, you get total loss or partial loss of plasmids. From my understanding of the situation, it is very difficult to make general statements on plasmid stability in continuous cultures.

C. SUBDEN: I think the data of Tubs and all reports so far have shown that if you look at brewing yeast and wine yeast, for that matter, you have high copy numbers of two micron DNA and you also have so called "killer" double-stranded RNA.

Q. BULL: I shouldn't do this, Peter (P. Williams), but do you have any thoughts?

C. P. WILLIAMS (Univ. College of North Wales): We don't know what those two microns are doing. As far as I know, it may be an advantage in that case for the cells to have them. As far as bacteria are concerned, I think Alan (A. Bull) is quite right that the results from different labs and different plasmids go up and down. I think in many cases, it is a problem of actually knowing what the roles of plasmids are, in general, in bacterial physiology. Some plasmids may well have some advantage to the cells which we don't know about, and some may have a severe disadvantage. I think that may place some account in selective pressures during long, continuous cultures.

Q. In relation to the continuous culture, I was wondering what some of the basic parameters are or might be that limits what can be done. I was thinking of the growth rate of organisms compared to the maximum velocity with which they actually metabolize a substrate. That is, suppose you take a yeast -- how many seconds does it actually take to start with a sugar molecule, get it through the wall, and make an ethanol molecule? I would think that those kinds of basic parameters would be some of the ones which would set the rate at which you must recycle and at which you must dilute. So, are there a body of studies of that kind that give us these numbers?

A. BULL: I think someone such as Art Koch has addressed this sort of problem.

Q. J. STAMER (N.Y. State Agri. Expt. Station): Bob Finn and Steinkraus had published on that subject five years ago. You'll find it in Biotechnology and Bioengineering. All of the statistics are in there.

Q. H.M. TSUCHIYA (Univ. of Minnesota): We've been working with *Aspergillus awamoi*. That is the USDA strain of fungal amylase which produces alpha amylase and glucamylase. The alpha amylase comes up very early. I'm speaking only of batch growth here. On the other hand, the glucamylase comes up maybe well towards the end, about the 80th hr. Therefore, I think that your information on the plug-flow reactor is very, very pertinent. You had a recycle in your plug-flow, didn't you?

A. BULL: Yes.

C. The Japanese apparently have optimized the growth of mold on semi-solid mash of wheat bran and soybeans. They operate a true plug-flow fermentation. It takes them only forty-eight hours to get glucamylase whereas it took us five days, batch-wise, to get fungal amylase going in Iowa.

A. BULL: Just a very brief comment on that. Yes, you're quite right. The schematic representation of plug-flow I showed incorporated a biomass recycle system. The reason it was shown in that way is as follows: if you have plug-flow, you've got to have continuous inoculation of the fermenter. One presumably convenient way of getting that continuous inoculation is to have a small biomass recycle to the beginning of the reactor.

THE OBLIGATE METHANE-OXIDIZING BACTERIA AND THEIR BIOTECHNOLOGICAL POTENTIAL

Roger Whittenbury and Howard Dalton
Department of Biological Sciences
University of Warwick
Coventry CV4 7AL, United Kingdom

INTRODUCTION

The properties and present taxonomic status of the obligate methane oxidizing bacteria are described. Methane-monooxygenase, the enzyme involved in the first step of the oxidation of methane to carbon dioxide, is discussed in detail with particular reference to its ability to insert oxygen into a wide range of compounds, such as ammonia, carbon monoxide, methanol, ethanol, alkanes, alkenes, dimethyl and diethyl-ether, alicyclic, aromatic and heterocyclic compounds. This widespread hydroxylase activity is a characteristic of all methane monoxygenases studied, though some are less catholic than others. The biotechnological potential of this enzyme is discussed and other potential biotechnological applications of methane oxidizers are mentioned.

Much of the biotechnology we hear about today is goal-oriented, strategically planned, and technologically assessed from the moment of inception, or so we are led to believe. In truth, of course, most biotechnological ventures are a mixture of preconceived ideas and serendipity, and, we suspect, serendipity is going to be a major driving force of future biotechnology. The examples discussed here are largely of the latter character, being based on our studies of obligate methane utilizing bacteria, and serve to illustrate that recombinant DNA techniques are not the sole technologies of biotechnology. These examples also point to a potential problem emerging in biotechnology, the danger of neglecting the need to develop an active research program on the physiology and biochemistry of microbes, by allowing too great a diversion of scarce resources and personnel towards the presently more glamorous molecular biological side of biotechnology. We are certain that in the short to medium-term microbes and their biochemical attributes are likely to be the source of most of the successful biotechnological ventures - and that this will only come about if research effort in the fundamental properties of these organisms receives greater encouragement and support than seems presently to be the case. Without this knowledge, cloners will have nothing to clone!

In support of this thesis, we describe in this article the obligate methane oxidizing bacteria, beginning with a description of them and a brief survey of other methane oxidizers and concluding with a discussion of their biotechnological potential, identified as a consequence of research on their biochemistry.

THE METHANE OXIDIZERS

The existence of methane oxidizing bacteria has been known for the best part of 100 years [23], but such organisms remained very much a minority interest until the early 1950s when Foster and his colleagues at Texas [7,15] reisolated strains of methane oxidizing bacteria thought to be similar to the *Bacillus methanicus* of Sohngen

[23]. They provided preliminary descriptions of their physiology, biochemistry, and morphology and, more importantly, as is now seen in retrospect, began to succinctly define some of the questions concerning their biochemical mechanisms; for example what is the relationship between co-oxidation and methane oxidation? A few further contributions appeared in the literature in the late 1950s and the 1960s [6,9], following the initial burst of activity of the Texas group, but no advances were made concerning the biochemistry of the methane oxidation.

All this changed abruptly towards the end of the 1960s. This change, characterized by a sudden flurry of research activity which has been maintained ever since, represents an early example of the influence of renewed interest in Biotechnology of the pre-recombinant DNA era. The objective in mind was "single-cell protein". Various single cell protein ventures were under development at the time, the most technically advanced being the yeast/liquid *n*-alkine process of British Petroleum. For many reasons hydrocarbons of the straight chain *n*-alkane type seemed ideal feedstocks on which to base single cell protein systems and, in particular, methane which is a very cheap carbon and energy sources in vast supply in many parts of the world, seemed a natural successor or alternate substrate to liquid *n*-alkanes. Such a possibility stimulated the research activities of investigators then beginning to explore the mechanism of methane oxidation and also led to the development in different parts of the world (the United Kingdom in particular) of new research groups concerned with the isolation and biology of new varieties of methane oxidizers with the aim of selecting the most suitable candidate for single cell protein production by continuous fermentation techniques. Technically and scientifically, a single cell protein project based on strains of *Methylococcus capsulatus* (first described by Foster and Davis, ref. 9) looked very promising. However, the new oil pricing policy introduced by OPEC countries in the early 1970s spelled the end of existing projects in the U.K.

based on direct utilization of hydrocarbons by microbes. Only one single-cell protein process of any size survives in the western world, that is the ICI bacterial process based on methanol produced catalytically from methane, and we understand that ICI have recently indicated that they do not now expect to develop new biomass producing plants based on this system. Fortunately, sufficient research momentum has been gained to survive such a catastrophe and the results accruing were of sufficient fundamental importance as to ensure the continuation of financial support. In addition, new biotechnological possibilities have now surfaced concerning the methane oxidizers and these appear to have greater promise than "single-cell protein". As a consequence, the research effort has notably increased. However, it is necessary to review the nature of methane oxidizers before further discussion of what these are.

At the present time three distinct groups (Table 1) of methane oxidizing microbes are known; the obligate methane utilizing bacteria, the facultative methane oxidizing bacteria, and the facultative methane utilizing yeasts. A tentative fourth group is the anaerobic methane oxidizing bacteria. However, defined cultures ('pure' or consortia) have yet to be described and, consequently, nothing more can be said about them at this juncture.

Although both groups of methane oxidizing bacteria possess a number of properties in common, they nevertheless appear to constitute distinctive types of bacteria which are not, taxonomically, closely related. The obligate methane oxidizers appear as unique organisms [4;5,32,33] while the facultative methane oxidizers appear more akin to certain types of facultative methanol utilizers [10] than to the obligate species.

The methane oxidizing yeasts are the least documented of the aerobic methane oxidizing microbes and will not be discussed further, the remainder of this article being concerned mainly with the obligate methane oxidizers.

Table 1

The Four Groups of Microbes which Oxidize Methane Important Features

THE OBLIGATE METHANE OXIDIZING BACTERIA
Growth occurs only with methane, methanol or formaldehyde as combined control and energy sources. Growth does not occur on formate (though both energy and ancillary carbon - as formate or CO_2 - is provided by formate).
THE FACULTATIVE METHANE OXIDIZING BACTERIA {18}
Growth occurs on a variety of organic compounds (e.g. ethanol, glucose, succinate, malate - but varies with strains) in addition to methane and methanol. Methylobacterium ethanolicum is an example. Methane oxidizing powers appear unstable in many strains, possibly on plasmids which may be lost. Now appears taxonomically {10} more clearly related to facultative methanol utilizers than to obligate methane utilizers.
THE ANAEROBIC METHANE UTILIZING BACTERIA {17,36}
No defined (single or multi-membered) cultures yet studied, but anaerobic enrichment cultures consume methane.
THE FACULTATIVE METHANE OXIDIZING YEASTS
Species of the genera Rhodotorula and Sporobolomyces grow slowly on methane but do not grow on methanol. Intermediates in methane oxidation seem to be those occuring in methane oxidation by bacteria. A methane hydroxylase is involved, as in bacteria. Microbodies seem to be the site of methane oxidation and contain large amounts of catalase in methanol peroxidation).
{See also references 16,34,35}

The Obligate Methane Utilizers

Following the publication of reliable procedures for enriching, isolating, and maintaining methane oxidizers [33] and preliminary descriptions of the properties of the new isolates [5,32,33], many investigators have successfully isolated and described obligate methane-oxidizers [11,29]. Their taxonomy, however, has proved to be a persistent problem up to the present day. A major difficulty in this context is the fact of their obligateness and consequently limited range of biochemical properties (certainly so far as their negative responses to those conventionally used biochemical tests) often employed in taxonomic studies of bacteria. Nevertheless, attempts have been made to define new genera and new species of those bacteria [21].

Despite the unresolved taxonomic situation, a diagnostic grouping scheme, first proposed by Whittenbury et al. [33] and subsequently modified on a number of occasions [4] following the emergence of additional information, has provided a basis for identification of types or groups of methane oxidizers of which there are presently three (Table 2a, 2b). In each case, these groups are probably composed of more than one genus and certainly a number of species. Final separation into taxa will depend upon the elucidation of molecular properties, such as nucleic acid studies (DNA/DNA and DNA/RNA hybridization, 16S and RNA oligonucleotide cataloging), sequencing of selected protein molecules, and the identification of differentiating or determinative wall and membrane components respectively considered along with characteristics determined by conventional techniques, but which, in isolation, have had limited taxonomic value to date.

Before discussing particular properties of biotechnological interest, certain of the features indicated in Tables 2a and b, other properties are amplified below.

Ecologically, these Gram negative, aerobic organisms are widespread, occurring in bodies of water and predominantly on sediment surfaces in lakes and ponds and in soil. Morphologically they are varied; coccal, vibroid, and rod forms being described. Some are motile. A major characteristic is the arrangement of the complex of intracellular membranes they all form [5]. Two arrangements occur: a "Type I", vesicular discs of membrane organized into bundles distributed throughout the cell; and a "Type II", pairs of membranes which extend throughout the cell running in parallel to the cytoplasmic membrane. Both arrangements can be seen in electron micrographs [5].

Table 2a

A Scheme for Categorizing Obligate Methane Oxidizers into Groups

CHARACTER	GROUP I (Type I)	GROUP II (Type II)
Membrane arrangement		
Vesicular discs (bundles)	+	-
Paired membranes aligned to cell	-	+
Resting stages		
Exospores or "lipid cysts"	-	+
Cysts (*Azotobacter*-like)	+	-
Major carbon assimilation pathways		
Ribulose monophosphate pathway (3-hexulose phosphate synthetase $+_{ve}$)	+	-
Serine pathway (hydroxypryruvate reductase $+_{ve}$)	-	+
Tricarboxylic acid cycle		
Complete	-	+
Incomplete (α-ketoglutarate dehydrogenase-ve)	+	-
Nitrogen salts (ammonium and nitrate)		
GS/GOGAT	+	+
ADH/GDH	+	-
Predominant fatty acid carbon chain length	16	18

GS = Glutamine synthetase

GOGAT = Glutamine-oxyglutamate amino transferase

ADH = Alanine dehydrogenase

GDH = Glutamate dehydrogenase

Resting stages [32] are probably formed by all strains. These may be cysts, morphologically indistinguishable from those formed by *Azotobacter* species, lipid cysts characterized by large lipid inclusion, and exospores, formed by a budding process at one pole. All these resting cells resist desiccation, but only the exospores are also resistant to heat (85°c for 15 min).

Table 2b

Sub-division of Group I Obligate Methane Oxidizers.

CHARACTER	Sub Group Ia (sub type Ia)	Sub Group Ib (sub type X)	Group II (Type II)
Autotrophic CO_2 fixation	-	+	-
Mol % G + C of DNA	50-54	62.5	62.5
Iso citrate dehydrogenase			
NAD, NAD(P) dependent	+	-	-
NAD dependent only	-	+	-
NAD(P) dependent only	-	-	+
Nitrogen fixation	-	+	+
Cell shape			
cocci	Some	+	-
rods	Some	-	Some
vibrios	-	-	Some
Growth at 45°	±	+	-
Named examples	*Methylomonas methanica*	*Methylococcus capsulatus*	*Methylosinus trichosporium*

Strains of methane-oxidizers may be pigmented (yellow, ochre, pink, or red). On encystment some form a brown pigment, others may release a water soluble pigment (sapphire, yellow, or brown). Growth temperature varies, some strains being thermophilic, growing at 45° to 55°C and failing to grow at 30°C. Many strains are sensitive to the normal oxygen content of air, growing microaerobically and many form extracellular polysaccharides.

Although all strains can use methanol as a sole carbon and energy source (in addition, all require exogenous carbon dioxide to initiate growth on methane or methanol), methanol can be toxic when supplied above trace concentrations. Many strains, however, give rise to methanol-tolerant mutants or can be "trained" to tolerate higher levels of methanol (e.g., 0.5% V/V). The biochemical basis of this mutation is not understood.

Carbon dioxide is an essential though minor carbon source, formaldehyde, formed via the oxidation of methane or methanol, or provided separately, is the major and essential carbon source. Acetate, formate, some amino acids, and many co-oxidizable substrates can serve as supplementary carbon sources [4]. If metabolized, co-oxidizable substrates (e.g., primary alcohols, alkanes, dimethyl- and diethyl-ether, alicyclic, aromatic, and heterocyclic compounds) and carbon dioxide may provide both supplementary energy and carbon but cannot be used as sole sources of energy and carbon, as will be discussed later.

Differences in the tricarboxylic acid (TCA) cycle occur among the obligate methane oxidizers; two groups of strains lack the enzyme α-keto-glutarate dehydrogenase, and therefore possess an incomplete cycle that only plays a biosynthetic role. Even though the remaining group possesses a complete TCA cycle, there is no evidence that this means that the cycle plays a role in energy production. Indeed, logic would indicate that the operation of an energy-producing TCA cycle in an organism which grows on a one-carbon compound is redundant. That such a capacity is inherent in these organisms, however, has led to speculation [12] on the potential benefits of co-oxidation (e.g., the fortuitous use of acetate).

However, the recent work of Shiskina and Trotsenko [22] on the reasons for obligateness (Tables 3,4) in both major metabolic types of obligate methane oxidizer clearly emphasizes their incapacity to use either acetate or pyruvate as potential energy sources and that acetate or pyruvate entering the TCA cycle (via Acetyl COA) most probably end up as lipids and amino acids.

One final comment on the nature of these organisms concerns the possession by Methylococcus capsulatus species of phosphoribulokinase and ribulosebisphosphate carboxylase [26]. Although carbon

Table 3

Enzymes of Intermediary Metabolism in Methylotrophs[c]

Enzyme	Obligate (I) *Methylomonas methanica*	Obligate (II) *Methylosinus trichosporium*	Facultative *Pseudomonas* AM1
Hexokinase	+	-	?
6-phosphogluconate dehydrogenase	+	-	?
Pyruvate kinase[a]	-	-	+
PEP synthetase	-	-	+
PEP carboxylase	+	+	-
Pyruvate dehydrogenase	+	-	+
α-Ketoglutarate dehydrogenase	-	+	+
Isocitrate lysase	-	-	-
Malate synthase	-	-	+[b]

[a]The absence of pyruvate kinase in both Type I and Type II obligate methylotrophs is seen to be very significant in that PEP cannot be converted to pyruvate, leading on to the fact that energy cannot be generated from compounds metabolized via the glycolytic sequence.

[b]This apparent activity (see ref. 22) is due to joint action of malyl-COA lyase and malyl-COA hydrolase.

[c]Abstracted from Shiskina and Trotsenko (22).

dioxide can be fixed by this autotrophic route, it has proved impossible to demonstrate autotrophic growth [30]. Theoretically, these organisms should, for instance, grow on formate which they oxidize, but they do not.

METHANE MONO-OXYGENASES

All bacteria possessing the ability to oxidize methane aerobically (i.e., facultative and obligate methane oxidizers) do so via

Table 4

Pyruvate and Acetate Metabolism in Obligate Methane Oxidizers[a]

Property	*Methylomonas methanica*	*Methylomonas trichosporium*
Uptake (μmol/h/mg protein)		
($3-^{14}C$) pyruvate + CH_4	0.32	0.30
− CH_4	0.10	0.11
($2-^{14}C$) acetate + CH_4	0.37	0.30
− CH_4	0.05	0.20
Rate of oxidation (μl O_2/h/mg protein)		
Pyruvate	17	13
acetate	0	4
methane	152	140
methanol	100	93

[a]Abstracted from Shishkina and Trotsenko (22).

methane mono-oxygenase, an energetically expensive oxygenation, in that a mole of reduced pyridine nucleotide or its equivalent is oxidized per mole of methanol formed without, to date, evidence of any useful energy production in the process [4]. The methanol formed is subsequently oxidized through to carbon dioxide. The most interesting feature, in the context of this article, is the ability of this enzyme, *in vivo* and *in vitro*, to insert oxygen in compounds other than methane [4].

This catholic property of oxygenation has been variously termed "co-metabolism" or "co-oxidation" and recently "fortuitous oxidation" [24] or "supplementary metabolism" [12] according to the purposes this activity may serve the organisms and determined in the minds of those espousing the terms.

Before commenting upon these claims, it is necessary to establish what the consequences are of such apparently illogical oxygenations, bearing in mind that formaldehyde and, therefore, in practice methane or methanol are essential carbon sources for growth. A judgement has been made [24] that they must be beneficial if there is an increase in biomass assayed over that occurring with the same amount of methane in the absence of the "co-oxidizable" compounds. At best, this is a crude and uncertain measure, in that yields on methane and methanol can be variable and difficult to standardize in the laboratory, for a variety of reasons. At worst it is an ambiguous measure, because explanations other than direct contributions to cell energy and carbon could account for the biomass increase. Direct assays concerning carbon assimilation and energy production are obviously nore informative. That carbon dioxide and acetate can be used as supplementary sources of carbon is well understood [4], but the possibility of energy contributions from co-oxidation has not been commented upon recently and, therefore, requires a restatement here. The most direct way [31] to determine whether or not ATP and reducing equivalents can result from co-oxidation has proved to be by assaying nitrogenase activity occurring as a direct consequence of the oxidation of such compounds.

In summary, a number of compounds tested, including hydrogen, ethane, and ethanol, led to the active reduction of analogues of dinitrogen in the absence of methane and methanol. Consequently, it was clear that in the case of *Methylosinus trichosporium*, for instance (an organism possessing a complete TCA cycle), ethane could be oxidized through to acetate with the formation of energy producing compounds, and that the acetate could be oxidized further and also be incorporated as a supplementary carbon source, but that growth (biomass increase) was dependent upon the presence of either methane or methanol. However, a problem for the methane oxidizers, of course, is that many co-oxidizable compounds, such as ammonia and ethane, compete with methane for the active site on methane mono-oxygenase, and that when significant amounts of either is present in the growth system [33] methane oxidation is inhibited or severely reduced depending upon the organism. Therefore, in situations where ethane is present at levels which, theoretically, could lead to a measurable contribution to growth, the paradox of methane uptake inhibition as a consequence of the ethane effect appears to negate the putative beneficial effect of ethane. Therefore, this one example serves to illustrate the doubtful value of pursuing the thesis that co-oxidation represents some special case of nutritional benefit conferred through evolutionary selection pressures. Firstly, it ignores the many co-oxidations which provide no putative benefit (e.g., oxidation of CO) or results in inhibition of growth (e.g., acetylene) and, secondly, it seems more reasonable to accept that methane mono-oxygenase is just one of a number of known "inefficient' enzymes (as regards lack of specificity for the key substrate) such as ribulosebisphosphate, carboxylase/oxygenase and nitrogenase. In neither of these two instances has a "beneficiary role" been argued for the lack of specificity; indeed, in the case of the role of ribulosebisphosphate carboxylase as an oxygenase, the evidence is more of organisms evolving mechanisms to reduce or compensate for the unwanted oxygenase role effect, rather than conserving the "inefficiency" for survival reasons.

The Properties of Methane Monoxygenase

The earliest studies on the nature of this enzyme were by Ribbons and his colleagues [19,20] on the strain of *Methylococcus capsulatus* isolated by Foster and Davis [9]. However, the most detailed studies have been carried on three other obligate methane oxidizers, a strain of *Methylomonas methanica* [3,8], and *Methylosinus capsulatus* (Bath) about which most is known [1,2], and

Table 5

Properties of Methane Mono-oxygenase

STRAIN	CHARACTERISTICS
Methylomonas methanica {3}	Particulate; NADH as electron donor; broad broad substrate specificity, but does not oxidize aromatic hydrocarbons stable at -70°C; cyanide sensitive; certain heavy metals, metal chelating agents and electron transport inhibitors inhibit activity.
Methylococcus capsulatus (Foster and Davis strain) {20}	Particulate; NADH as electron donor; ethane oxidized (no other information about other hydrocarbon oxidations); cyanide sensitive; metal chelating agents are inhibitory.
Methylococcus capsulatus (Bath) {25}	Soluble; NADH as electron donor, very wide substrate specificity; stable at -70°C, cyanide insensitive, insensitive to most inhibitors (C_2H_2 and 8-OH Quinoline are inhibitory).
Methylosinus trichosporium OB3b	Particulate {27}; soluble {25}; ascorbate {27} as electron donor, ascorbate {25} not an electron donor; NADH as an electron donor; some alkanes oxygenated {26}, very wide substrate specificity {25}; cyanide sensitive {27}, cyanide insensitive {25}; unstable on freezing {27}, stable on freezing {25}, metal chelators inhibitory {27}, metal chelators not inhibitory {25}. Partial explanation for this contradictory evidence proposed by Higgins et al. {13}.

Methylosinus trichosporium OB 3b [25,27,28].

As can be seen (Table 5), the methane mononxygenases from these three strains are not identical and there are also conflicts of evidence to be resolved; for example, whether ascorbate can substitute for reduced NAD as an electron donor in Methylosinus trichosporium [28] and whether or not the enzyme in this organism is particulate or soluble [25,28]. In the latter instance, it now appears that growth conditions [13] may influence this property, though it cannot be ruled out that two enzymes may exist, one or the other being induced or derepressed in response to control mechanisms influenced by growth conditions. Most of the work on the properties of the components of the oxygenase has been on that of Methylococcus capsulatus (Bath) as shown in Table 6.

The Biotechnological Potential of Methane Monoxygenase

Having discovered that methane oxidizers possessed this amazing capacity to oxygenate a vast range of compounds including ammonia and carbon monoxide, we then became aware that the ability to insert molecular oxygen into certain compounds with the production of one or, occasionally, two oxygenated products recoverable before further oxidation, was attractive industrially, should ever prove feasible to harness the process at substantial cost savings in relation to existing or proposed processes. This, then, is an example of potential biotechnology being an after-thought rather than a stimulus to research. At present it is far too soon to make any categorical judgements about the future commercial success of the process. Questions concerning the use of whole cells, cloned cells, or enzyme extracts, whether immobilization of cells or extracts will be the answer, or whether whole cells in batch or continuous culture will be involved, all need to be explored. Clearly, methanol is likely to be preferred to methane as a feedstock to produce the active catalyst (cells or enzymes) though, of course, cloned cells, containing the relevant enzymes, will lead to a wider choice of feedstock. A complication is the need for this enzyme to be driven by an electron donor, that is, a reducing source has to be continually added or regenerated. Whether this might be direct electric current, derived from the feedstock itself, or added specifically in the form of a reduced compound able to regenerate reduced NAD, is a question to be resolved bearing in mind the economics of the particular process and the state of the art at the time. In addition, a technical assessment has to be made, and the judgement of its

Table 6

Properties of Components (Resolved by DEAE Cellulose Chromatography) of Methane-mono-oxygenase from Methylococcus Capsulatus (Bath) (1,2)

Properties	Component A	Component B	Component C
Mol. Wt.	220,000	∿15,000	44,500
Metal	2Fe	-	2Fe
2nd Prosthetic group	-	-	1FAD
Acid labile sulfur	not detected	-	2S
Core extrusion of Fe_2 S_2 cluster	+	-	+
Activity	None	None	NAD(P)H electron acceptor reductase

commercial potential continually reviewed, in relation to existing and putative processes.

One example of an application being explored is the hydroxylation of propylene to propylene oxide (Table 7), which, if compared, for instance, with the Cetus process looks attractive, if only because of its relative simplicity and because the process is not hazarded by potential marketing problems occurring with other products of the process. The yields indicated here for the methane mono-oxygenase process are in no sense a representation of the final level of efficiency. Obviously means of developing the process are being explored and such matters as whole-cell performance versus enzyme-extract performance, under a variety of conditions, including immobilization, coupled with studies on how to present the substrate for oxygenation (whether under pressure and in what form) and whether or not the cells can be gentically modified, are some examples of investigations in progress. There are, of course, a number of examples of biological processes being improved over the years, often by empirical means rather than by pre-planned research

Table 7

Propylene to Propylene Oxide by Whole Cells and Cell-free Extracts of Obligate Methane Oxidizing Bacteria

Strains	Whole cell (WC) or cell-free (CF)	Rate (nmoles/min/mg protein)	Reference
Methylococcus	WC	36	(24)
capsulatus (Bath)	CF soluble	83	
Methylococcus capsulatus CRL MI	WC	42.7	(14)
Methylosinus	WC	13.6-93.3	
trichosporium OBBb	CF soluble	26	(12)
	CF particulate	18	

strategies, and the production, salicylic acid from naphthalene (Table 8) by pseudomonads is a pertinent one in the context of this discussion.

Bulk chemical production, of course, is only one of the possibilities of methane-mono-oxygenase exploitation. Preparation of cells or enzymes, as methane monoxygenase agents, may find applications, for instance, in assays, the purification of effluents, and the removal or detoxification of specific substances such as chlorinated hydrocarbons. Obviously, these are just a few examples of applications under active consideration.

OTHER BIOTECHNOLOGICAL ROLES FOR METHANE OXIDIZERS

As our core of knowledge of this group of organisms increases, it becomes a reasonable proposition to regard them as primary resources in themselves, and to begin to explore exploitable facets of their biology not necessarily related directly to methane-mono-oxygenase, bearing in mind that methanol as well as methane will support their growth. So, in conclusion, we list just a few

Table 8

Production of Salicyclic Acid from Naphthalene

Organism	Yield (G/L)	Conditions	Year
Pseudomonas arvilla	0.65		1955
Pseudomonas aeruginosa	9.3	Initial pH 8.0 high phosphate Ca^{++}, Cu^{++} and Fe^{++} required	1957
Pseudomonas aeruginosa	25.6	1.5% $CaCO_3$ added pH control used various growth factors added	1967
Pseudomonas fluorescens	30	Na_2SO_4 added	1967
Pseudomonas fluorescens	206	Production via semi continuous dialysis culture	1970

examples of potential applications.

1. Polymer production, including polysaccharides, for various industrial purposes;
2. Monomer productions, including amino acids and citric acid;
3. Nitrification agents in effluent disposal and denitrification agents that are possibly driven by methane formed by methanogenesis;
4. A source of, or recipient of, genes; these organisms are amenable to gene manipulation techniques.

REFERENCES

1. Colby, J., and H. Dalton, 1978. Resolution of methane monooxygenase of *Methylococcus capsulatus* (Bath) into three

components. Purification and properties of Component C, a flavoprotein. Biochem. J. 171:461-468.

2. Colby, J., and H. Dalton. 1979. Characterization of the second prosthetic group of the flavoenzyme NADH acceptor reductase (Component C) of the methane mono-oxygenase from Methylococcus capsulatus (Bath). Biochem. J. 177:903-908.

3. Colby, J., H. Dalton, and R. Whittenbury. 1976. An improved assay for bacterial methane mono-oxygenase: Some properties of the enzyme from Methylomonas methanica. Biochem. J. 151:459-462.

4. Colby, J., H. Dalton, and R. Whittenbury. 1979. Biological and biochemical aspects of microbial growth on C_1 compounds. Ann. Rev. Microbiol. 33:482-517.

5. Davies, S.L., and R. Whittenbury. 1970. Fine structures of methane and other hydrocarbon oxidizing bacteria. J. Gen. Microbiol. 61:227-232.

6. Davis, J.B., V.F. Coty, and J.P. Stanley. 1964. Atmospheric nitrogen fixation by methane-oxidizing bacteria. J. Bacteriol. 88:468-472.

7. Dworkin, M., and J.W. Foster. 1956. Studies on Pseudomonas methanica (Sohngen) nov. comb. J. Bacteriol. 72:646-659.

8. Ferenci, T., T. Strom, and J.R. Quayle. 1975. Oxidation of carbon monoxide and methane by Pseudomonas methanica. J. Gen. Microbiol. 91:29-94.

9. Foster, J.W., and R.H. Davis. 1966. A methane-dependant coccus, with notes on classification and nomenclature of obligate, methane-utilizing bacteria. J. Bacteriol. 91:1924-1931.

10. Green, P.N., and I.J. Bousfield. 1982. A taxonomic study of some Gram-negative faultatively methylotrophic bacteria. J. Gen. Microbiol. 128:623-638.

11. Hazeu, W., W. M. Batenburg-van der Egte, and J.C. de Bruyn. 1980. Some characteristics of Methylococcus mobilis sp. nov. Arch. Microbiol. 124:211-220.

12. Higgins, I.J., D.J. Best, and R.C. Hammond. 19812. New findings in methane-utilizing bacteria highlight their importance in the biosphere and their commercial potential. Nature (London) 286:561-564.

13. Higgins, I.J., D.J. Best, R.C. Hammond, and D. Scott. 1981. Methane-oxidizing bacteria. Micorobiol. Rev. 45:556-590.

14. Hou, C.T., R.N. Patel, A.I. Laskin, and N. Barnabe. 1980. Microbial oxidation of lower n-alkanes by resting suspensions of various methylotrophic bacteria, and the effect of methane metabolites. FEMS (Fed. Eur. Microbiol. Soc.) Microbiol. Letts. 9:267-270.

15. Leadbetter, E.R., and J.W. Foster. 1958. Studies on some methane-utilizing bacteria. Arch. Microbiol. 30:91-118.

16. Lynch, M.J., A.E. Wopat, and M.L. O'Connor. 1980. Characterization of two new facultative methylotrophs. Appl. Environ. Microbiol. 40:400-407.

17. Panganiban, A.T., T.E. Patt, W. Hart, and R.S. Hanson. 1979. Oxidation of methane in the absence of oxygen in lake water samples. Appl. Environ. Microbiol. 37:303-309.

18. Patt, T.E., G.C. Cole, J. Bland, and R.S. Hanson. 1974. Isolation and characterization of bacteria that grow on methane and organic compounds as sole sources of carbon and energy. J. Bacteriol. 120:955-964.

19. Ribbons, D.W. 1975. Oxidation of C_1 compounds by particulate fractions from Methylococcus capsulatus. Distribution and properties of methane-dependent reduces nicotinamide adenine dinucleotide oxidase (methane hydroxylase). J. Bacteriol. 123:1351-13463.

20. Ribbons, D.W., and J.M. Michaeover. 1970. Methane oxidation by cell free extracts of Methylococcus capsulatus. FEBS Lett. 11:41-44.

21. Romanowskaya, V.A., Y.R. Malushenko, and V.N. Bogachenko. 1978. Corrected diagnoses of genera and species of methane assimilating bacteria. Microbiologiya 47:120-130.

22. Shishkina, V.N., and Y.A. Trotsenko. 1982. Multiple enzymic lesions in obligate methanotrophic bacteria. FEMS (Fed. Eur. Microbiol. Soc.) Microbiol. Lett. 13:237-242.

23. Söhngen, N.L. 1906. Über Bakterien welhe Methan als Kohlenstoffnahrung und Energiequelle Gebrauchen. Zentrabl. Bacteriol. Parasitenk. Infektionskr. Hyg. Abt. II 125:513-517.

24. Stirling, D.I., and H. Dalton. 1979. The fortuitous oxidation and cometabolism of various carbon compounds by whole-cell suspensions of Methylococcus capsulatus (Bath). FEMS (Fed. Eur. Microbiol. Soc.) Microbiol. Lett. 5:315-318.

25. Stirling, D.I., and H. Dalton. 1979. Properties of the methane mono-oxygenase from extracts of Methylosinus trichosporium OB3b and evidence of its similarity to the enzyme from Methylococcus capsulatus (Bath). Eur. J. Biochem. 96:205-221.

26. Taylor, S.C., H. Dalton, and C.S. Dow. 1981. Ribulose 1, 5-bisphosphate carboxylase/oxygenase and carbon assimilation in Methylococcus capsulatus (Bath). J. Gen. Microbiol. 122:89-94.

27. Tonge, G.M., D.E. F. Harrison, and I.J. Higgins. 1977. Purification and properties of the methane mono-oxygenase system from Methylosinus trichosporium OB3B. Biochem. J. 161:333-344.

28. Tonge, G.M., D.E.F. Harrison, C.J. Knowles, and I.J. Higgins, 1975. Properties and partial purification of the methane-oxidizing enzyme from Methylosinus trichosporium. FEBS Lett. 58:293-299.

29. Trotsenko, Y.A. 1976. Isolation and characterization of obligate methanotrophic bacteria, p. 329-336. In H.G. Schlegel, G. Gottschalk, and N. Pfennig (eds.), Symposium on microbial production and utilization of gases (H_2, CH_4, CO), Göttingen. Akademic der. Wissenschaften, Göttingen.

30. Whittenbury, R. 1980. The interrelationship of autotrophy and methylotroph as seen in Methylococcus capsulatus (Bath), p. 181-190. In H. Dalton (ed.), Microbiol growth on C_2 compounds. Heyden, London.

31. Whittenbury, R., J. Colby, H. Dalton, and H.C. Reed. 1976.

Biology and ecology of methane oxidizers, p. 281-292. In. H-G. Schleger, G. Gottschalkf, and N. Pfennig (eds.), Symposium on microbiol production and utilization of gases (H_2, CH_4, CO), Göttingen. Akademic der Wissenschaften, Göttingen.

32. Whittenbury, R., S.L. Davies, and J.F. Davey. 1970. Exospores and cysts formed by methane utilizing bacteria. J. Gen Microbiol. 61:219-228.

33. Whittenbury, R., K.C. Phillips, and J.F. Wilkinson. 1970. Enrichment, isolation and some properties of methane-utilizing bacteria. J. Gen. Microbiol. 61-205-218.

34. Wolf, H.J., and R.S. Hanson. 1979. Isolation and characterization of methane-utilizing yeasts. J. Gen. Microbiol. 114-187-194.

35. Wolf, H.J., and R.S. Hanson. 1980. Identification of methane-utilizing yeasts. FEMS (Fed. Eur. Microbiol. Soc.) Microbiol. Lett. 7:177-179.

36. Zehnder, A.J.B., and T.D. Brock. 1979. Methane formation and methane oxidation by methanogenic bacteria. J. Bacteriol. 137:420-432.

BIODEGRADATION AND ENZYME TECHNOLOGY
CHAIRMAN'S OVERVIEW

F. William Tuominen
Henkel Corporation
Minneapolis, Minnesota 55413

From my personal perspective on the interfaces of science and technology and of academia and industry, the essence of biotechnology is the construction and use of catalytic systems whose structures are determined by a genetic bluprint. This definition seems appropriate whether one deals with isolated enzymes, cells, or organisms. The uses of biotechnology, as other technology, are driven by need (real or perceived) fulfillment.

There is no need here to review the massive amounts of knowledge (scientific and technological) that is foundational to the topics of enzymology and biological degradation. Instead, we should reflect on the basic fundamentals which make enzymes and enzymatic pathways a topic of continuing interest: high catalytic activity; a high degree of specificity relative to non-biologically derived systems; mild reaction conditions. Most impressive of all is the coupling of energetically exothermic and endothermic reactions to build life as we know it -- a highly improbable condition for molecules from a thermodynamic perspective.

Earlier, the use of enzymatic catalysis at commerical scale was limited by instability, the absence of re-use schemes and less costly alternatives. Enzyme and cell immobilization have done much to improve the cost-competitive posture of biocatalysts. This has allowed engineers to design a number of practical configurations for reactors. Dr. Chibata and his group have been at the forefront of this interface between science and technology. In his paper, he discusses specific examples of practical commercial systems.

"What has biotechnology done for us lately" is a common question, especially by technical skeptics. For certain, the number of pronounced commercial successes is low relative to the immense array of possibilities. In this society, success is often decreed only when a need and a capability to fulfill the need are properly coupled. Many of our capabilities in biotechnology are looking for needs. In other cases, biocatalysts cannot displace more cost-effective technologies. Many important uses for enzymes, however, are not broadly communicated and often not obvious even to enzymologists. Alexander Klibanov discusses some specific examples in his paper on unconventional uses.

My favorite example of little-known uses for enzymes is in the hydraulic fracturing of oil and gas wells. Nearly all of the new wells which are drilled in the USA are stimulated for accelerated rates of production. Hydraulic (pressure) fracturing is the most common method used. The system consists of high-pressure pumping of water, sand, and an alkoxylated polysaccharide (e.g., hydroxypropyl guar gum - a polygal actomannan). The whole process depends on destroying, through well-timed hydrolase action, the viscosifying polymer. This leaves the sand "down-hole" (when the pressure is released) to maintain the resultant formation fractures in an open condition. The net result is an accelerated rate of production.

The paper of Peter Williams also deals with an underground topic -- soil microorganisms. The catabolic activities of these organisms are of course foundational to the ecosystem. Understanding the genetic factors governing their activities under natural conditions is important. It is as important to understand these biological factors in light of the variety of synthesized chemicals which today make contact with the soil.

As a representative of Henkel -- a company which is heavily dependent on renewable raw materials (fats, oils, and polysaccharides) -- I would like to finish with a comment on the interface of biotechnology and sunlight. It is clear that the historic interplay between soil, water, air, and agronomic crops will be challenged by a number of factors. The direct capture of light energy by biological systems is the most practical and economic way to generate such highly reduced molecules as fatty acids and fatty alcohols. Having the capability of doing this without intensive land use should be a goal. In my opinion, efforts could be intensified on cutting edges of science and technology of photosynthetic systems.

INDUSTRIAL PRODUCTION OF OPTICALLY ACTIVE COMPOUNDS USING IMMOBILIZED BIOCATALYSTS

Ichiro Chibata
Research Laboratory of Applied Biochemistry
Tanabe Seiyaku Co., Ltd.
16-89, Kashima-3-chome, Yodogawa-ku
Osaka, Japan

INTRODUCTION

Since the late 1970s, biotechnology has been noticed with respect to problems of natural resources and energy; it is a comprehensive term combining the techniques of fermentation technology, enzyme engineering, genetic engineering, and so on. In this field, enzyme engineering technology, such as bioreactors using the actions of immobilized enzymes and microbial cells, is one of the main focal topics.

Since the beginning of the 1960s we have been studying immobilized enzymes and have succeeded in their industrialization. This technique is considered to be very promising in the future for the production of useful compounds. Thus, this paper discusses the immobilization of enzymes and microbial cells and their industrial applications.

Enzymes are biological catalysts, and participate in many chemical reactions occurring in living things. Unlike ordinary chemical catalysts, enzymes have the ability to catalyze a reaction under very mild conditions in neutral aqueous solutions at ambient temperatures and pressures, and with very high substrate specificity. However, enzymes are produced by organisms for their own requirements, and not for utilization by human beings. Therefore, although enzymes are efficient and effective catalysts, they are not always ideal catalysts for practical applications. Some of the advantages of enzymes may even be disadvantages in practical use as catalysts. Namely, enzymes are generally unstable and cannot be used in organic solvents or at elevated temperatures. Also, it is technically very difficult to recover active enzymes from the reaction mixture for reuse.

To eliminate these disadvantages inherent in ordinary enzymes, and in order to obtain superior catalysts for applications, two approaches have been investigated. One is the synthetic approach, using recently developed techniques of organic synthesis and polymer chemistry to synthesize catalysts having enzyme-like activities. Another approach is the "modification" of enzymes produced by organisms. Immobilization of enzymes is a part of this approach.

The definition of immobilized enzymes is, "...enzymes, physically confined or localized in a certain defined region of space with retention of their catalytic activities, and which can be used repeatedly and continuously." Immobilized microbial cells can be defined by replacing the word "enzymes" with "cells" in the definition.

If active and stable water-insoluble enzymes, that is, immobilized enzymes, are prepared, most of the above disadvantages are eliminated, and it becomes possible to use enzymes conveniently in the same way as ordinary solid catalysts used in synthetic chemistry. In addition, because enzymes can catalyze specific reactions under mild conditions, application of immobilized enzymes in the chemical industry can reduce energy requirements. Therefore, the expected advantages of using immobilized enzymes are as follows:

(1) Stability of enzymes is improved

(2) A catalyst can be tailor-made for specific use

(3) Enzymes can be reused

(4) Continuous operation becomes practical

(5) In the continuous operation, reactions require less space

(6) Better control of reaction is possible

(7) Higher purity and yield of products is possible

(8) Saving resources and less pollution is expected.

The first attempt to immobilize an enzyme to improve its properties for a particular application was made in 1953. Grubhofer and Schleith of Heidelberg immobilized enzymes such as carboxypeptidase, diastase, pepsin, and ribonuclease by using diazotized polyaminopolystyrene resin. Only a few additional papers were published on immobilized enzymes in the 1950s. In the 1960s, Katchalski-Katzir and his co-workers at the Weizmann Institute of Science, Israel, carried out extensive studies on immobilization techniques, and on the enzymatic, physical, and chemical properties of immobilized enzymes.

Also, since the early 1960s, we have investigated immobilized

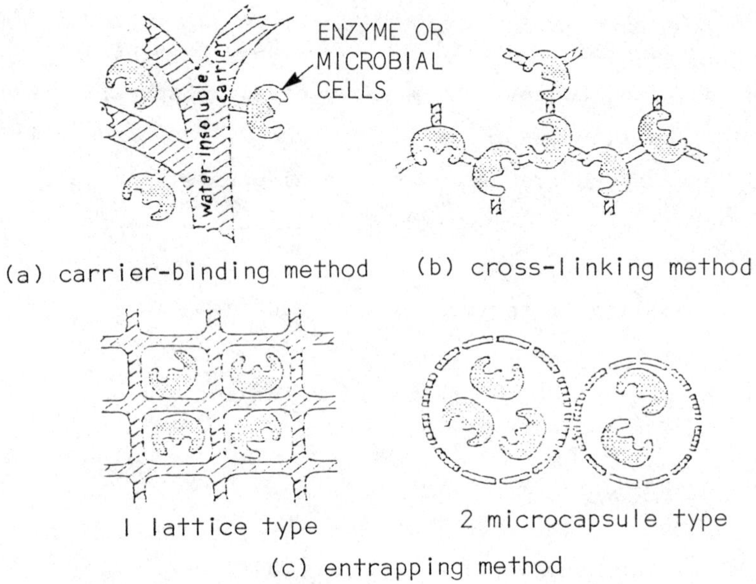

Fig. 1. Schematic diagrams of immobilized enzymes and immobilized microbial cells.

enzymes with the aim of utilizing them for continuous industrial production. And in 1969, we succeeded in the industrialization of a continuous process for the optical resolution of DL-amino acids using immobilized aminoacylase. This was the first industrial application of immobilized enzymes in the world.

From the late 1960s, science and technology has been aiming at more efficient utilization of enzyme activity, and specificity has been termed "Enzyme Engineering", a rapidly developing field.

A large number of methods have been reported concerning immobilization techniques. These methods can be classified into three basic categories (as shown in Fig. 1):

1) Carrier-binding method: the binding of enzyme to water-insoluble carriers via physical, ionic, or covalent binding;

2) Cross-linking method: without using water-insoluble carrier, intermolecular cross-linking of enzymes by means of bifunctional or multifunctional reagents such as glutaraldehyde;
3) Entrapping method: incorporating enzymes into the lattice of a gel matrix or enclosing the enzymes in a semi-permeable polymer membrane.

For immobilization of cells, the entrapping method has been most extensively investigated so far. These immobilizations should be carried out under very mild conditions to avoid the inactivation of enzymes.

Today, applications of immobilized systems are extending to a variety of fields such as analytical, medical, food processing, biomass conversion, energy generation, and so on. This is a new and typical multidisciplinary science and technology. In this paper, our main applications or immobilized systems for continous bioconversions are reviewed.

Immobilized Aminoacylase for Optical Resolution of Racemic Amino Acids

Utilization of L-amino acids for medicine and food has been developing rapidly in recent years. For the industrial production of L-amino acids, fermentation and chemical synthesis are considered to be promising methods. However, chemically synthesized amino acids are optically inactive racemic mixtures of L- and D-isomers. To obtain natural L-amino acid from the chemically synthesized DL-form, optical resolution is necessary.

Among the many optical resolution methods, the enzymic method using mold aminoacylase developed by us is one of the most advantageous procedures, yielding optically pure L-amino acids.

A chemically synthesized acyl-DL-amino acid is asymmetrically hydrolyzed by aminoacylase to give L-amino acid and unhydrolyzed acyl-D-amino acid as follows:

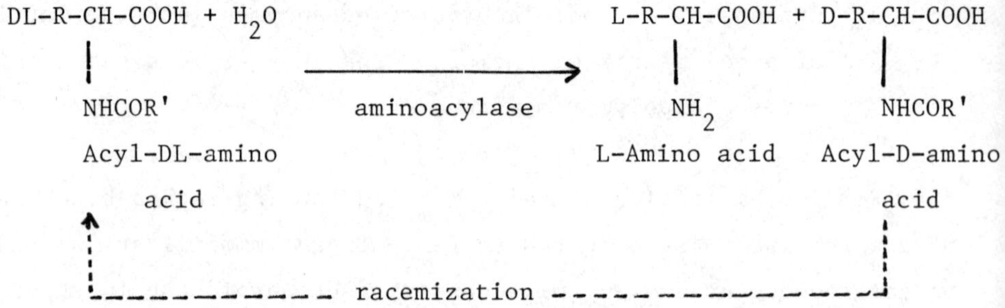

The two products are easily separated by the difference in their solubilities. Acyl-D-amino acid is racemized, and reused for the resolution procedure.

From 1953 to 1969, this enzymatic resolution method was employed by the Tanabe Seiyaku Co. for the industrial production of several L-amino acids. The enzyme reaction was carried out batchwise by incubating a mixture containing substrate and soluble enzyme. However, this procedure had some disadvantages inherent to batch processes using soluble enzymes. For instance, in order to isolate L-amino acid from the reaction mixture, we had to remove enzyme protein by pH and/or heat treatments. These treatments resulted in an uneconomical loss of enzyme. In addition, as a complicated purification procedure was necessary to remove contaminating proteins and coloring substances, the yield of L-amino acid was lowered. Also, much labor was necessary for batch operation.

To overcome these drawbacks and to improve this procedure, we extensively studied the continuous optical resolution of DL-amino acids using immobilized aminoacylase. When we started this study in the early 1960s, reports on enzyme immobilization were very few and there were practically no reports on application of immobilized enzymes for production purposes. Therefore, we studied a variety of methods for immobilization of aminoacylase. As a result, relatively active and stable immobilized aminoacylases were obtained by ionic binding to DEAE-Sephadex [1,2], covalent binding to iodoacetylcellulose [3], and entrapment in polyacrylamide gel lattice [4]. Furthur, to select the most suitable preparation for industrial purposes, the properties of these immobilized aminoacylases were compared [5]. Finally, we chose the immobilized aminoacylase prepared by ionic binding to DEAE-Sephadex for the industrial production of L-amino acids. Because preparation is easy, the activity is high and stable, and regeneration of deteriorated immobilized enzyme is possible.

Further, we carried out chemical engineering studies and designed an enzyme reactor system for continuous production of L-amino acids with immobilized aminoacylase as shown in Figure 2 [5,6]. Substrate, acetyl-DL-amino acid solution, is continuously charged into the enzyme column at a constant flow rate through a filter and a heat exchanger. During passage through the column, the enzyme reaction occurs. The effluent is concentrated, and L-amino acid is crystallized. Acetyl-D-amino acid contained in the mother liquor is racemized by heating in a racemization tank and reused for optical resolution. This system is automatically controlled and operated.

In the immobilized enzyme process, the overall production cost was more than 40% lower than that of the conventional batch process using the soluble enzyme. Savings of enzyme and labor costs are the main contributors, as well as the increase of product yield due to easy isolation of L-amino acids from the reaction mixture. Although DEAE-Sephadex is a relatively expensive carrier, production cost is not greatly affected by the cost of the carrier, because it can be used for a very long period. Since 1969, we have been industrially operating several series of enzyme reactors in our plants for the production of L-methionine, L-valine, L-phenylalanine, and so on.

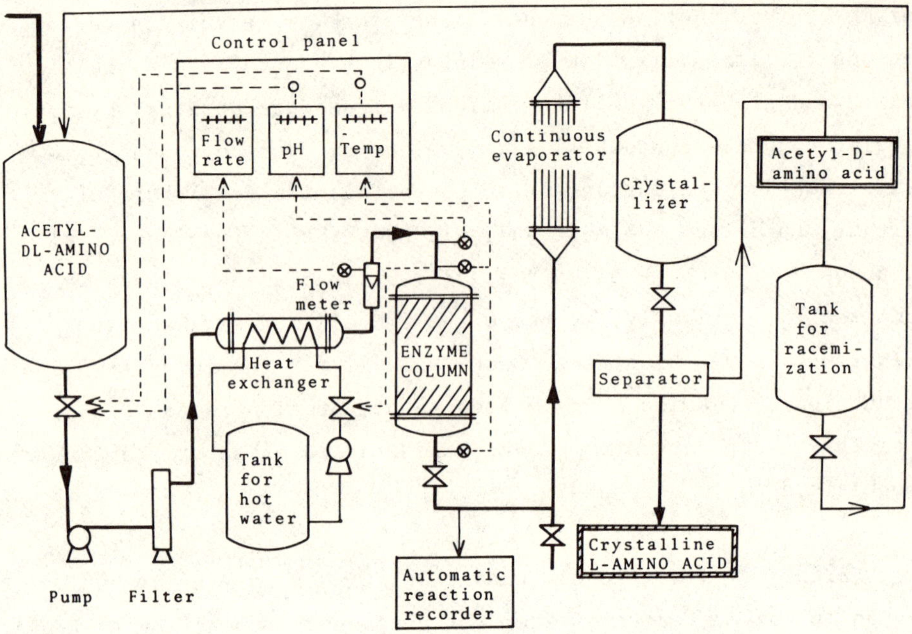

Fig. 2. Flow diagram for continuous production of L-amino acid by immobilized aminoacylase.

Production of L-Aspartic Acid by Immobilized Escherichia Coli

Following the industrialization of optical resolution by immobilized aminoacylase, we attempted the continuous asymmetric synthesis of L-aspartic acid by immobilized aspartase. L-Aspartic acid is used for medicines and food additives. From 1960 to 1973, we had industrially produced L-aspartic acid from ammonium fumarate using the action of aspartase as follows:

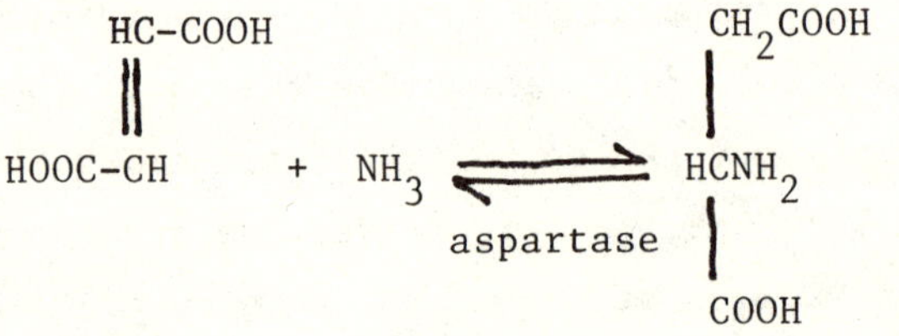

Fumaric acid

L-Aspartic acid

This asymmetric reaction has been carried out using a batch procedure, which has disadvantages for industrial purposes, just as in the case of the native aminoacylase process. Thus, we studied the continuous production of L-aspartic acid with immobilized aspartase [7]. As the aspartase is an intracellular enzyme, it was necessary to extract the enzyme from microbial cells before immobilization . Extracted intracellular enzymes are generally unstable, and most of the immobilization methods we tried resulted in low activity and poor yield. Although entrapment in polyacrylamide gel lattice gave relatively active immobilized aspartase, its operational stability was not sufficient for the industrial production of L-aspartic acid. We considered that if the whole microbial cells could be immobilized directly, these disadvantages might be overcome. From these points of view, we studied the immobilization of whole microbial cells [8]. Reports on immobilization of whole microbial cells were very scarce at that time, so we tried various methods for immobilization of *Escherichia coli*. Among these methods the most active immobilized *E. coli* cells were obtained by entrapping the cells in polyacrylamide gel lattice. To prepare the most efficient immobilized microbial cells, the type and concentration of bifunctional reagents for cross-linking and the concentration of acrylamide monomer were investigated. As a result, optimum conditions of the immobilization of *E. coli* were decided [8]. *E. coli* cells collected from cultured broth were suspended in physiological saline. To this suspension were added acrylamide monomer, BIS, β-dimethylaminopropionitrile, and potassium persulfate. The mixture was allowed to stand at below 40°C for 10-15 min, and the resulting stiff gel was made into granules of approximately 3 mm.

Figure 3 shows the structure of cells entrapped in acrylamide gel lattice. Small molecular weight substrate and product can pass through the gel lattice, but high molecular weight aspartase protein does not leak out from the gel lattice.

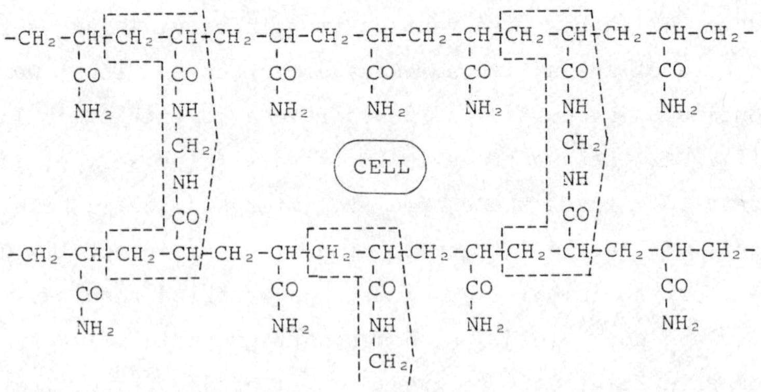

Fig. 3. Chemical structure of polyacrylamide gel.

A comparison of the operational stability of various preparations is shown in Fig. 4. Immobilized cells are stable, and the half-life was estimated to be 120 days. Therefore, it is clear that the immobilized cell system is advantageous for industrial purposes.

Using a column packed with these immobilized E. coli cells, conditions for continuous production of L-aspartic acid from ammonium fumarate were investigated in detail, and the aspartase reactor system was designed [9,10]. The system is essentially the same as that for the immobilized aminoacylase system. That is, a solution of ammonium fumarate containing $MgCl_2$ is passed through the immobilized E. coli column at a flow rate of SV=0.6. The effluent is adjusted to pH 2.8 with sulfuric acid and then cooled at 15°C. By this simple procedure pure L-aspartic acid can be obtained without recrystallization in very high yield, over 95%. When a 1000 liter column is used, theoretically the yield of L-aspartic acid is 1915 kg/day and about 60 tons/month.

A comparison of the costs for production of L-aspartic acid by the conventional batch process using intact cells and the continuous process using immobilized cells is shown in Fig. 5.

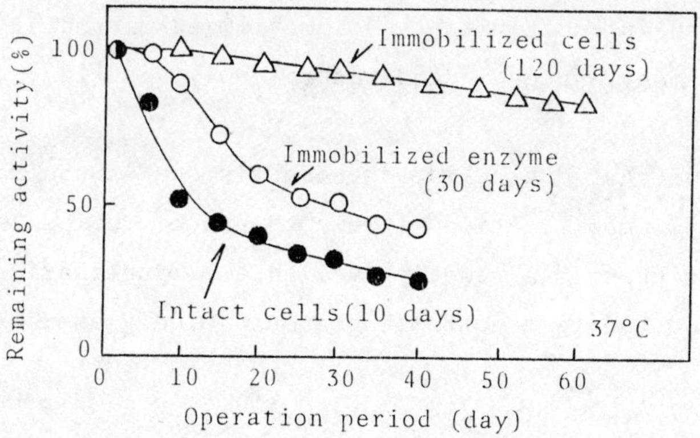

Fig. 4. Operational stability of various aspartase preparations.

The overall production cost of the immobilized cell system is about 60% of that of the conventional batch process using intact cells. Furthermore, the procedure employing immobilized cells is advantageous from the standpoint of waste treatment. Therefore, it is clear that this new technique is very efficient and superior to the conventional fermentative or enzymic batch technique. We have been industrially operating this new system in our plant for automatic and continuous production of L-aspartic acid since the autumn of 1973. This is considered to be the first industrial application of immobilized microbial cells.

New Immobilization Method -- k-Carrageenan

As stated above, the polyacrylamide gel method is advantageous for immobilization of microbial cells and for industrial application. However, there are some limitations in this method. That is, some enzymes are inactivated during the immobilization procedure by the action of the acrylamide monomer, β-dimethylaminopropionitril, or by potassium persulfate. Therefore, this method is not always satisfactory for immobilization of enzymes and microbial cells. Thus, in order to find a more general immobilization technique and to improve the productivities of immobilized microbial cell systems, we screened many synthetic and natural polymers [11].

We found that "kappa-carrageenan" is one of the most suitable matrices for immobilization of enzymes and microbial cells. Kappa-carrageenan is a readily available polysaccharide isolated from seaweeds and is a nontoxic compound widely used as a food additive.

Carrageenan becomes a gel under mild conditions. It gels by cooling as in the case with agar, and by contact with various gel-inducing agents such as metal ions, ammonium ion, various amines, and water-miscible organic solvents.

Therefore, taking into consideration the characteristics of the enzyme-protein and the kind of substrate and product, we can choose the most suitable procedure for immobilization of microbial cells. In our experience, the procedures of cooling and/or contacting with an aqueous solution containing K^+ or NH_4^+ are very easily carried out for gelation, and as these conditions are very mild, immobilized preparations having high activity can be obtained [12].

The immobilization procedure of microbial cells using carrageenan is as follows [12]. A cell suspension is warmed at $37^\circ \sim 50^\circ C$, and carrageenan dissolved in physiological saline is also warmed at $37^\circ \sim 60^\circ C$. Both are mixed, and the mixture is cooled and/or contacted with an aqueous solution containing a gel-inducing agent. After this treatment, the gel is granulated in suitable particle size. If the operational stability of immobilized cells is not satisfactory, the immobilized cells are treated with hardening agents such as glutaraldehyde and hexamethylenediamine. As a result, stable immobilized cells can be obtained.

By this simple procedure many kinds of microbial cells and enzymes are successfully entrapped into gel-lattice.

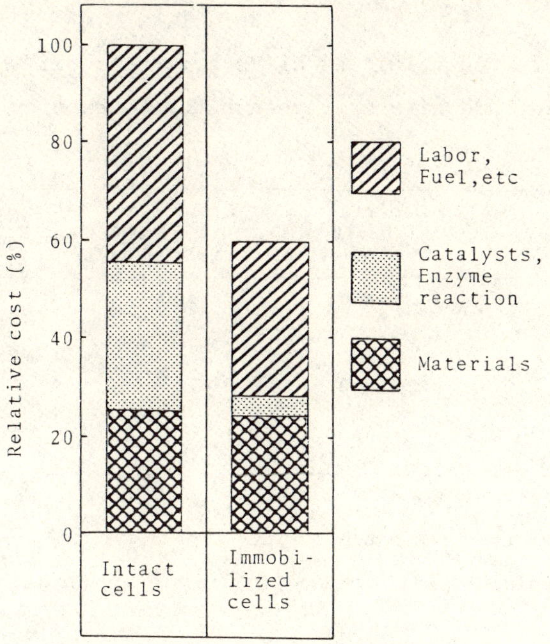

Fig. 5. Comparison of cost for production of L-aspartic acid.

A further advantage of this method using carrageenan is that various shapes of immobilized preparations, such as cubic, bead, and film types, can be easily tailored for particular application purposes. For instance, the bead type can readily be prepared by dropping the mixture of cell suspension and carrageenan solution into a stirred solution containing a gel-inducing reagent such as KCl.

As carrageenan was found to be a useful matrix for immobilization of microbial cells, we extensively studied this carrageenan method to improve the previously industrialized L-aspartic acid production using immobilized E. coli cells by the polyacrylamide gel method [13]. It was found that the operational stability of immobilized E. coli cells with carrageenan was greatly increased by a hardening treatment with glutaraldehyde and hexamethylenediamine;

Table 1

Comparison of Productivities of Escherichia coli Immobilized with Polyacrylamide and with Carrageenan for Production of L-Aspartic Acid

Immobilization method	Aspartase activity (unit/g cells)	Stability at 37°C (half-life, day)	Relative productivity
Polyacrylamide	18,850	120	100
Carrageenan	56,340	70	174
Carrageenan (GA)	37,460	240	397
Carrageenan (GA+HMDA)	49,400	680	1,498

GA: glutaraldehyde, HMDA: hexamethylenediamine

Productivity = $\int_0^t E_0 \exp(-kd \cdot t)\,dt$

E_0=initial activity, kd=decay constant, t=operational period

these immobilized cells are very stable, with a half-life of 680 days.

Table 1 shows a comparison of productivities of E. coli cells immobilized with polyacrylamide and with carrageenan for production of L-aspartic acid. When the productivity of the immobilized preparation with polyacrylamide was taken as 100, that of immobilized cells with carrageenan had hardened with glutaraldehyde and hexamethylenediamine was 1500. As this carrageenan method is apparently more advantageous than the polyacrylamide method, in 1978 we changed to this new method for the industrial production of L-aspartic acid.

Production of L-Malic Acid by Immobilized Brevibacterium ammoniagenes

Following the production of L-aspartic acid, in 1974 we succeeded in the third industrial application, namely, asymmetric synthesis of L-malic acid from fumaric acid by immobilized microbial cells [14,15]. L-Malic acid is an essential compound in cellular metabolism and is mainly used in the pharmaceutical field.

We investigated continuous production of L-malic acid from fumaric acid by following fumarase reaction using immobilized microbial cells.

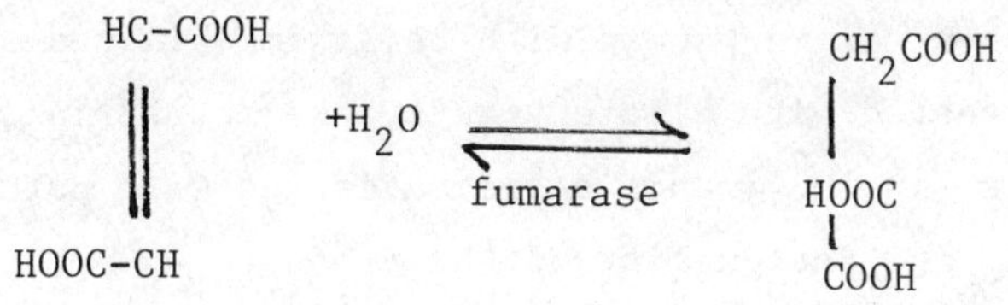

Fumaric acid L-Malic acid

Several microorganisms giving high fumarase activity were immobilized by the polyacrylamide gel method and their activities were investigated. _Brevibacterium ammoniagenes_ showed the highest activity per unit weight of cells; also per unit volume of culture medium. Therefore, we employed this microorganism for the production of L-malic acid.

However, when immobilized _B. ammoniagenes_ was used for the production of L-malic acid from fumaric acid, some by-products were formed. Namely, besides unreacted fumaric acid, considerable accumulation of succinic acid was observed in the reaction mixture. Although fumaric acid can be easily separated by acidifying the reaction mixture, industrial separation of succinic acid from L-malic acid is very difficult. Therefore, the point of success for industrial production of pure L-malic acid is the prevention of succinic acid formation during the enzyme reaction. We tried various methods to suppress succinic acid formation, and found that treatment of immobilized cells with detergents such as deoxycholic acid, bile acid, and bile extract was effective. These detergent treatments not only suppressed succinic acid formation but also markedly enhanced L-malic acid formation by the immobilized B. ammoniagenes cells. This result indicates that the permeability barrier of the cell membrane for substrate and/or product was removed by these detergent treatments.

We then studied the conditions for the production of L-malic acid using a column packed with cells immobilized by polyacrylamide gel and treated with bile extracts. We industrialized this production system in 1974, and we are satisfied with both economical efficiency and the quality of the product.

Then, as in the case of production of L-aspartic acid, we tried to improve the productivity for L-malic acid using cells immobilized with carrageenan [16,17]. In this case, we screened again the microorganisms having higher fumarase activity, and Brevibacterium flavum was found to have higher enzyme activity after immobilization with carrageenan, compared with the former B. ammoniagenes. The stabilities were also studied, and the productivities are compared in Table II.

When the productivity of B. ammoniagenes immobilized with polyacrylamide was taken as 100, that of B. flavum immobilized with carrageenan was 897. Therefore, it is evident that the carrageenan method is more advantageous than the conventional polyacrylamide method. We changed from the polyacrylamide method to the carrageenan method in 1977.

Further, we found that the heat stability of fumarase activity of B. flavum increased when immobilized with carrageenan in the presence of polyethylenimine [18]. As shown in Table II, the productivity of B. flavum immobilized with carrageenan and polyethylenemine increased to 21 times that of B. ammoniagenes immobilized

Table 2

Comparison of L-Malic Acid Productivity of Various Immobilized Preparations

Microbial cells and immobilization method	Operation temperature (°C)	Fumarase activity (μmole/h/ml of gel)	Operational stability (Half-life; days)	Relative productivity (%)
B. ammoniagenes Polyacrylamide	37	530	53	100
B. flavum Polyacrylamide	37	610	94	273
κ-Carrageenan	37	900	160	897
κ-Carrageenan + Polyethyleneimine	37	980	243	1587
"	45	1420	165	2073
"	50	1670	128	1992
"	55	2160	74	1730

$$\text{Productivity} = \int_0^t E_0 \exp(-Kd \cdot t)\,dt \quad \begin{cases} E_0 = \text{Initial fumarase activity} \\ Kd = \text{Decay constant} \\ t = \text{Operational period} \end{cases}$$

with polyacrylamide. Thus, in 1980 the industrial production system of L-malic acid was changed to this improved method.

It is difficult to get direct evidence of the mechanism of stabilization by immobilization with carrageenan. But generally, enzymes binding to particles and membranes are more stable than free and soluble forms. Carrageenan interacts with cells and helps to keep the bound state of the enzyme. Actually, lysis of the cells is retarded by immobilization with carrageenan. Polyethyleneimine is supposed to increase interaction of carrageenan with cells and enzymes.

Production of L-Alanine by Immobilized Microbial Cells

Following the two industrial applications of immobilized microbial cells for production of L-aspartic acid and L-malic acid, we have been studying continuous production of L-alanine from L-aspartic acid using immobilized microbial cells [19,20]. L-Alanine is a useful amino acid not only as a medicine but also as a food additive because of its good taste. It has been industrially produced from L-aspartic acid in our plant since 1965 by a batchwise enzyme reaction using L-aspartate β-decarboxylase of *Pseudomonas dacunhae*. The enzyme reaction proceeds as follows:

$$\begin{array}{ccc} COOH & & \\ | & & \\ CH_2 & \xrightarrow[\beta\text{-decarboxylase}]{\text{L-Asparate}} & CH_3 \\ | & & | \\ CHNH_2 & & CHNH_2 + COH2 \\ | & & | \\ COOH & & COOH \end{array}$$

L-Aspartic acid L-Alanine

Thus, we studied immobilized *P. dacunha* cells having high L-aspartate β-decarboxylase to establish an efficient continuous process for L-alanine production. Relatively stable and active immobilized cells were obtained by immobilization of *P. dacunhae* cells with carrageenan and following hardening treatment with glutaraldehyde.

In the continuous production system using immobilized *P. dacunhae*, one of the problems is the evolution of CO_2 gas during the L-asparate β-decarboxylase reaction. It is not efficient to perform this reaction using a conventional column system at normal pressure, because the evolution of CO_2 gas makes it difficult to obtain complete plug-flow of substrate solution and the pH of the reaction mixture increases within the column as the reaction progresses. Therefore, we investigated the most advantageous reactor system using immobilized *P. dacunhae* for continuous production of L-alanine, and designed a closed column reactor which performs the enzyme

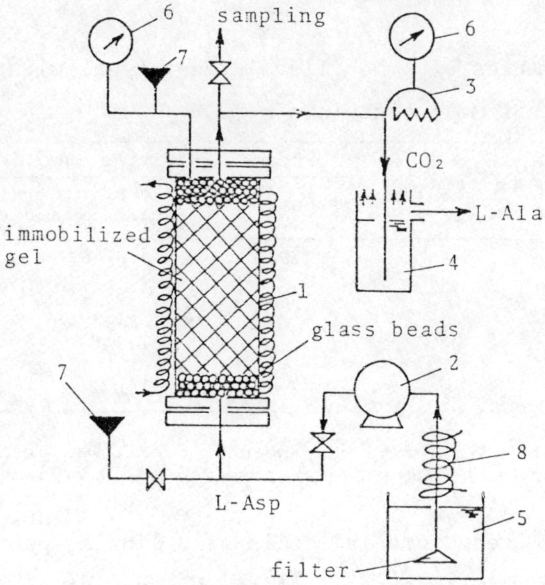

Fig. 6. Closed column reactor for production of L-alanine. 1: Reactor 2: Plunger pump 3: Pressure control valve 4: Receiver 5: Substrate tank 6: Pressure gauge 7: Safety valve 8: Heat exchanger

reaction at high pressure, such as 10 kg/cm^2. This reactor is shown in Fig. 6. By using this reactor, since liberated CO_2 gas is dissolved into the reaction mixture, complete plug-flow of substrate solution is obtained and the pH of reaction mixture is not much changed.

The efficiency of immobilized cells for production of L-alanine in the closed column system at high pressure was much higher than that in the conventional column system at normal pressure. The stability of immobilized cells in both systems was similar. It is apparent that the closed column reactor is advantageous for the reaction evolving CO_2.

The method described above involved continuous enzyme reactions

Table 3

Enzyme Activities of Immobilized Preparations with or without pH-Treatment of Microorganisms

Microorganism	pH-treatment*	Enzyme activities (μmole/hr g of gels)			
		Aspartase	L-Aspartate β-decarboxylase	Alanine racemase	Fumarase
E.coli	-	7,510	—	89.4	1,310
	+	7,470	—	<1	1.4
P.dacunhae	-	—	1,140	28.0	745
	+	—	1,030	<0.3	<0.5

*Before immobilization with carrageenan, *E.coli* was treated at pH 5.0 and 40°C for 1 hr, and *P.dacunhae* was treated at pH 4.75 and 30°C for 1 hr.

using immobilized microbial cells of a single species for production of L-alanine from L-aspartic acid. We then considered that if immobilized *E. coli* having aspartase activity, and immobilized *P. decunhae* having L-asparate β-decarboxylase were to be employed in a single reactor, L-alanine would be more efficiently produced from ammonium fumarate [21]. Thus, we investigated the conditions for production of L-alanine from ammonium fumarate using immobilized microbial cells of two organisms. However, as shown in the following equations, *E. coli* and *P. dacunhae* have alanine racemase and fumarase.

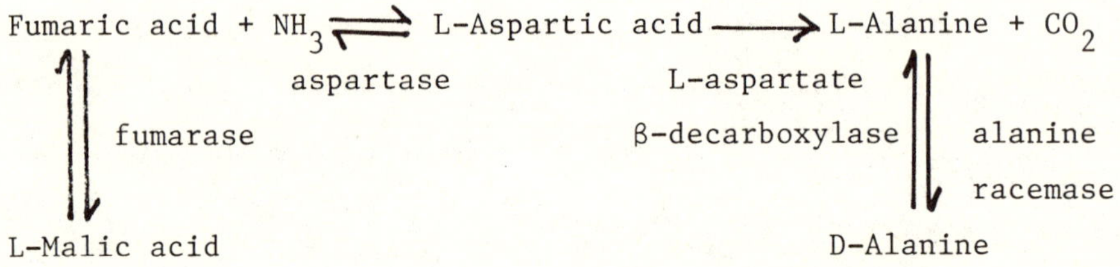

Therefore, when the two types of immobilized microbial cells were used in a single reactor for production of L-alanine from

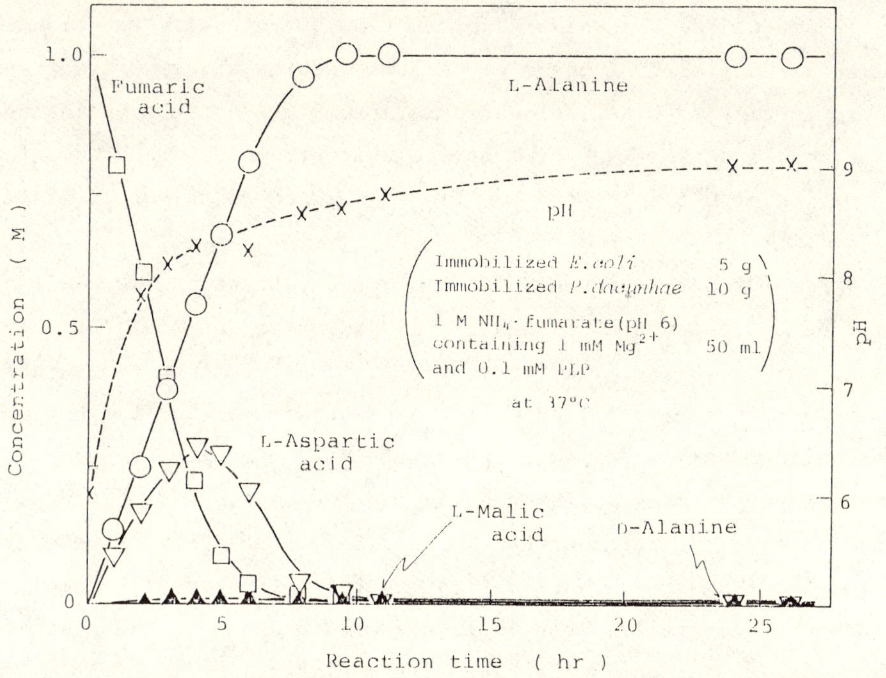

Fig. 7. Time-course of L-alanine production by batchwise reaction using two pH-treated immobilized microbial cells.

ammonium fumarate, D-alanine and L-malic acid were formed as by-products.

Thus, for effective production of L-alanine, it was necessary to prevent the actions of these undesirable enzymes. So, we tried various procedures for removal of these enzymes. It was found that when E. coli was treated at pH 5.0 and 40°C for 1 hour and P. dacunhae at pH 4.75 and 30°C for 1 hour, respectively, before immobilization with kappa-carrageenan, the aspartase of E coli and L-asparate β-decarboxylase of P. dacunhae were not decreased but the alanine racemase and fumarase of two immobilized microbial cells were almost completely inactivated as shown in Table III.

Time-course of L-alanine production by batchwise reaction using immobilized microbial cells of the two species after pH treatment is shown in Fig. 7. L-Aspartic acid is accumulated at the beginning of reaction, and then L-alanine is stoichiometrically produced. The formation of D-alanine and L-malic acid is completely suppressed.

For further improvement of L-alanine production, we co-immobilized *E. coli* and *P. dacunhae* cells in carrageenan at the same time. However, the efficiency of L-alanine formation using the mixture of two immobilized cell types was higher than that of co-immobilized cells. This difference of efficiency may be due to micro-environmental differences in the two systems. Influences include the inhibition of L-aspartate β-decarboxylase by L-aspartic acid, and a discrepancy of optimal pH for both enzymes. Namely, microenvironmentally these influences are greater in the case of co-immobilization than in the case of the mixture.

Thus, we are now studying conditions for continuous production of L-alanine from ammonium fumarate using the mixture of two immobilized cell types, and are going to industrialize this L-alanine production system in the near future.

Industrial Application of Immobilized Biocatalysts

In this paper our applications of immobilized systems for chemical processes have been presented. At present, it is said that the six systems shown in Table 4 are industrialized in the world. Namely, besides our systems for optical resolution of DL-amino acid, and for production of L-aspartic acid and L-malic acid, three immobilized systems, glucose isomerase, penicillin amidase and β-galactosidase are used in industry. The continuous production of high fructose syrup by immobilized glucose isomerase is becoming one of the major fields of application of immobilized systems. Further,

Table 4

Current Applications of Immobilized Enzymes and Immobilized Microbial Cells in Industry

Enzymes and microorganisms	Application	Operating since
Aminoacylase	Optical resolution of DL-amino acid	1969
Glucose isomerase	Isomerization of glucose to fructose	(1973)
Penicillin amidase	Production of 6-APA	(1973)
Escherichia coli (Aspartase)	Production of L-aspartic acid	1973
Brevibacterium ammoniagenes (Fumarase)	Production of L-malic acid	1974
β-Galactosidase	Hydrolysis of lactose	1977

6-aminopenicillanic acid is produced from penicillin using immobilized penicillin amidase. 6-Aminopenicillanic acid is an important intermediate for semisynthetic pencillins. Also low lactose milk is produced by immobilized β-galactosidase. In the near future, many other immobilized systems are expected to be industrialized.

Immobilized Living Microbial Cells

In this paper continuous enzyme reactions using immobilized microbial cells for production of L-aspartic acid, L-malic acid and others have been described. These reactions are primarily catalyzed by a single enzyme and the immobilized cells are in a dead state, though the enzyme in immobilized cells is in an active and stable state. However, many useful compounds, especially those produced by fermentation methods, are usually formed by multi-step reactions catalyzed by many kinds of enzymes in living microbial cells. Also these reactions often require generation of ATP and other co-enzymes. If immobilized cells are kept in a living state, they may be applied for these multi-enzyme reactions.

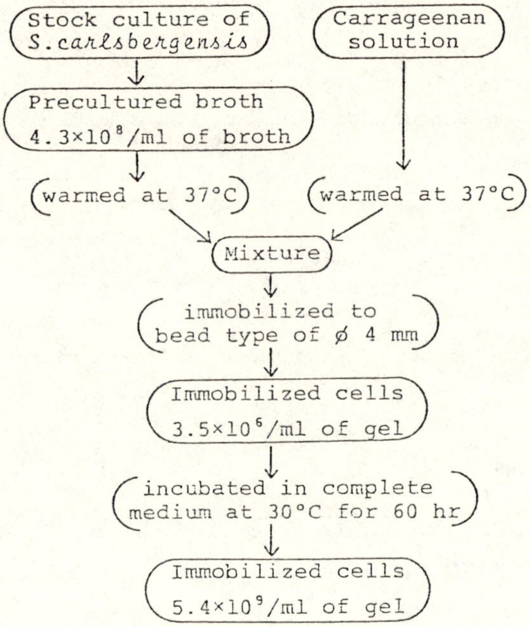

Fig. 8. Immobilization method of yeast cells using carrageenan.

From these standpoints, we have studied ethanol production as a model system using immobilized living cells [22,23]. We found that ethanol can be continuously and efficiently produced by using living yeast cells immobilized with carrageenan.

Figure 8 shows the immobilization method for the yeast, Saccharomyces carlsbergensis (1) Harvesting of yeast cells was not necessary. Precultured broth was directly mixed with carrageenan solution at a ratio of below 5% and made into immobilized cells of the bead type. (2) These gels, containing a small amount of cells, were incubated in complete medium on a rotary shaker at 30°C. After 60 hours incubation, the numbers of living cells in gel increased to 1000 fold that of the gel before incubation. The growth of cells in gel was compared with that of free cells on complete medium and the results are shown in Fig. 9. Both growth rates were similar in the initial phase. Free cells reached full growth at 30 hours. On the

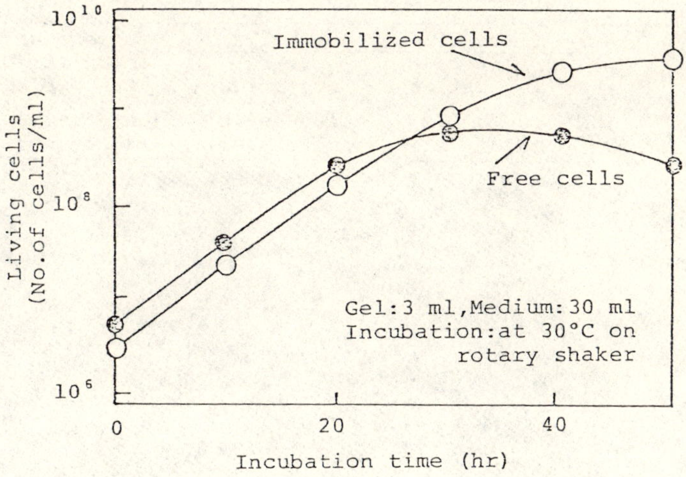

Fig. 9. Comparison of growth of free and immobilized yeast cells.

other hand, the immobilized yeast cells showed better growth than free cells. After 60 hours of incubation, the numbers of living cells in gel reached 10 fold the number of free-growing cells.

To explain the reason for this higher growth of yeast cells in gel than free cells in the conventional culture method, we considered that in gel (1) microbial cells can select suitable environmental conditions and (2) cells may be well protected from environmental changes in gel by the buffer action of the carrageenan gel.

Photographs in Fig. 10 depict a gel bead and a slice of a gel bead. Before incubation, the gel bead looks clear because it contains a small number of cells. After incubation, the appearance of the gel bead changed and is similar to that of a gel homogeneously entrapping a large number of harvested cells. However, the slice of gel after incubation showed the formation of a thin layer of condensed yeast cells near the surface of the bead, and cells were not observed at the center of the bead. Therefore, these immobilized cells forming a condensed thin layer near the surface of the

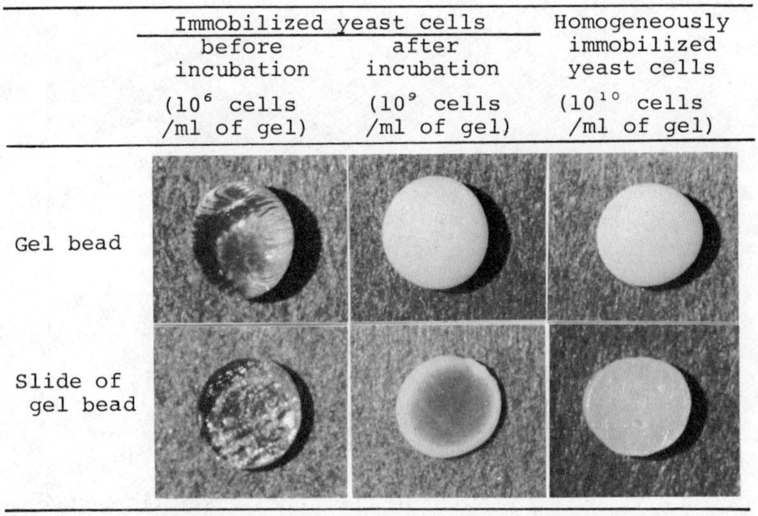

Fig. 10. Photographs of immobilized yeast cells in gel.

gel bead were expected to show efficient catalytic activities in enzyme reactions.

Figure 11 shows a scanning electron micrograph of living yeast cells immobilized with carrageenan.

We studied ethanol production using a column packed with these immobilized living yeast cells. A typical pattern of continuous production of ethanol by immobilized yeast cells is shown in Fig. 12.

In the operation, steady state was maintained for longer than 90 days. Some release of cells from the gel occurs as shown in this figure. However, the number of cells in the effluent is as low as $10^{6\sim7}$, while the cells in gel were maintained at high levels, $10^{9\sim10}$. Therefore, it is clear that most of alcohol is produced by the cells in gel. Gel beads keep their shape after 90 days operation. For constant production of higher concentrations of ethanol, it was necessary to increase step-wise the concentration of glucose.

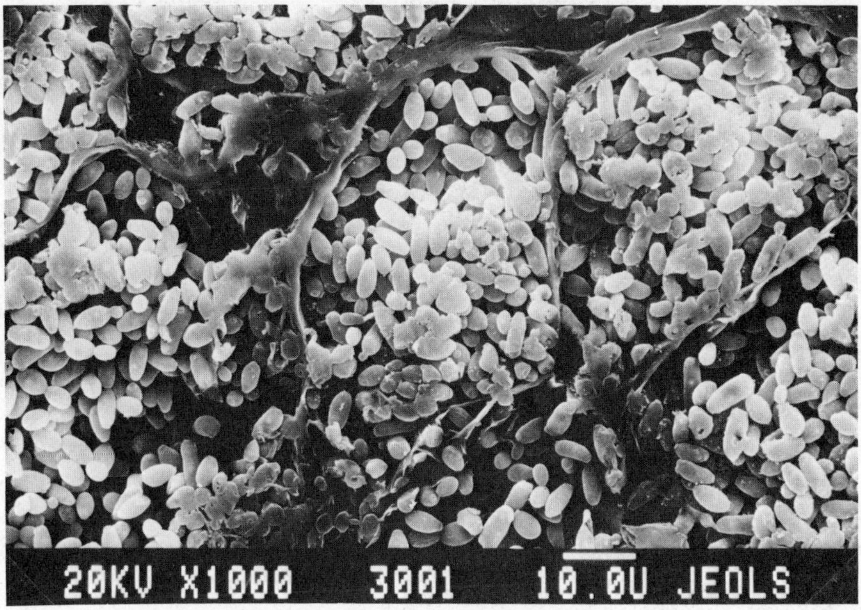

Fig. 11. Electron micrograph of immobilized living yeast cells.

Namely, in the initial stage (0∿5 days) 100 mg glucose/ml, and in the middle stage (5∿10 days) 150 mg/ml were used. In the stationary stage, 200 mg glucose/ml (20%) were used, and we could continuously produce high concentrations of ethanol such as 100 mg/ml (12.7 volume %) for over 90 days at short retention times, e.g., 3 hours.

This immobilized living yeast cell system is being further investigated by domestic alcohol industries with respect to optimum operation and scale up, and it promises to become a useful technique for industrial production of ethanol.

Besides ethanol production, applications of this type of immobilized living cell system are now extending. That is, it is being applied to multistep reactions such as production of alcohols, organic acids, amino acids, vitamins, steroids, antibiotics, and enzymes, and also to hydrogen and methane generation.

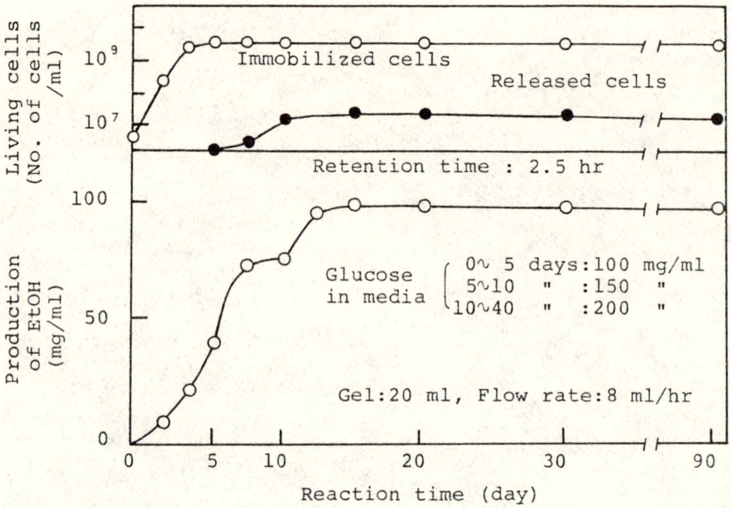

Fig. 12. Pattern of continuous production of high concentrations of ethanol using a column packed with immobilized yeast cells.

Very recently, in addition to the immobilization of enzymes and microbial cells, immobilization of plant and animal cells have been reported. Immobilized plant cells are considered to be advantageous catalysts for production of medicines originating from plants, and are used for transformation of natural products. Immobilized animal cells will be used for biological sensors, extracorporeal shunt systems, and production of useful biomaterials.

CONCLUSION

As stated above, the techniques that began with immobilized enzymes have developed to immobilized microbial cells, immobilized living microbial cells, and further to immobilized plant and animal cells. These immobilized systems are applied in a variety of fields and play a very important role in enzyme engineering in the field of biotechnology.

Recently, genetic engineering as well as enzyme engineering has been paid special attention as being among the most promising techniques in biotechnology. Genetic engineering and enzyme engineering are not competing technologies, but should cooperate with each other to further progress. Fundamentally, genetic engineering cannot be an independent production technology. To be an efficient production technology, it should be combined with fermentation technology, enzyme engineering, and further with isolation and purification process technologies.

If a novel microorganism having desired characteristics is produced by genetic engineering and used for immobilized enzyme and immobilized living microbial cell technology, this will be a very promising production technology.

Therefore, we are convinced that if cooperation among scientists and engineers in a variety of fields related to biotchnologies is accelerated, biotechnology will contribute to the future welfare of human beings.

REFERENCES

1. Tosa, T., T. Mori, N. Fuse, and I. Chibata. 1966. Studies on continuous enzyme reactions. I. Screening of carriers for preparation of water-insoluble aminoacylase. Enzymologia 31:214-224.
2. Tosa, T., T. Mori, and I. Chibata. 1969. Studies on continuous enzyme reactions. Part VI. Enzymatic properties of the DEAE-Sephadex-aminoacylase complex. Agr. Biol. Chem. 33:1053-1059.
3. Sato, T., T. Mori, T. Tosa, and I. Chibata. 1971. Studies on immobilized enzymes. IX. Preparation and properties of

aminoacylase covalently attached to halogenoacetylcelluloses. Arch. Biocehm. Biophys. 147:788-796.

4. Mori, T., T. Sato, T. Tosa, and I. Chibata. 1972. Studies on immobilized enzymes. X. Preparation and properties of aminoacylase entrapped into acrylamide gel-lattice. Enzymologia 43:213-226.

5. Chibata, I., T. Tosa, T. Sato, T. Mori, and Y. Matsuo. 1972. Preparation and industrial application of immobilized aminoacylases. Proc. IV. IFS: Ferment. Technol. Today: 383-389.

6. Tosa, T., T. Mori, and I. Chibata. 1971. Studies on continuous enzyme reactions. VIII. Kinetics and pressure drop of aminoacylase column. J. Ferment. Technol. 49:522-528.

7. Tosa, T., T. Sato, T. Mori, Y. Matsuo, and I. Chibata. 1973. Continuous production of L-aspartic acid by immobilized aspartase. Biotech. Bioeng. 15:69-84.

8. Chibata, I., T. Tosa, and T. Sato. 1974. Immobilized aspartase-containing microbial cells: Preparation and enzymatic properties. Appl. Microbiol. 27:878-885.

9. Tosa, T., T. Sato, T. Mori, and I. Chibata. 1974. Basic studies for continuous production of L-aspartic acid by immobilized E. coli cells. Appl. Microbiol. 27:886-889.

10. Sato, T., T. Mori, T. Tosa, I. Chibata, M. Furui, K. Yamashita, and A. Sumi. 1975. Engineering analysis of continuous production of L-aspartic acid by immobilized E. coli cells in fixed beds. Biotech. Bioeng. 17:1797-1804.

11. Takata, I., T. Tosa, and I. Chibata. 1977. Screening of matrix suitable for immobilization of microbial cells. J. Solid-Phase Biochem. 2:225-236.

12. Tosa, T., T. Sato, T. Mori, K. Yamamoto, I. Takata, Y. Nishida, and I. Chibata. 1979. Immobilization of enzymes and microbial cells using carrageenan as matrix. Biotech. Bioeng. 21:1697-1709.

13. Nishida, Y., T. Sato, T. Tosa, and I. Chibata. 1979. Immobilization of *E. coli* cells having aspartase activity with carrageenan and locust bean gum. Enzyme Microb. Technol. 1:95-99.

14. Yamamoto, K., T. Tosa, K. Yamashita, and I. Chibata. 1976. Continuous production of L-malic acid by immobilized *Brevibacterium ammoniagenes* cells. European J. Appl. Microbiol. 3:169-183.

15. Yamamoto, K., T. Tosa, K. Yamashita, and I. Chibata. 1977. Kinetics and decay of fumarase activity of immobilized *Brevibacterium ammoniagenes* cells for continuous production of L-malic acid. Biotech. Bioeng. 19:1101-1114.

16. Takata, I., K. Yamamoto, T. Tosa, and I. Chibata. 1979. Screening of microorganisms having high fumarase activity and their immobilization with carrageenan. European J. Appl. Microbiol. Biotech. 7:161-172.

17. Takata, I., K. Yamamoto, T. Tosa, and I. Chibata. 1980. Immobilization of *Brevibacterium flavum* with carrageenan and its application for continuous production of L-malic acid. Enzyme Microb. Technol. 2:30-36.

18. Tosa, T., I. Takata, and I. Chibata. 1982. Stabilization of fumarase activity of *Brevibacterium flavum* cells by immobilization with carrageenan and polyethyleneimine. Enzyme Eng. 7 (in press).

19. Yamamoto, K., T. Tosa, and I. Chibata. 1980. Continuous production of L-alanine using *Pseudomonas dacunhae* immobilized with carrageenan. Biotech. Bioeng. 22:2045-2054.

20. Takamatsu, S., K. Yamamoto, T. Tosa, and I. Chibata. 1981. Stabilization of L-aspartate β-decarboxylase activity of *Pseudomonas dacunhae* immobilized with carrageenan. J. Ferment. Technol. 59:489-493.

21. Sato, T., S. Takamatsu, K. Yamamoto, I. Umemura, T. Tosa, and I. Chibata. 1982. Production of L-alanine from ammonium

fumarate using two types of immobilized microbial cells. Enzyme Eng. 7 (in press).

22. Wada, M., J. Kato, and I. Chibata. 1979. A new immobilization of microbial cells. European J. Appl. Microbiol. Biotechnol. 8:241-247.

23. Wada, M. J. Kato, and I. Chibata. 1980. Continuous production of ethanol using immobilized growing yeast cells. European J. Appl. Microbiol. Biotechnol. 10:275-287.

UNCONVENTIONAL CATALYTIC PROPERTIES OF CONVENTIONAL ENZYMES: APPLICATIONS IN ORGANIC CHEMISTRY

Alexander M. Klibanov
Laboratory of Applied Biochemistry
Department of Nutrition and Food Science
Massachusetts Institute of Technology
Cambridge, Massachusetts 02139

ABSTRACT

The major objective of this paper is to stress that enzymes, in addition to their "normal" reactions (reflected in their names), often can catalyze other, sometimes quite different processes. The latter, although unimportant for the enzyme-producing organism, can be very valuable for biotechnological applications. The examples of "unnatural" catalytic activities of common enzymes that are considered, taken from the author's recent studies, include: (i) reduction of aromatic compounds catalyzed by glucose oxidase; (ii) prochiral and enantiomeric stereospecificity of galactose oxidase in the oxidation of non-sugar, three-carbon alcohols; (iii) selective hydroxylation of aromatic compounds catalyzed by peroxidase; (iv) geometrically and positionally specific oxidation of aromatic aldehydes catalyzed by xanthine oxidase.

It is pointed out that along with conventional bacterial screening, a "chemical screening", i.e., the search for new, unconventional catalytic activities for known enzymes, can be beneficial.

I. INTRODUCTION

More than 2,000 different enzymes have been described in the literature [1]. Of these, about 200 are commercially available (most of them in milligram or gram quantities), and of these two hundred, only 16 are available in industrial amounts (kilograms) [2].

It is quite clear from the aforementioned data that if one is to employ an enzyme as a catalyst in a practical process, e.g. in preparative organic synthesis, it would be highly desirable if this enzyme is one of the sixteen or at least one of the two hundred. In such a case the enzyme can simply be purchased from a commercial supplier, as opposed to its laborious and time-consuming fermentative (or, even worse, animal or plant) production with no guarantee that the sought-after enzyme will be found and will meet the requirements of the future process. The very fact that a given enzyme is commercially available usually implies that it is sufficiently active, stable, and easy to handle.

The only objection this rather obvious reasoning is likely to raise is the following: What if none of the commercially available enzymes is capable of catalyzing the reaction one is interested in? It would seem then that a search for a new enzyme becomes inevitable.

At this point it appears necessary to make a general comment concerning the substrate specificity of enzymes. There is a vast misunderstanding among researchers, especially non-enzymologists, with respect to what enzymes can and cannot do. This confusion is often caused by taking the names of enzymes literally and in the absolute sense. For example, if an enzyme is called ascorbate oxidase, this simply means that it can oxidize ascorbic acid with O_2 and that this reaction is probably a physiological function of this enzyme. The above name certainly does not mean that this enzyme cannot catalyze other reactions.

Despite the obviousness of this logic, it is usually not implemented in biotechnological strategy. Suppose one aims at finding an enzyme that can oxidize phenol(s). It is highly unlikely that one will test ascorbate oxidase to achieve this goal. The latter sounds almost ridiculous: to use ascorbate oxidase for oxidation of phenol(s). However, it turns out that actually this might not be such a bad idea, since, in fact, ascorbate oxidase does catalyze the oxidation of a number of different phenols [3].

The major thrust of this paper is to promote biotechnological applications of such "unnatural", non-physiological, catalytic properties of enzymes. Using examples from our recent studies, it will be demonstrated that these properties, although perhaps unimportant for the organism that produced the corresponding enzyme, can be very valuable in biotechnology, in particular in preparative organic syntheses.

II. GLUCOSE OXIDASE FOR THE PREPARATIVE REDUCTION OF AROMATIC COMPOUNDS

Glucose oxidase (EC 1.1.3.4) catalyzes the oxidation of β-D-glucose with molecular oxygen to produce D-gluconolactone (which is subsequently non-enzymatically hydrolyzed to D-gluconic acid) and H_2O_2 (Fig. 1)[4,5]. This enzyme is currently manufactured in commercial quantities [2] because of its extensive use in the food industry [6].

From the viewpoint of a chemist, neither of the products of the glucose oxidase-catalyzed reaction (gluconic acid and hydrogen peroxide) is a coveted target and hence it would seem that glucose oxidase has a very limited, if any, potential for the chemical indus-

GLUCOSE OXIDASE

(EC I.I.3.4)

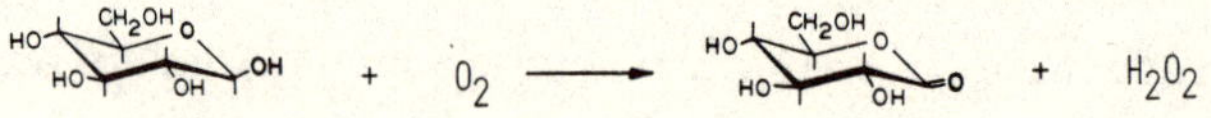

D-GLUCOSE D-GLUCONOLACTONE

MECHANISM:

$$E\cdot FAD + \text{GLUCOSE} \longrightarrow E\cdot FADH_2 + \text{GLUCONOLACTONE}$$

$$E\cdot FADH_2 + O_2 \longrightarrow E\cdot FAD + H_2O_2$$

Fig. 1. The reaction catalyzed and mechanism of glucose oxidase.

try. This feeling persists if one reads text books on enzymology [5,7], all of which assert that glucose oxidase is an extremely specific enzyme. This specificity is the reason for the wide use glucose oxidase has found in clinical and chemical analyses for selective determination of glucose in the presence of other compounds [8,9].

These statements concerning the specificity, although correct, are somewhat misleading. Glucose oxidase, while indeed very specific with respect to the electron donor (D-glucose), is not specific at all with respect to the electron acceptor (O_2). For instance, molecular oxygen in this reaction can be replaced by some artificial dyes, in particular indophenols [10].

Glucose oxidase from *Aspergillus niger* has a high catalytic activity, is fairly stable (at least in the absence of H_2O_2) and is inexpensive. The reducing substrate, D-glucose, is manufactured on a large scale from starch and is cheap. Therefore it occurred to us that if O_2 can be replaced by another electron acceptor, the reduction of which will result in a commercially important product, such a process can be of practical interest.

REDUCTION OF BENZOQUINONE TO HYDROQUINONE

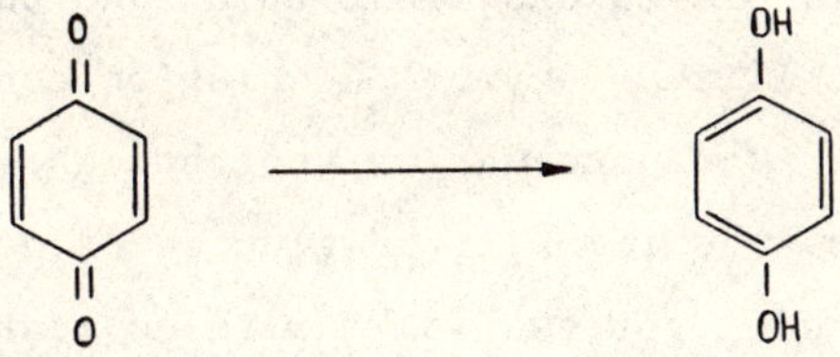

ENZYMATIC REDUCTION

BENZOQUINONE + D-GLUCOSE $\xrightarrow{\text{GLUCOSE OXIDASE}}$ HYDROQUINONE + D-GLUCONOLACTONE

- EFFICIENCY
- STOICHIOMETRY
- YIELD

Fig. 2. Glucose oxidase-catalyzed conversion of benzoquinone to hydroquinone.

We have illustrated this approach by the glucose oxidase-catalyzed production of hydroquinone (which is used in industry as a photographic developer and as an inhibitor of autoxidation and polymerization) from benzoquinone (Fig. 2)[11]. It has been found that (i) the rate of the glucose oxidase-catalyzed oxidation of D-glucose under anaerobic conditions in the presence of 10 mM benzoquinone as an electron acceptor is 3 times as high as that under air in the absence of benzoquinone (the "normal" reaction, see Fig. 1). That is, benzoquinone is a very effective replacement for O_2 in the glucose oxidase catalysis; (ii) one molecule of hydroquinone is produced per one molecule of glucose consumed, i.e., the enzyme catalyzes a stoichiometric reduction of benzoquinone by glucose; (iii) the yield of hydroquinone in the enzymatic reaction (Fig. 2) is nearly 100%.

To make the production of hydroquinone preparative, we covalently attached glucose oxidase to alumina and packed a small column with the immobilized enzyme. A solution containing 0.1 M glucose and 0.1 M benzoquinone was passed through the column under anaerobic conditions. The immobilized glucose oxidase column was operated in this fashion for two weeks with no measurable decline in its catalytic efficiency and produced more than a hundred grams of hydroquinone [11].

It should be stressed that the enzymatic reduction of benzoquinone is just one example of the aforementioned approach. A number of substituted quinones (many of which, such as vitamin K derivatives, have biomedical applications) can replace O_2 in the glucose oxidase-catalyzed reaction, as well as various aromatic nitro compounds, e.g. nitrobenzene which is reduced to nitrosobenzene (H.H. Freedman, personal communication).

III. GALACTOSE OXIDASE FOR THE STEREOSPECIFIC OXIDATION OF ALIPHATIC COMPOUNDS

Galactose oxidase (EC 1.1.3.9) is even more striking than glucose oxidase in terms of the diversity of the reactions catalyzed. This enzyme is specific with respect to neither electron acceptor (O_2) nor electron donor (D-galactose).

In its "normal" reaction, Dactilium dendroides galactose oxidase oxidizes D-galactose with molecular oxygen to D-galactohexodialdose and H_2O_2 (Fig. 3) [12]. Again, as in the case of glucose oxidase, this normal reaction is of no interest from the standpoint of the chemical industry.

Fortunately, in addition to D-galactose, galactose oxidase can also oxidize a number of non-sugar, aliphatic and aromatic alcohols

GALACTOSE OXIDASE
(EC 1.1.3.9)

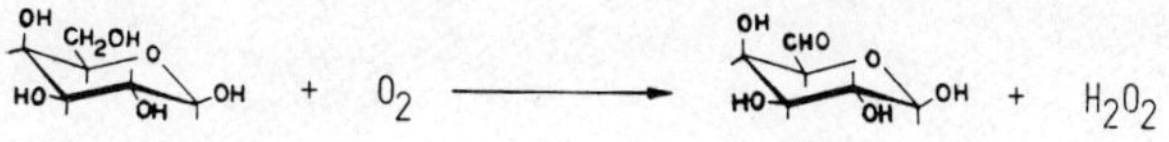

D-GALACTOSE D-GALACTO-HEXODIALDOSE

"UNNATURAL" REACTION:

ALIPHATIC OR AROMATIC ALCOHOL + O_2 → ALDEHYDE + H_2O_2

EXAMPLES OF ALCOHOLS OXIDIZED BY GALACTOSE OXIDASE:

1,3-PROPANEDIOL	2-METHYLENE-1,3-PROPANEDIOL
GLYCEROL	HYDROXYPYRUVATE
HYDROXYACETONE	SALICYL ALCOHOL
DIHYDROXYACETONE	3,4-DIMETHOXYBENZYL ALCOHOL
GLYCOLALDEHYDE	HYDROXYACETOPHENONE

Fig. 3. "Normal" and "unnatural" reactions catalyzed by galactose oxidse.

(some of which are listed in Fig. 3) to the corresponding aldehydes [12]. This reaction, although not breathtaking, might be useful because many alcohol-oxidizing chemical catalysts carry out the oxidation all the way to the acids instead of stopping at the aldehydes.

The "unnatural" reaction shown in Fig. 3 would really be attractive if galactose oxidase catalyzed the oxidation of alcohols <u>stereo-specifically</u>, since nearly all conventional chemical catalysts fail to do that and there is a great demand for optically active compounds in the specialty chemicals area. Bearing this in mind, we have examined stereospecificity of the enzyme in the oxidation of simple three-carbon alcohols [13].

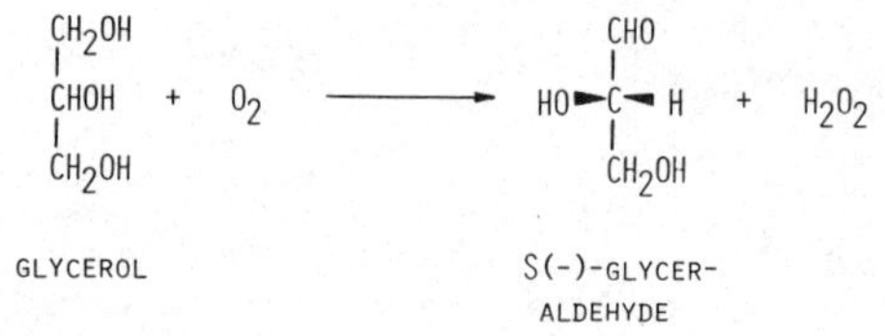

Fig. 4. Prochiral specificity of galactose oxidase. Galactose oxidase-catalyzed oxidation of glycerol to S (-) [L(-)] glyceraldehyde.

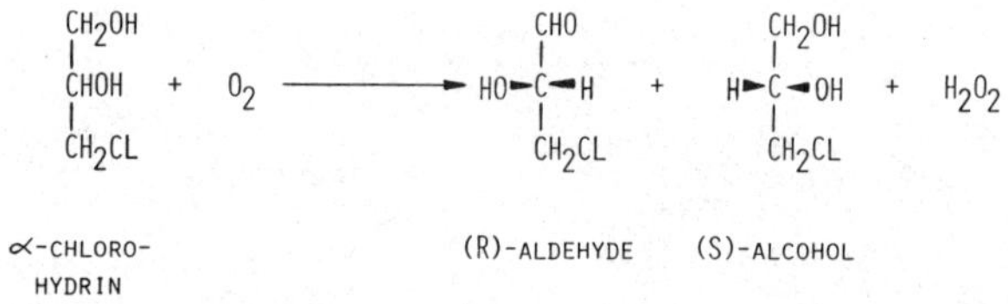

Fig. 5. Enantiomeric specificity of galactose oxidase. Galactose oxidase-catalyzed oxidation of 1-chloro-2,3-propanediol to the corresponding aldehyde. Only the R alcohol reacts with the enzyme.

The simplest alcohol substrate of galactose oxidase possessing a prochiral carbon is glycerol. For this reason, glycerol was chosen to reveal whether the enzyme will oxidize it to glyceraldehyde asymmetrically. A mixture containing 2 M glycerol, galactose oxidase and catalase (to decompose H_2O_2 formed in the reaction) was incubated at 4°C under air for 3 weeks after which time 105 mM glyceraldehyde was produced. Measurement of its optical rotation indicated that it was optically pure S(-)glyceraldehyde (Fig. 4). That is, galactose oxidase exhibits absolute prochiral specificity.

In order to elucidate the enantiomeric stereospecificity of the enzyme, the enzyme-catalyzed oxidation of 3-chloro-1,2-propanediol and 3-bromo-1,2-propanediol was studied. In contrast to glycerol, the C2 atom in these two alcohols is chiral. The enzymatic reaction conditions were the same as for glycerol. On the basis of both the experimental data obtained and conformational analysis, it was concluded that galactose oxidase reacts only with the R isomer of 3-halo-1,2-propanediol (Fig. 5).

Hence, due to the dissymmetric environment of its active center, the enzyme stereoselectively oxidizes even its "unnatural" substrates.

IV. PEROXIDASE FOR THE SELECTIVE HYDROXYLATION OF AROMATIC COMPOUNDS

Horseradish peroxidase (EC 1.11.1.7) catalyzes oxidation of various phenols and aromatic amines with H_2O_2 to form polyaromatic products and water [14]. This enzyme is widely used in biotechnology, in particular in enzyme immunoassays and in clinical analyses (where it is coupled to a variety of other oxidases which form H_2O_2 as a product, thereby affording easy colorimetric detection). Recently, we have developed a process using peroxidase for the removal of phenols, aromatic amines, and other toxic organics from industrial aqueous effluents [15,16].

In the late fifties, Mason and coworkers discovered that in addition to peroxidation of phenols and aromatic amines, horseradish peroxidase can also catalyze hydroxylation of aromatic compounds in the presence of dihydroxyfumaric acid and molecular oxygen (e.g., see Fig. 6)[17]. Unfortunately, the yields of enzymatic hydroxylation were rather low and, even more importantly, several different products were formed in each reaction. This lack of specificity led Mason's group [17,18] and others [19] to the conclusion that the peroxidase-catalyzed hydroxylation proceeds via a free radical mechanism which is responsible for multiple products.

We were not convinced by the above conclusions and re-examined the reaction in Fig. 6, initially using L-tyrosine as a model. In

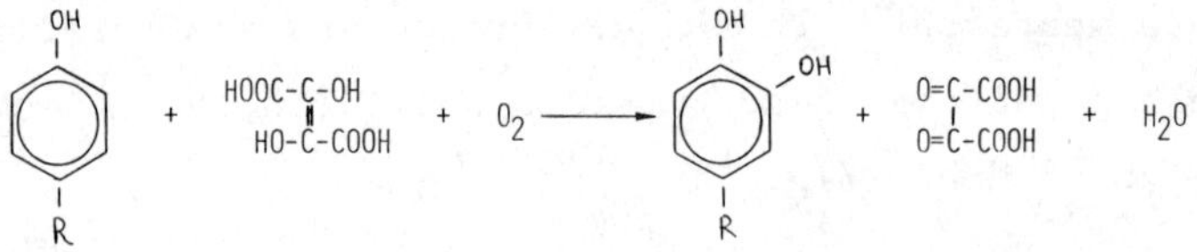

Fig. 6. Peroxidase-catalyzed hydroxylation of p-substituted phenols in the presence of dihydroxyfumaric acid and molecular oxygen.

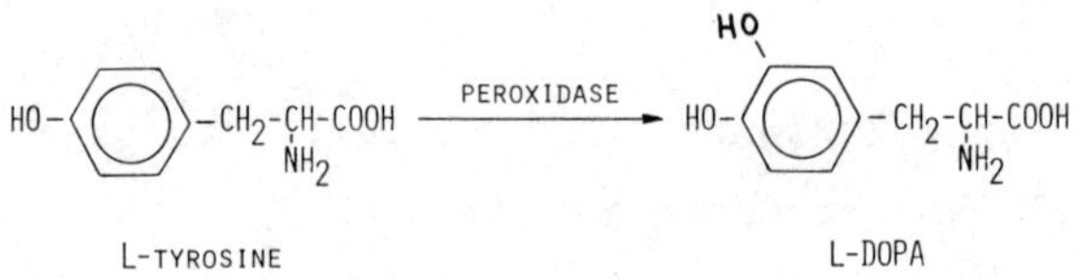

Fig. 7. Peroxidase-catalyzed conversion of L-tyrosine to L-DOPA.

agreement with the literature results, a yield not exceeding 50% was obtained and several different products were detected. However, we also found that even in the absence of peroxidase, the hydroxylation takes place and its rate is comparable with that of the enzymatic reaction.

It occurred to us that maybe this non-enzymatic hydroxylation is responsible for the lack of selectivity of the overall process. Therefore, we undertook a search for conditions to eliminate the non-enzymatic hydroxylation by O_2 and dihydroxyfumaric acid.

We discovered [20] that a simple reduction in temperature from 25^oC to 0° nearly completely stops the non-enzymatic hydroxylation, while the rate of the enzymatic reaction is affected only slightly. Peroxidase-catalyzed hydroxylation of L-tyrosine at 0^oC (Fig. 7) was facile and specific: 70% conversion was achieved after 3 hrs with L-3,4-dihydroxy-phenylalanine (L-DOPA) being the only product.

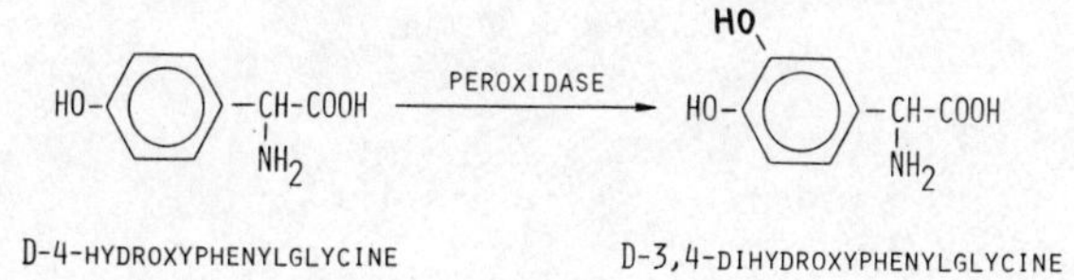

Fig. 8. Peroxidase-catalyzed conversion of D-4-hydroxyphenylglycine to D-3,4-dihydroxyphenylglycine.

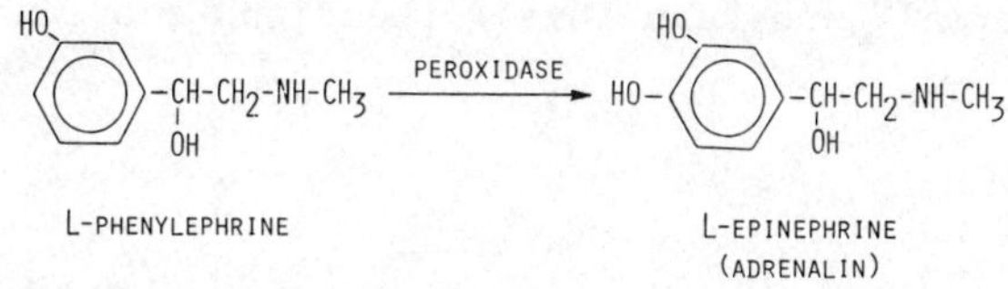

Fig. 9. Peroxidase-catalyzed conversion of L-phenylphrine to L-epinephrine.

To assess the generality of the peroxidase hydroxylation, we carried out the reaction in Fig. 6 with D(-)-4-hydroxyphenyglycine (an important intermediate in the synthesis of semisynthetic antibiotics). Again, after a 3 hr reaction at $0^{o}C$, up to 70% conversion was obtained with D(-)-3,4-dihydroxyphenylglycine being the only product (Fig. 8).

In both of the above examples (Figs. 7 and 8), peroxidase catalyzed the hydroxylation of _para_ substituted aromatic compounds at the _meta_ position. It was of obvious interest to find out the direction of enzymatic hydroxylation in the case of _meta_ substituted aromatic compounds. To address this problem, we studied peroxidase-catalyzed hydroxylation of L-phenylephrine (Fig. 9). Ninety minutes after the beginning of the reaction, about 50% of the substrate was converted to a single product, L-epinephrine (Fig. 9). That is, exclusive hydroxylation at the _para_ position took place.

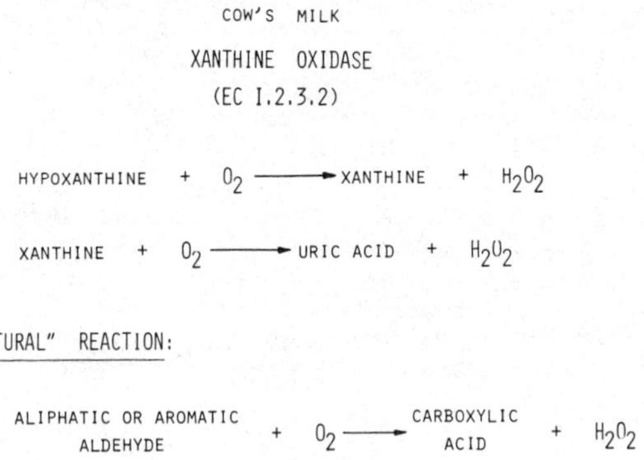

Fig. 10. "Normal" and "unnatural" reactions catalyzed by xanthine oxidase.

The ability to selectively hydroxylate aromatic compounds seems to be a general feature of peroxidase: lactoperoxidate from milk and yeast cytochrome c peroxidase also convert L-tyrosine to L-DOPA in the reaction shown in Fig. 6 [20].

Selective hydroxylation of aromatic compounds is a difficult task in preparative organic chemistry. Therefore the simple and efficient hydroxylation catalyzed by peroxidase could be quite useful to preparative transformations of various pharmaceuticals and fine chemicals.

V. XANTHINE OXIDASE FOR THE GEOMETRICALLY AND REGIO-SPECIFIC OXIDATION OF ALDEHYDES

The natural function of cow's milk xanthine oxidase (EC 1.2.3.2) is to oxidize hypoxanthine and xanthine by O_2 to form uric acid and H_2O_2 (Fig. 10)[21]. In 1938, Booth discovered that the enzyme is also capable of doing something quite different - oxidizing a number of aliphatic and aromatic alcohols to the corresponding carboxylic acids [22].

Such oxidations, of course, can be carried out by chemical catalysts as well. Hence the enzymatic process can be of interest for preparative organic conversions only if it involves some unique features missing in chemical catalysts, e.g. selectivity. We have discovered that xanthine oxidase indeed exhibits both geometric (*cis*/*trans*) and regio (positional) specificity in the oxidation of aromatic aldehydes.

a. Geometric Specificity of Xanthine Oxidase in the Oxidation of Arylacroleins [23]

Separation of *cis* and *trans* isomers of unsaturated compounds is a classical problem in organic chemistry. Functional properties (e.g. biological or pharmaceutical activities, odor, etc.) of geometric isomers are, generally speaking, different, since they are determined by the molecular geometry.

In order to take advantage of the properties of the geometric isomers of unsaturated, in particular β-arylacrylic compounds, one should be able to readily prepare both the *cis* and *trans* isomer separately. Unfortunately, nearly all conventional chemical syntheses of, for example, cinnamic compounds will yield almost exclusively *trans* isomers. A mixture of *trans* and *cis* iosmers can be produced by ultraviolet irradiation of a solution of the *trans* isomer. However, separations of such mixtures are very laborious, time-consuming, and inefficient and therefore not applicable on a large scale.

It occurred to us [23-25] that enzymes might be used for the preparative separation of *trans* and *cis* isomers of β-arylacrylic compounds. It is well established that active centers of most enzymes represent narrow clefts (openings). It is unlikely then that geometric isomers will fit into such an opening equally well

TRANS CIS

ALDEHYDE	$RATE_{TRANS}/RATE_{CIS}$
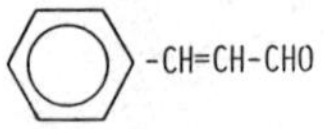 CINNAMALDEHYDE	42
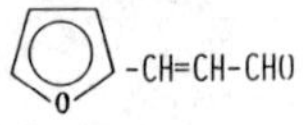 β-(2-FURYL)ACROLEIN	130

Fig. 11. Cis/Trans specificity of xanthine oxidase in the oxidation of β-arylacroleins.

and both in the correct way. Therefore one can expect different reactivities of cis and trans isomers to a given enzyme. This, in turn, can be a basis for the enzymatic separation: since one of the isomers will be enzymatically converted to a new chemical functionality, it should be easy to separate it from the unreacted, second isomer.

We verified the above approach in xanthine oxidase-catalyzed oxidation of cis and trans isomers of two β-arylacroleins, cinnamaldehyde and β-(2furyl)acrolein. In both cases, the trans isomer is oxidized by the enzyme about 2 orders of magnitude faster than its cis counterpart (Fig. 11).

This geometric specificity of xanthine oxidase can be used for preparation of the pure cis isomer from its commercially available trans counterpart, as exemplified by cinnamaldehyde: trans-cinnamaldehyde is irradiated with UV light, then the resultant mixture of

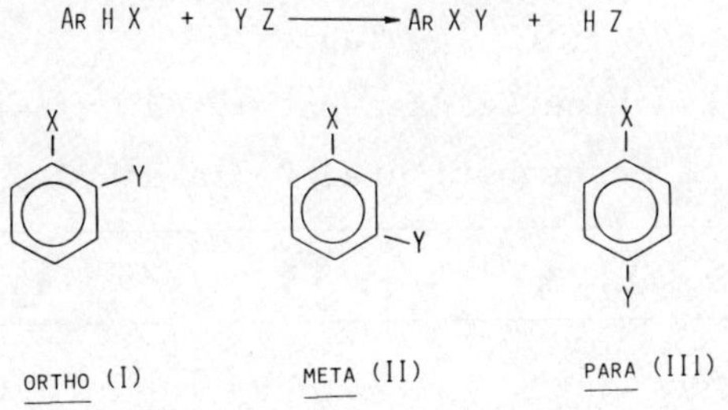

Fig. 12. The introduction of a second substituent into a mono-substitutde benzene ring resulting in the production of a mixture of ortho, meta and para isomers.

geometric isomers is treated by the enzyme and the trans-cinnamic acid produced is adsorbed on an anionexchanger, followed by extraction of the remaining cis-cinnamaldehyde with ether.

b. Positional Specificity of Xanthine Oxidase in Oxidation of Substituted Benzaldehydes [26]

The introduction of a second substituent into monosubstituted benzene rings (e.g. in the reaction ArXH + YZ → ArXY + HZ) usually results in the production of a mixture of positional isomers, ortho, meta, and para (I, II, and III, respectively) (Fig. 12). Preparative separation of such isomers, in particular ortho from meta and ortho from para (which is often of greater practical significance) is in many cases rather difficult because most of their physicochemical properties (e.g. boiling points, solubilities, etc.) are not sufficiently different.

It occurred to us that enzymes could be used for the separation of positional isomers. The rationale for this approach is as follows. Consider that an enzyme reacts with group X in I, II, and III. Simple steric considerations suggest that, at least in the

Table 1

Xanthine Oxidase-catalyzed Oxidation of Monosubstituted Benzaldehydes [26]

Benzaldehyde	$rate_{para}/rate_{ortho}$
fluoro-	0.7
chloro-	4
bromo-	11
iodo-	133
methoxy-	2
ethoxy-	14
propoxy-	34

case of a bulky Y, such an enzymatic reaction will be hindered in I, but not in II or III, due to the proximity of the second substituent (Y). Leaving electronic effects aside, this should result in different reactivities to the enzyme of I and II or III which, in turn, can be the basis for their separation: since one of the isomers will be preferentially converted by the enzyme to a new chemical functionality, it should be easy to separate it from the other isomer. That is, in fact, the enzymatic treatment transforms the problem of separation of positional isomers of a given chemical entity to the much easier problem of separation of two different chemical entities.

This rationale was confirmed in our studies on the reactions of xanthine oxidase with substituted benzaldehydes: we found that due to steric reasons the enzyme oxidizes *p*- (or *m*-) substituted benzaldehydes much faster than their o-counterparts in the case of bulky substituents.

Table 1 shows the initial rates of xanthine oxidase-catalyzed oxidation of p- and o-substituted halobenzaldehydes. One can see that while for fluorobenzaldehyde the rates of the two isomers are comparable, upon further increase in the size of the halogen atom the para/ortho specificity factor greatly increases to exceed two orders of magnitude for iodobenzaldehyde. Comparison of the data for Cl-, Br-, and I-benzaldehydes indicates that this regiospecificity of xanthine oxidase is due to diminishing reactivity of the o-isomer (as opposed to increasing reactivity of its p-counterpart). The observed positional specificity of the enzyme is not brought about by electronic effects since it takes place not only with electron-withdrawing halogen substituents but also with electron-donating alkoxy ones (Table 1).

Positional specificity of xanthine oxidase is truly remarkable in the oxidation of nitrobenzaldehydes: whereas para and meta nitrobenzaldehydes are enzymatically oxidized at the same rates (stressing once again a relative insignificance of electronic factors), the oxidation rate for ortho nitrobenzaldehyde is at least two and a half orders of magnitude lower. It is imperative for the observed regiospecificity that a bulky substituent be in close proximity to the carbonyl group. This conclusion follows from the fact that in contrast to nitrobenzaldehyde, nitrocinnamaldehyde (which has an electronic structure similar to that of the former but in which the carbonyl moiety is separated from the benzene nucleus by a vinylene group) exhibits virtually no regiospecificity in the reaction with xanthine oxidase: p- and o-isomers have approximately the same reactivity.

Simple steric considerations suggest that a diminished reactivity of ortho (in comparison with meta or para) substituted benzaldehydes should be really profound only in interactions with a bulky reagent such as the active center of an enzyme but not with relatively small substances. We have tested this by studying the oxidation of o-, m-, and p-nitrobenzaldehydes by hydrogen peroxide (which at acidic pH is known to oxidize aromatic aldehydes to the corresponding carboxylic acids). In complete agreement with our model, ortho nitrobenezaldehyde reacts with H_2O_2 at the same rate as meta nitrobenzaldehyde, with the para isomer being only about twice as reactive as the other two.

We employed the regiospecificity of xanthine oxidase described above for the separation of a mixture of positional isomers. As an example, we have chosen a mixture of m-nitrobenzaldehyde (80%) and o-nitrobenzaldehyde (20%) which is routinely produced by the direct nitration of benzaldehyde, the procedure used industrially. A solution containing the above mixture and xanthine oxidase was stirred under air for 1 hr. Then the nitrobenzaldehydes remaining were extracted and analyzed gas-chromatographically. This assay showed that more than 99% of m-nitrobenzaldehyde disappeared whereas the concentration of onitrobenzaldehyde did not change appreciably. That is, the treatment of a mixture of o- and m-NO_2-benzaldehydes with the enzyme converts it to a mixture of o-NO_2-benzaldehyde and m-NO_2-benzoic acid which can easily be separated by differential extraction.

VI. CONCLUDING REMARKS

In all of the examples discussed above, we took advantage of the ability of enzymes to catalyze "unnatural" reactions, often quite different from their "normal", physiological reactions reflected in their names. There is no doubt that this ability is not limited to the four enzymes considered herein but represents a rather general phenomenon. Recognition of this fact will greatly expand the arsenal of approaches at a biotechnologist's disposal. The existence of multiple activities of a given enzyme implies that in order to catalyze a new reaction one does not have to necessarily employ a new enzyme - sometimes a good look at one's "own backyard", at commercially available enzymes, can be extremely beneficial. Finally, the aforesaid indicates that along with conventional bacterial screening, it might be worthwhile to carry out a "chemical screening" to systematically seek novel, unconventional activities for known enzymes.

ACKNOWLEDGMENTS

The author is a recipient of the Henry L. Doherty Professorship.

REFERENCES

1. Enzyme Nomenclature. 1979. Academic Press, New York.
2. Schmid, R.D. 1979. Oxidoreductases present and potential applications in technology. Process Biochem. 14(6):27.
3. Dawson, C.R., 1966. Ascorbate oxidase: a review. In J. Peisach, P. Aisen, and W.E. Blumberg (eds.), The Biochemistry of Copper, pp 305-337. Academic Press, New York.
4. Bright, H.J. and D.J.T. Porter. 1975. Flavoprotein oxidases, chapter 7. In P.D. Boyer (ed.), The Enzymes, 3rd ed., vol. 12. Academic Press, New York.
5. Whitaker, J. R. 1972. Principles of enzymology for the food sciences, chapter 21. M. Dekker, New York.
6. Scott, D., 1975. Applications of glucose oxidase, chapter 19. In G. Reed (ed.), Enzymes in Food Processing, 2nd ed. Academic Press, New York.
7. Dixon, M. and E.C. Webb,, 1979. Enzymes, 3rd ed., pp. 243-244. Academic Press, New York.

8. Carr, P.W. and L.D. Bowers, 1980. Immobilized enzymes in analytical and clinical chemistry, chapter 5. Wiley, New York.
9. Guilbault, G.G., 1980. Immobilized enzymes as analytical rea gents. Appl. Biochem. Biotechnol. 7:85-98.
10. Keilin, D. and E.F., Hartree, 1948. Properties of glucose oxidase. Biochem. J. 42:221-229.
11. Alberti, B.N. and A.M. Klibanov, 1982 . Preparative production of hydroquinone from benzoquinone catalyzed by immobilized glucose oxidase. Enzyme Microb. Technol. 4:47-49.
12. Hamilton, G.A., J. DeJersey and P.K. Adolf, 1973. Galactose oxidase: the complexities of a simple enzyme, pp. 103124. In T.E. King, H.S. Mason, and M. Morrison (ed.), Oxidases and related redox systems, vol. 1. University Park Press, Baltimore.
13. Klibanov, A.M., B.N. Alberti, and M.A. Marletta, 1982. Stereospecific oxidation of aliphatic alcohols catalyzed by galactose oxidase. Biochim. Biophys. Acta, submitted for publication.
14. Saunders, B.C., A.G. HolmesSiedle, and B.P. Stark, 1964. Peroxidase. Butterworth, London.
15. Klibanov, A.M., B.N. Alberti, E.D. Morris, and L.M. Felshin, 1980. Enzymatic removal of toxic phenols and anilines from waste waters. J. Appl. Biochem. 2:414-421.
16. Alberti, B.N. and A.M. Klibanov, 1981. Enzymatic removal of dissolved aromatics from industrial aqueous effluents. Biotechnol. Bioeng. Symp. 11:373-379.
17. Mason, H.S., I. Onopryenko, and Buhler, D. 1957. Hydroxylation: the activation of oxygen by peroxidase. Biochim. Biophys. Acta 24:225-226.
18. Buhler, D. and H.S. Mason, 1961. Hydroxylation catalyzed by peroxidase. Arch. Biochem. Biophys. 92:424-437.
19. Daly, J.W. and D.M. Jerina, 1970. Aerobic aromatic hydroxylation catalyzed by horseradish peroxidase: absence of NIH shift. Biochim. Biophys. Acta 208:340-342.

20. Klibanov, A.M., Z. Berman, and B. N. Alberti,, 1981. Preparative hydroxylation of aromatic compounds catalyzed by peroxidase. J. Amer. Chem. Soc. 103:6263-6264.

21. Massey, V., 1973. Ironsulfur flavoprotein hydroxylases, pp. 301-360. In W. Lovenberg (ed.), Ironsulfur proteins, vol. 1. Academic Press, New York, New York.

22. Booth, V.H., 1938. The specificity of xanthine oxidase. Biochem. J. 32:494-502.

23. Klibanov, A.M. and P.P. Giannousis, 1982. Geometrically specific oxidation of β-arylacroleins catalyzed by xanthine oxidase: the preparative potential. Biotechnol. Lett. 4:57-60.

24. Klibanov, A.M. and E.H. Siegel, 1982. Geometric specificity of porcine liver carboxyl esterase and its application for the production of cis-arylacrylic esters. Enzyme Microb. Technol. 4:172-174.

25. Klibanov, A.M. and P.P. Giannousis, 1982. Geometric specificity of alcohol dehydrogenases and its potential for separation of trans and cis isomers of unsaturated aldehydes. Proc. Natl. Acad. Sci. USA 79:3462-3465.

26. Pelsy, G. and A.M. Klibanov, 1982. Remarkable positional (regio) specificity of xanthine oxidase and some dehydrogenases in the reactions with substituted benzaldehydes. Biochemistry 21:submitted for publication.

DISCUSSION

Q. J.E. TREND (3M Company): At what point does this type of approach become cost-effective vs. the traditional view? Admittedly these are just examples but have you made any study of this problem? When does it become cost-effective to get the additional enzyme purity, and at what point, at what level of purity does it become cost-effective to use this approach?

A. KLIBANOV: Well, I think that if the traditional approach is cost-effective then this approach is going to be cost-effective as well because you don't do here anything in addition to what you usually do, just take the same enzyme of the same purity, put it in the same chemical reactor (or slightly different), and just go ahead. It is a question that does not have much to do with the purity of the enzyme, it has something to do with the process, but the chances are that if the traditional application is O.K., then this application is going to be O.K. too.

Q. R. LOVRIEN: (University of Minnesota): Have you looked at the effects of various solvents on some of these enzymes in that some of the products, or some of the reactants that one might want to use often tend to be soluble only in organic solvents but enzymes might not be compatible with these solvents or perhaps with the corresponding aqueous-organic mixtures.

A. KLIBANOV: This certainly is a very important point, you are absolutely right. Many of the substrates with which we have dealt are very poorly soluble in water and I think that, in general, if in the future we are to use enzymes as catalysts in preparative organic syntheses, we will have to solve this problem. Certainly we have looked into this aspect and, in fact, we are actively involved at this time in using enzymes in biphasic systems, water + water-immiscible organic solvents, something like water-chloroform or water plus benzene. In this case what you do is put your enzyme in water, where it feels real good and it doesn't want to go to the organic solvent, and you put your substrates in the organic phase from where they can easily diffuse to water, undergo chemical conversion, and then diffuse back to the organic solvent. I feel that it is really a very promising approach and we will widely employ it in the future.

CORRELATION BETWEEN SPONTANEOUS PHENOTYPIC CHANGES IN *PSEUDOMONAS* STRAINS WITH CHANGES IN THE STRUCTURE OF CATABOLIC PLASMIDS: EXPERIENCES WITH TOL PLASMIDS

Peter A. Williams, Patricia A. Cane, David J. Jeenes, and Roger W. Pickup

Department of Biochemistry and Soil Science

University College of North Wales

Bangor, Gwynedd LL57 2UW, Wales, United Kingdom

It is part of the traditional lore of microbiology departments, handed down by word of mouth but largely unrecorded in the literature, that bacteria, isolated from the environment for their ability to perform particularly interesting metabolic functions, often show an infuriating instability. The usual version of the story is that a strain, originally obtained by selective enrichment on some esoteric compound as sole carbon source, could no longer grow on that compound after sitting on a slope for several months. In other versions, instability was a regular occurrence and part of a routine laboratory practice would be to reisolate the original strain from a selective medium. Occasionally a promising sequence of publications on a particularly interesting strain became abruptly terminated due to the failure to resuscitate it from its premature functional demise.

The discovery that many bacteria contained extrachromosomal DNA in the form of replicons called plasmids, occurred in the 1960's [23]. Furthermore it became apparent that plasmids were not essential for the host cell's viability and could also carry a variety of

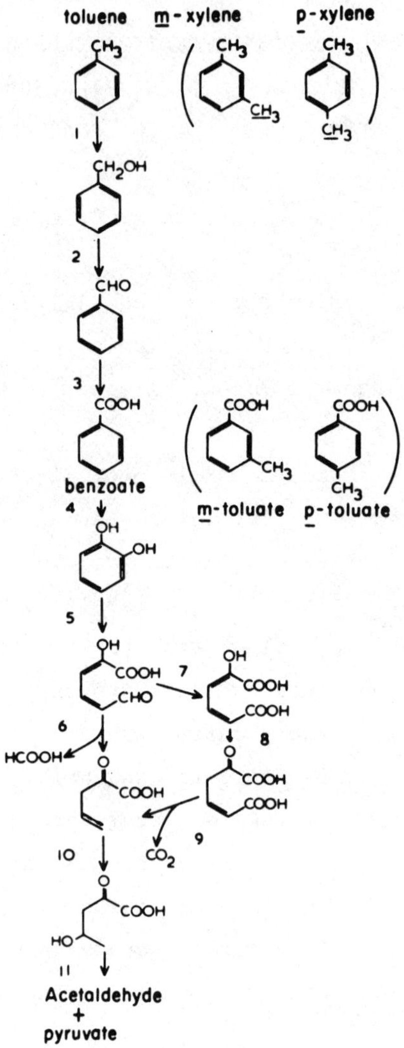
toluene
m-xylene
p-xylene
CH3
CH2OH
CHO
COOH
benzoate
m-toluate
p-toluate
OH
COOH
CHO
HCOOH
CO2
HO
1
2
3
4
5
6
7
8
9
10
11
Acetaldehyde
+
pyruvate

genes which could confer a characteristic phenotype on the host cell. Failure of a plasmid to replicate during cell division could therefore lead to variants in the population which had lost the particular function encoded on the plasmid. The frequency of occurrence of plasmid loss could be drastically increased in the laboratory by a variety of conditions such as exposure to chemicals such as acridine orange, ethidium bromide, or Mitomycin C, or by elevated growth temperatures, but often occurred spontaneously at a low, but detectable, frequency. Thus the occurrence of plasmid encoded characters gives at least one potential explanation for genetic loss of certain functions. Subsequent investigations have shown that specific DNA sequences, the insertion sequences (IS) and transposons, are important vectors in promoting a wide variety re-organization of DNA structures, and that plasmids are particularly susceptible to such modifications [13,49]. Changes in phenotype may not be produced exclusively by plasmid loss, but may also be the

←

Fig. 1. The complete catabolic pathway encoded by TOL plasmids. Strains carrying TOL plasmids can utilize any of the twelve compounds (hydrocarbons, alcohols, aldehydes, and carboxylic acids) as sole carbon sources; for simplicity, the alcohol, aldehydes, and later metabolites of the xylenes have been omitted, but their methyl groups are unmodified throughout the pathway. The enzymes involved are: 1, xylene oxidase; 2, benzyl alcohol dehydrogenase; 3, benzaldehyde dehydrogenase; 4, toluate oxidase; 5, catechol 2,3-oxygenase; 6, 2-hydroxymuconic semialdehyde (2-HMS) hydrolase; 7, 2-HMS dehydrogenase; 8, 4-oxalocrotonate tautomerase; 9, 4-oxalocrotonate decarboxylase; 10, 2-oxopent-4-enoate hydratase; 11, 4-hydroxy-2-oxovalerate aldolase.

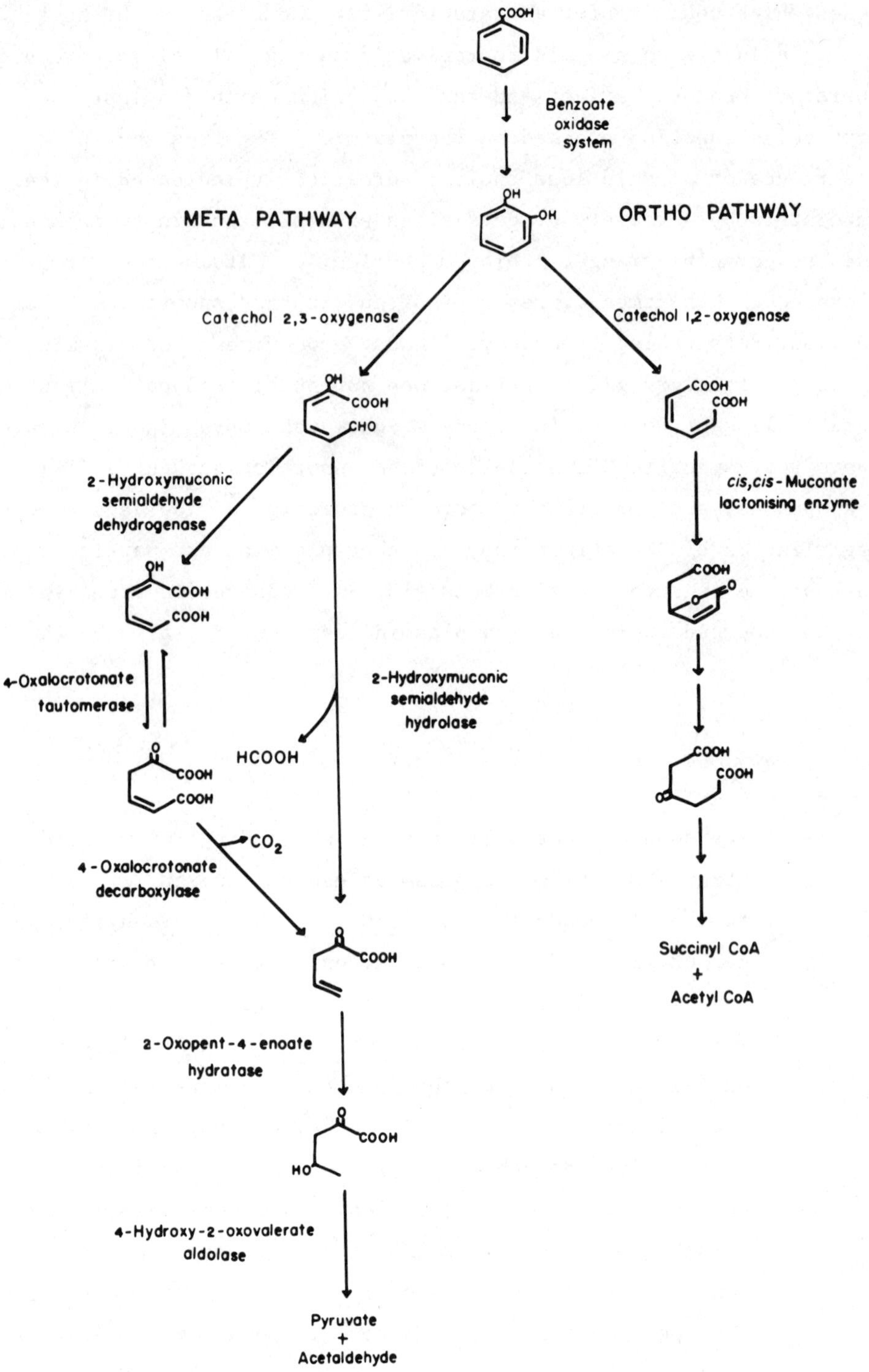

Benzoate
oxidase
system
META PATHWAY
ORTHO PATHWAY
Catechol 2,3-oxygenase
Catechol 1,2-oxygenase
2-Hydroxymuconic
semialdehyde
dehydrogenase
cis,cis-Muconate
lactonising enzyme
4-Oxalocrotonate
tautomerase
2-Hydroxymuconic
semialdehyde
hydrolase
HCOOH
CO2
4-Oxalocrotonate
decarboxylase
Succinyl CoA
+
Acetyl CoA
2-Oxopent-4-enoate
hydratase
4-Hydroxy-2-oxovalerate
aldolase
Pyruvate
+
Acetaldehyde

result of structural modifications resulting from the action of transposons or IS-like sequences.

This paper describes some of the phenotypic changes associated with plasmid-mediated catabolism which we have described in our laboratory over the past several years. All have been achieved by the selective pressure of growth of the host strains on particular carbon sources and may simply be examples of many of the anecdotal experiences of phenotypic changes which have occurred over the years in many other laboratories.

Catabolic Plasmids

The first published reports of the occurrence of genes for catabolic pathways on plasmids all came from the laboratory of I.C. Gunsalus in Urbana. He and his co-workers reported that in various strains of *Pseudomonas*, the catabolism of salicylate [10], camphor [47], octane [11], and naphthalene [22] were determined by plasmids: these were referred to as SAL, CAM, OCT, and NAH respectively. The early papers relied exclusively on genetic evidence, conjugal transfer between distinguishable strains, and irreversible loss of the ability to grow on the particular compound, either spontaneously at

←

Fig. 2. The alternative routes for the metabolism of benzoate by TOL plasmid-carrying *Pseudomonas* strains. The *meta* pathway is determined by the TOL plasmid and the *ortho* pathway is chromosomally encoded. TOL$^+$ strains have two benzoate (toluate) oxidase genes with plasmids and chromosomal locations. Due to differences in regulation of the two pathways, TOL$^+$ strains utilize only the *meta* pathway for growth on benzoate, but the *ortho* pathway in cured or mutant strains supports a faster growth rate.

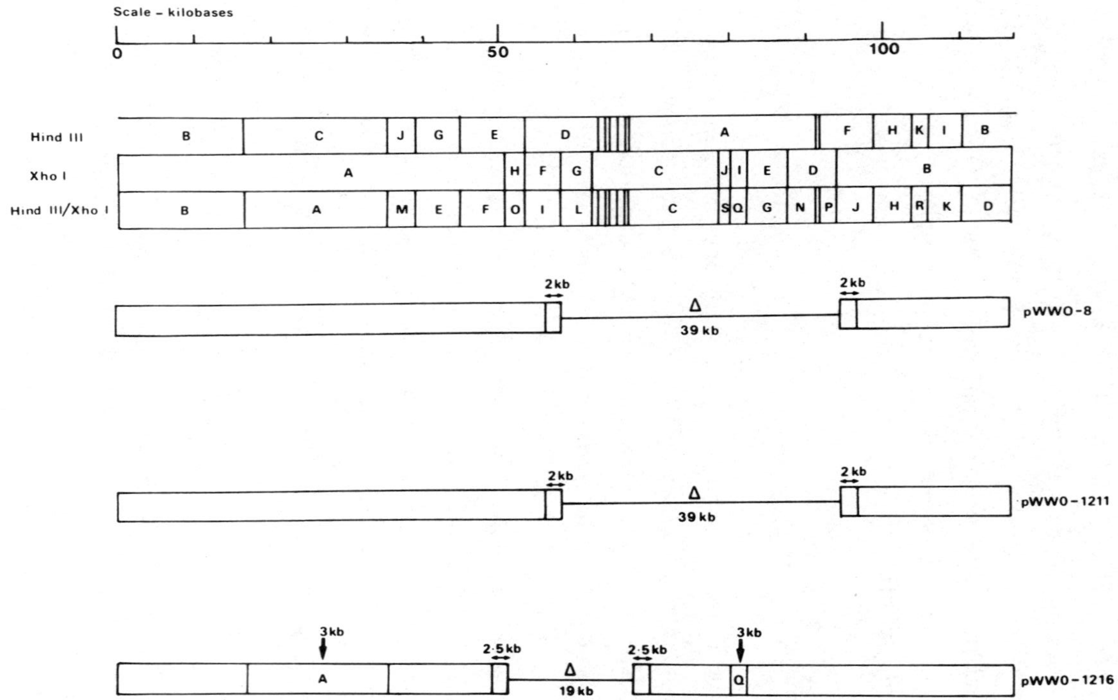

Fig. 3. A restriction map of the TOL plasmid pWWO and some of its derivatives. The map is drawn in a linear form from the XhoI site between fragments XhoI-A and XhoI-B. The derivative plasmids are: (a) pWWO-8 from the 'benzoate-cured' strain PaW8. (b) pWWO 1211 from the constructed halobenzoate-utilizing strain WR211. It is indistinguishable from pWWO-8, but the missing TOL genes are integrated into the chromosome. (c) pWWO-1216 from the constructed halobenzoate utilizer WR216. The horizontal double arrows represent the error in determining the ends of the deletions. The vertical arrows represent insertions in the specified Hind III-XhoI fragments.

low frequency or induced by increasing concentrations of Mitomycin C. Thus at this stage, proof of the existence of a catabolic plasmid relied partially on loss of the phenotype.

The TOL Plasmid

In 1974 three laboratories, including our own, independently reported genetic evidence for the existence of a plasmid in *Pseudomonas putida* mt-2 coding for utilization of three aromatic carboxylic acids, benzoate, *m*-toluate, and *p*-toluate [39,52,55]. This plasmid was called TOL and was subsequently shown to code for the complete metabolism of three hydrocarbons toluene, *m*-xylene, and *p*-xylene [57] of which benzoate, *m*-toluate, and *p*-toluate respectively are metabolites (Fig. 1). Williams and Murray [52] showed that the catabolic phenotype conferred by TOL could be selected against by growth of its host on benzoate-minimal medium for about 20 generations. Although benzoate is a metabolite on the plasmid determined pathway and is degraded by it through catechol and the *meta* pathway, virtually all fluorescent *Pseudomonas spp*. have an alternative chromosomal pathway: benzoate is first converted to catechol but this is further metabolized by the *ortho* or β-ketoadipate pathway [42] (Fig. 2). The reason for the selection of derivatives of *P. putida* mt-2 which have irreversibly lost the plasmid coded pathway and which grow on benzoate by the alternative chromosomal route was attributed by Williams and Murray [52] to two factors: (a) differences in the regulation of the two pathways [41, 56] resulting in the chromosomal pathway not being expressed when the plasmid pathway is functional and (b) a faster growth rate on benzoate of segregants using the chromosomal route. Both factors combine to make growth on benzoate a strong selection for derivatives without the plasmid pathway. Because of the identity of strains derived from benzoate selection with strains produced by exposure to Mitomycin C, the treatment became known in our laboratory as 'benzoate curing'. At first we thought that it resulted exclusively in total loss of the plasmid, renamed as pWWO; however, when it became possible to physically isolate plasmid DNA from PaW1 (P. putida mt-2 wild type) and its derivatives, we rapidly learned that benzoate curing did not always lead to total elimination of pWWO: in a survey of ten independently isolated strains, phenotypically identical, five had lost all plasmid DNA and five had smaller plasmids, all of which were identical deleted variants of pWWO [3]. Mapping of pWWO [18] and of pWWO-8, the deleted variant [19] showed that the deletion involved loss of a 39 kb region from the 117 kb plasmid (Fig. 3). The facility of occurrence of this specific deletion has been shown to be due to a direct repeat of about 1.4 kb at the termini of the deletion, one copy of which is retained in pWWO-8 [36]; the deletion presumably results from reciprocal recombination between the two identical sequences. None of the plasmid determined catabolic enzymes can be detected in PaW8, a derivative of PaW1 which contains the 78 kb deleted plasmid pWWO-8. Subsequent analysis of the physical location of the xyl genes (the structural and regulatory genes of the TOL pathway) from insertion and deletion mutants [25,26,38] and by cloning restriction fragments of into recombinant plasmids [26,29,30] has further substantiated that all the genes so far located lie within the two 1.4 kb repeats, and are thus lost when the 39 kb segment is deleted.

It appears that pWWO forms recombinant plasmids with the IncPI plasmid RP4 (RP1) very readily in vivo. These have been constructed in a number of laboratories [12,31,37] and, in fact, the elegant recombinant DNA analyses by Nakazawa's group have been carried out using pTN2, an RP4::TOL recombinant, rather than on pWWO. The early estimates of the size of the recombinants based on sucrose gradient centrifugation indicated that they contained a piece of pWWO DNA of about 60 kb. [12, 20]. However, analysis from restriction digests has proved this to be incorrect in some cases [36]. pTN2 does contain a 56 kb piece of pWWO DNA which includes the 39 kb region but extends on either side of it [29,38]. We have strong reasons to believe that this same 56 kb segment can behave like a transposon or, at least, can be involved in transposon-like recombination (see below). However, this region is not exclusively involved in recombination with RP4. There are other sites on pWWO which can be involved, since different lengths of pWWO are incorporated in different RP4::TOL plasmids [36]; they all include the 39 kb region.

pWWO in Strain Construction: The Halobenzoate Utilizers

The *xyl* genes of pWWO have a potential application in strain construction since they encode a sequence of non-specific enzymes converting hydrocarbon growth substrates through interesting intermediates to central metabolites [34,57] and thus ultimately to cell mass and CO_2. The genes could be manipulated to construct strains which convert hydrocarbons to intermediates of commercial value or alternatively which have an extended range of growth substrates for the biodegradation of otherwise recalcitrant waste products of industry. Two alternative approaches are possible. Recombinant DNA technology could be used, and Timmis and his coworkers have used this approach to clone the entire *meta* pathway catabolic sequence on to a high expression promiscuous vector [26]. On the other hand, pWWO itself is conjugative, even derepressed for transfer in some hosts [8]; it can also participate in intergeneric transfer into *E. coli* although the catabolic genes are not significantly expressed in this host [5,12,31]. Knackmuss and his co-workers have used conjugation of pWWO to construct a *Pseudomonas* strain with an increased capacity for totally degrading halosubstituted benzoic acids. Strain WR1 (*Pseudomonas* sp. B13) was isolated by selective enrichment on 3-chlorobenzoate (3CB) as sole carbon source [17]. Chlorinated aromatic substrates are degraded by a unique pathway, which we call the chlorocatechol pathway. In the initial steps, 3CB is converted to 3-chlorocatechol, the ring of which is opened by a catechol 1,2-oxygenase as in the *ortho* pathway. However the chlorocatechol pathway then diverges from the *ortho* pathway, and the next step eliminates the chlorosubstituent as inorganic chloride as a result of lactonisation [17,27,28).

WR1 cannot degrade chlorobenzoates other than 3CB because of the restricted substrate specificity of its benzoate 1,2-dioxygenase for only 3CB and benzoate [44]. However pWWO encodes an isofunctional enzyme with a much broader substrate specificity [see refs. 44,52, and Fig. 1). By conjugal transfer of pWWO into WR1, Reineke and Knackmuss were able to select derivatives capable of growing on 4-chlorobenzoate (4CB) and even 3,5-dicholorobenzoate [45] using the pWWO encoded non-specific toluate 1,2-dioxygenase for the first step and the resident chlorocatechol pathway to complete the catabolism [28,45,46]. Two derivatives of WR1 are relevant here. WR211 is a transconjugant derived by direct transfer of pWWO into WR1, selecting for ability to grow on the TOL substrate m-toluate ($Mtol^+$)[45]. It no longer grows on the hydrocarbon substrates, typified by m-xylene (Mxy^-), and grows on 3CB but not on 4CB. Selection for growth on 4CB gives a high frequency of $4CB^+$ derivatives of WR211, one of which, WR216, was maintained [45]; all such $4CB^+$ segregants of WR211 become $Mtol^-$ as a direct result of their acquisition of $4CB^+$ [32,45]. Examination of the plasmid DNA in WR211 (Fig. 3) has shown that four different events appear to have taken place [33]:

(a) Transfer of pWWO into WR1;

(b) A transposition-like integration of a 56 kb segment of pWWO DNA (identical to the 56 kb segment found in the RP4::TOL recombinant pTN2 [38] into the chromosome;

(c) Deletion of 39 kb segment from pWWO, leaving a 78 kb cryptic plasmid indistinguishable from pWWO-8 [19];

(d) An insertion of about 3 kb into the regulator gene xylR

in the 56 kb segment of pWWO in the chromosome, causing the Mxy$^-$ phenotype of WR211.

The evidence for the above relies on the elimination of the resident cryptic plasmid by either of the IncP9 resistance plasmids, R2 or pMG18, without effecting any change in the catabolic phenotype of the host. In addition, the R plasmid is able to rescue the chromosomal 56 kb segment (containing the additional 3 kb xylR insert) as a recombinant R::TOL plasmid by mating with another Pseudomonas and selecting for Mtol$^+$ transconjugants. The 39 kb region between the 1.4 kb direct repeats (plus the xylR insert) deletes readily from the R::TOL recombinants if the host strains are grown in benzoate minimal medium containing antibiotic to retain the resistance function. The net result is to leave in the R plasmid a residual 17 kb segment of pWWO DNA, made of two regions from each end of the 56 kb joined by a single copy of the 1.4 kb direct repeat. This 17 kb segment will be discussed later.

In selecting for 4CB$^+$ derivatives of WR211, it is necessary that the plasmid meta pathway is no longer expressed. The reason is that the first enzyme of the meta pathway, catechol 2,3-oxygenase, has a high affinity for 4-chlorocatechol, the metabolite of 4CB, which it converts into non-productive metabolites. WR211 is thus unable to convert sufficient 4CB into the productive chlorocatechol pathway to support growth. Only if the meta pathway is blocked, preferably at catechol 2,3-oxygenase, can 4CB serve as a growth substrate [32,46].

In selecting WR216 from WR211 by plating on 4CB minimal agar plates, the plasmid DNA undergoes an inexplicably complex structural change (Fig. 3). One feature of this change which can be explained is the acquisition of a 3 kb insertion in xylE, the structural gene for catechol 2,3-oxygenase, which not only inactivates that enzyme but exerts a polar effect on the expression of the next genes in the operon, xylF and xylG [32]. Less explicably the plasmid regains a large amount of the chromosomally integrated pWWO DNA but deletes a further section. The net result is that the plasmid in WR216 is larger than in its parent WR211 by about 20 kb, having a deletion of only 19 kb staggered relative to the deletion in the plasmid of WR211 (Fig. 3). It has also acquired a second insertion of about 3 kb in a region remote from the catabolic genes.

The particular structural changes in the pWWO derived plasmids when Reineke and Knackmuss selected WR211 and WR216 [45] are not the only ones which achieve the same phenotypic results. We have recorded a variety of different insertions and deletions in the plasmids of strains phenotypically identical to WR211 and WR216 (unpublished data). What is surprising to us is that none of the strains we have isolated by essentially the same procedures used by Reineke and Knackmuss [45] appear to have point mutations. This seems to indicate that, at least in the background of WR1, structural changes are occurring spontaneously at a frequency considerably higher than point mutations. In particular we have recorded a very large number of insertions of between 3 - 3.5 kb into different sites in the plasmid. Although we have not mapped these sequences, none of them have cutting sites for EcoRI, Hind III, and XhoI, and may well be copies of the same sequence found in the plasmids of WR 211 and WR216 (Fig. 3). Recent results have indicated that at least some of these inserts are copies of a 3.4 kb region of pWWO itself which has all the properties of an insertion sequence and is able to transpose into other regions of the plasmid giving rise to mutants (P.R. Lehrbach and P. Broda, personal communication).

pWWO DNA In A Naphthalene Catabolic Plasmid

The 17 kb of pWWO residual in the R::TOL plasmids after benzoate selection (see above) has turned up in an entirely different context but one which implies that it has the capability to act as a transposable element able to produce mutations.

PaW340 is a plasmid-free Trp^-Str^r derivative of PaW1 constructed by Dr. C.J. Duggleby as a P. putida strain useful as both a recipient and a donor for plasmids. We have used it in this context for several years. In particular we have recently used it as a recipient for a naphthalene catabolic plasmid pWW60-1, transferred out of Pseudomonas sp. NCIB 9816 which contains two plasmids. Strain NCIB 9816 has been featured prominently and somewhat controversially in the literature on microbial naphthalene catabolism. This is partly due to the inability of different laboratories to agree on exactly how the naphthalene was being degraded [2,15,51]. Thus it is a prime example of strain instability.

PaW701 is a transconjugant of PaW340 containing pWW60-1. It converts naphthalene via salicylate to catechol which is then further metabolized by the ortho pathway (Fig. 4). The metabolic pathway appears by a hybrid pathway using plasmid genes to convert the naphthalene through salicylate to catechol and chromosomal genes for metabolism of the catechol by the ortho pathway. Thus transfer of pWW60-1 into a mutant blocked in the ortho pathway no longer exhibits growth on salicylate. The strain does grow very poorly on naphthalene utilizing pyruvate formed from oxidation of the first ring [9].

PaW701 possesses a low constitutive catechol 2,3-oxygenase activity which is determined by pWW60-1 but the meta pathway is not functional. Thus PaW701 does not grow on 2-methylnaphthalene since the ortho pathway can only metabolize catechol, whereas the meta pathway is nonspecific and will oxidize catechol and methyl substituted catechols. In the presence of 2-methylnaphthalene, PaW701 accumulates metabolites in solution which indicates that partial metabolism occurs through the constitutive catechol 2,3-oxygenase

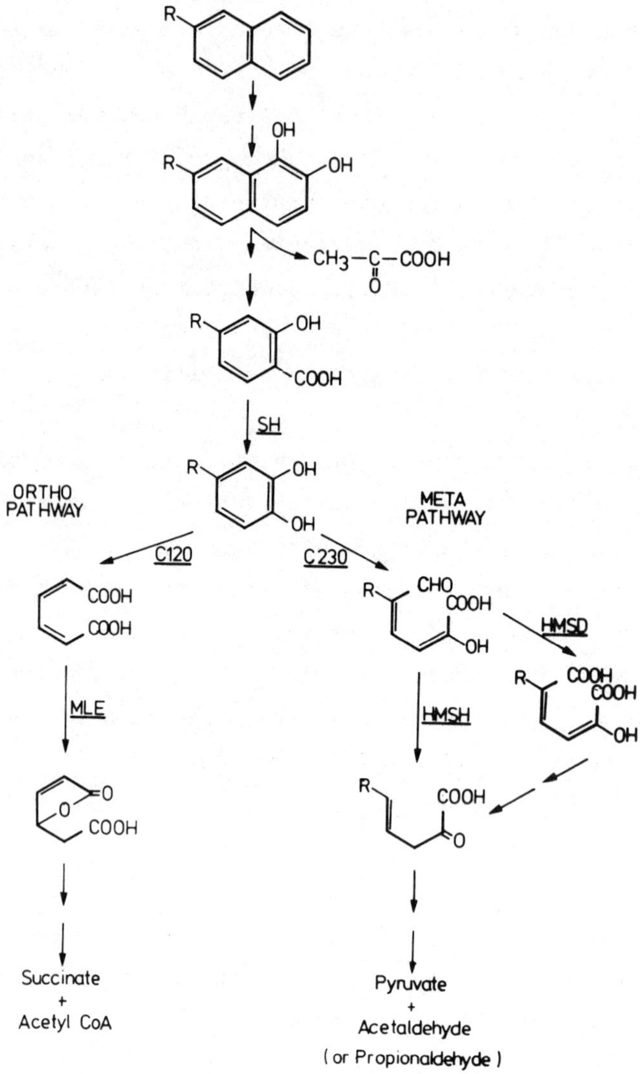
R
OH
OH
$CH_3-C-COOH$
O
R
OH
COOH
SH
R
OH
OH
ORTHO PATHWAY
META PATHWAY
C120
C230
COOH
COOH
R
CHO
COOH
OH
HMSD
R
COOH
COOH
OH
MLE
HMSH
O
O
COOH
R
COOH
O
Succinate
+
Acetyl CoA
Pyruvate
+
Acetaldehyde
(or Propionaldehyde)

until an unidentified brown product with λ_{max}=440 nm accumulates which appears to be toxic to the cells. It is possible to select mutants of PaW701 which grow on 2-methylnaphthalene. Two classes have been identified. Class A mutants are blocked at salicylate hydroxylase and accumulate salicylate from naphthalene and 4-methylsalicylate from 2-methylnaphthalene. They grow poorly on both substrates, presumably using the pyruvate from oxidation of the first ring, but the enzymic block stops formation of the toxic brown product from 2-methylnaphthalene. The plasmids in all Class A mutants contain an insertion at different sites in one of the restriction fragments, presumably the one which contains either the salicylate hydroxylase gene or a regulatory gene controlling its expression. In all the 13 class A mutants examined the insertion which inactivates this gene is 17 kb. From its Hind III and XhoI restriction sites and its ability to hybridize with pWWO it appears to be identical to the 17 kb unit derived from pWWO and described above. This implies that the same events which gave rise to the R::TOL deleted plasmid, i.e., insertion of the 56 kb transposon-like unit followed by excision of the central 39 kb, took place in PaW340 between pWWO and its chromosome before the plasmid was lost.

The second class of mutants able to grow on 2-methylnaphthalene, class B, of which there were two representatives, grew on

←

Fig. 4. The alternate pathways for naphthalene catabolism in *Pseudomonas putida* PaW710 and its mutants. PaW701 utilizes the *ortho* pathway but has uninduced levels of catechol 2,3-oxygenase (C23O). Class A mutants do not express salicylate hydroxylase (SH), accumulate salicylate and grow on the pyruvate released from oxidation of the first ring. Class B mutants used the *meta* pathway which is fully inducible.

salicylate and 4- and 5- methysalicylates (Fig 4). In both strains the meta pathway is fully inducible and is utilized for growth on all the substrates. In both mutants the complete pathway is plasmid determined since transconjugants of them are phenotypically and biochemically identical to the donors. Their plasmids have undergone a small deletion of 1.2 - 1.6 kb in a region very close to the sites of insertions in the class A mutants. pWW60-1 appears to be a plasmid which carries the full metabolic pathway from naphthalene to central metabolites via the meta pathway, but has acquired an insertion which blocks the complete expression of the meta pathway. It can only determine naphthalene metabolism in a cell which has a chromosomal pathway for assimilating catechol, as in PaW701 which has the ortho pathway. Selection for growth of 2-methylnaphthalene can result in deletion of the postulated insertion allowing the recovery of expression of the meta pathway as in class B mutants.

The proximity of the sites of insertion in class A mutants and the deletions in class B mutants is made clearer by the demonstration by Yen and Gunsalus [60], even though on a different naphthalene catabolic plasmid nah7, that the salicylate hydroxylase gene is the first gene of a transcriptional unit, the second is catechol 2,3-oxygenase and the subsequent genes are the rest of the meta pathway. The genes for salicylate hydroxylase and catechol 2-3,oxygenase on nah7 are close if not adjacent to one another. The same physical organization on pWW60-1 would explain the observed results.

Other TOL Plasmids

An interesting and, as yet, unexplained aspect of plasmids is the selective pressure which maintains a particular phenotypic character linked to an extrachromosomal replicon as opposed to becoming integrated into the bacterial chromosome. The phenotypic character could equally be drug resistant in clinical isolates of virtually any enteric bacterium or opportunistic pathogen, tumorigenicity in Agrobacterium, or equally of certain metabolic pathways in Pseudomonas. We have proposed for a number of years that many of the peripheral catabolic pathways in saprophytic soil bacteria will prove to be plasmid determined [53]. Certainly as microbial biochemists have become more aware of the ubiquitous role of plasmids, a wider range of catabolic plasmids have been described. However our original argument for expecting a widespread occurrence of such plasmids relied upon the proposition that it was advantageous to the microbial population as a whole that genes which were only required intermittently needed to be maintained in only a small number of individuals in the population if plasmid-coded. These strains would, however, be capable of disseminating their plasmids by conjugation or mobilization, should their acquisition become advantageous. In retrospect this argument seems weak because it raised selective advantage to the population above advantage to the individual cell and perhaps even more important, in the light of recent discussions about selfish genes [16, 40], it ignores selective pressures on individual plasmids.

Early in our investigations, we isolated a number of bacteria from soil using selective enrichment on m-toluate as a sole carbon source [54]. The genes for the complete TOL pathway were shown to be plasmid coded in all the isolates [20,54]. Subsequently we have isolated at least fifty independent $Mtol^+$ strains from soils of diverse geographical origins. Only a few did not contain TOL plasmids. Other laboratories have also isolated TOL plasmids [35,59]. The same situation also appears to apply to naphthalene where plasmid coding appears to be the rule [6,7,14,19,21,22] rather than the exception [61]. Other pathways have not yet been subject to the same degree of investigation at least in the published literature. It is difficult to see a convincing reason why toluene/xylene or naphthalene catabolism in Pseudomonas should be plasmid coded while the catabolism of phenol and the cresols (which shares the meta pathway in common with both the toluene and naphthalene pathways) should be chromosomally determined, at least in the P. putida strain which has been most thoroughly studied [4].

The TOL plasmids, although encoding an identical sequence of reactions, are a heterogeneous group as far as their structure is concerned. Most are very large and produce restriction enzyme digests of a formidable complexity [20,43]. The original TOL plasmid pWWO from P. putida mt-2 is by chance almost the smallest we have found.

Benzoate selection has produced an interesting class of derivatives of some of the other TOL^+ strains. Growth on benzoate of three of the original isolates (Pseudomonas sp. MT14, P. putida MT15 and P. putida MT20) strongly selects against the wild type. After only one cycle (15 to 20 generations) there is 100% loss of the TOL phenotype [54]. Two classes of segregants were found at about equal frequency:

(a) Strains with the phenotype which would be expected if the entire plasmid were lost (characterized as $Mxy^-Mtol^-Ben^+$);

(b) A second class, called the B3 mutants, which no longer grew on m- or p-toluate but did grow on the primary hydrocarbon substrates which were metabolized by the same pathway as in the wild type. They also grew on benzoate, using the chromosomal ortho pathway which accounted for their selection on benzoate. They are routinely phenotypically characterized as $Mxy^+Mtol^-Ben^+$.

Genetic investigation of one B3 mutant of P. putida MT20 indicated that its plasmid had deleted a regulator gene xylS (originally referred to as R2). The gene product was a positive regulator protein which, with the carboxylic acids as inducers, was responsible for induction of the lower part of the plasmid pathway [58]. The development of an improved procedure for isolating large catabolic plasmids [50] has allowed physical corroboration of these conclusions. The plasmid in MT20, pWW20, is 270-280 kb in size, whereas in a number of independently isolated B3 mutants, the plasmids were smaller after having undergone deletions ranging from 90 kb to 100 kb. Unlike the specific 39 kb deletion from pWW0, the termini of the deletions varied from strain to strain [43]. All have deleted a common core of fragments of about 70-80 kb, but the deletions extend from one or the other end of this core. *xylS* must lie within the deletion core and must be physically separate from the rest of the catabolic pathway genes which are on the residual plasmid.

The situation is similar in *Pseudomonas* sp. MT14 which also forms B3 mutants, except that it is complicated by the presence of another large catabolic plasmid (Pickup, Lewis, and Williams, unpublished results). The TOL plasmid in MT14, pWW14, is very similar to pWW20, and is about 270 kb in length. The B3 mutants of MT14 have a large deletion of 105 kb in pWW14. However, MT14 also contains pWW17, a 280 kb plasmid, which determines both the ability to utilize phenylacetic acid by an undetermined pathway, and codes for resistance to inorganic mercury. A surprising feature is that growth of MT14 on benzoate can result in changes in the phenotype determined by pWW17. It can undergo a large deletion of about 95 kb which results in loss of the ability to grow on phenylacetate but without loss of mercury resistance. Growth in benzoate results in a heterogeneous mixture of segregants since both plasmids can undergo a deletion as specified above or can be totally lost from the cell. There are, therefore, nine different derivatives of MT14 ranging from the wild type with both plasmids intact (Mxy^+ $Mtol^+$ Ben^+ Paa^+ Hg^r) to the plasmid-free strain (Mxy^- $Mtol^-$ Ben^+ Paa^- Hg^s). In any one benzoate selection experiment the relative abundance of the possible segregants varies considerably and it took us three such experiments to isolate one clone of each type.

We do not know why growth on benzoate selects for deletion in or loss of pWW17 from MT14 and we have not been able to show that the same events occur in the segregant of MT14 which contains only pWW17. pWW17 appears to be stably maintained during growth in either benzoate or nutrient broth and growth in benzoate does not appear to be a biochemical selection for loss of the Paa^+ phenotype. It seems likely that deletion or loss of pWW17 may be a direct result of the deletion or loss occurring in the TOL plasmid pWW14 for which benzoate is a potent counterselective agent.

A TOL plasmid which also segregates strains on benzoate is pDK1, a 180 kb plasmid studied by Kunz and Chapman [35]. _P. putida_ HS1, the host of pDK1, segregated three classes of mutants after growth on benzoate: (i) Seemingly cured strains which had lost the complete TOL phenotype but which still retained a 30kb plasmid, pDKC1; (ii) Mutants unable to grow on the methyl substituted substrates but able to grow on toluene. These had lost the _meta_ pathway enzymes, but retained the top part of the pathway; toluene was degraded by the early enzymes as far as benzoate which was then further degraded by the chromosomal _ortho_ pathway. The plasmid in one such mutant was 120 kb; (iii) The third class of segregants were unable to grow on all the hydrocarbons, but could grow on the carboxylic acids. They appear to have a deletion in the genes for the early enzymes of the plasmid pathway but retained the _meta_ pathway; one such derivative contained a 150 kb plasmid. It is the selection for this class of segregants which is inexplicable.

No restriction digest of pDK1 or its deleted variants has been published, so it is not possible to draw any conclusions about their structural relationships. The evidence strongly indicates that pDK1 is constructed in modules, consisting of separate elements coding for the *meta* pathway and for a conjugative replicon. Although it is not possible to say whether there is any homology between pDK1 and pWW0, it is of interest to note that the two halves of the pathway on pDK1 segregate separately, and on pWW0 both are regulated as different operons [56] and are physically separated [25,26,29,30].

We have been investigating a 107 kb TOL plasmid, pWW53, which shows some similarities in behavior with pDK1. Using selection on benzoate, the host strain *Pseudomonas* MT53 segregates two different classes of mutants, typified by MT53-1 (Mxy^-Mtol^+) and MT53-2 (Mxy^-Mtol^-). All the mutants similar to MT53-2 appear to be totally cured of their plasmid DNA. However strains like MT53-1, all contain an identical 75 kb plasmid, pWW53-1, indicating a loss of a specific 32 kb region of the 107 kb plasmid (Fig. 5). As with the similar derivatives of *P. putida* HS1, there is no clear reason why MT53-1 type variants should be selected, but biochemical analysis shows they have much reduced expression of the *meta* pathway enzymes (10% of wild type) and consequently grow slowly on *m*-toluate. Continuous culture of MT53 on limiting benzoate has shown that MT53-1 type variants overgrow the wild type cells in the early stages of growth, but that they are later lost as totally cured strains take over the population. This implies that the deletion leading to the Mxy^-Mtol^+ phenotype is a more frequent event than loss of the plasmid, and that on benzoate medium they have a growth rate between the slower wild type and the faster cured strains.

Because pWW53 is nonconjugative, it is therefore easy to set up experiments to form RP4::pWW53 cointegrate plasmids by mating RP4 into MT53, and then mating out from the MT53 (RP4, pWW53). A significant proportion of kanamycin resistant transconjugants are $Mtol^+$. The amount of pWW53 DNA incorporated in the recombinant plasmids we have examined varies from 85 kb to 30 kb in pWW53-4. The 30 kb of pWW53 present in pWW53-4 is common to all the recombinants (Fig. 5). It is of particular interest that pWW53-4 shares very little DNA in

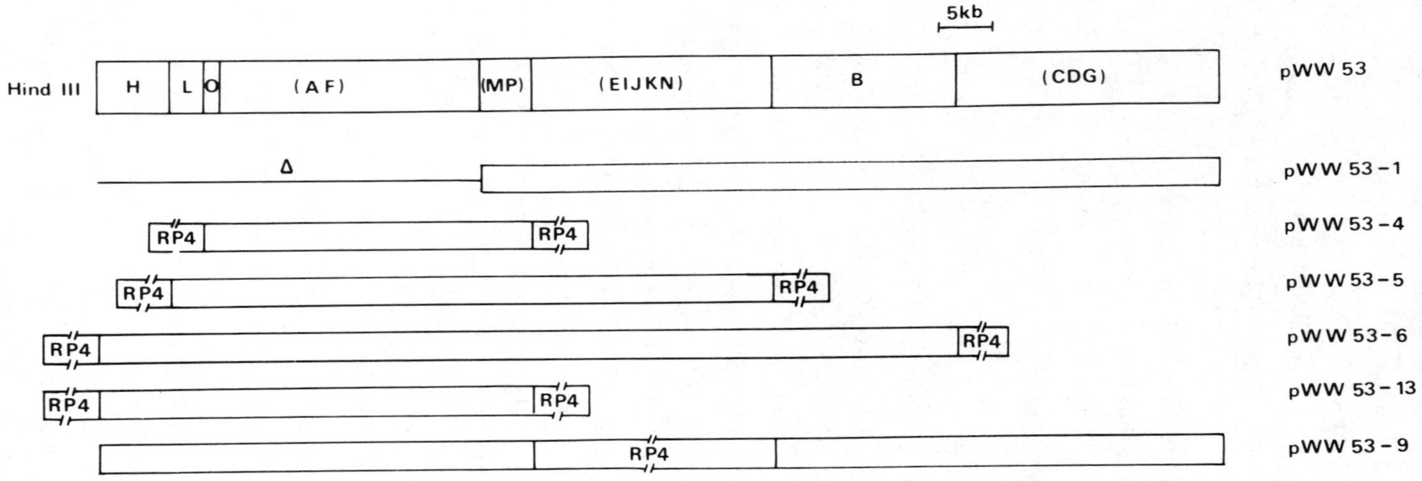

Fig. 5. Partial digest map of Hind III fragments of the TOL plasmid pWW53. pWW53 confers the ability to grow on all the TOL specific substrates, as do all the RP4::pWW53 cointegrate plasmids (pWW53-4, pWW53-5, pWW53-13, pWW53-9) which consist of the specified region of pWW53 integrated into RP4. pWW53-1 is a deleted plasmid derived from pWW53 during benzoate selection. It confers the ability to grow only on the carboxylic acid substrates (m-toluate, p-toluate, and benzoate) and the meta pathway enzymes are expressed to a lower extent than in pWW53 cells.

common with pWW53-1, the deleted plasmid conferring the $Mxy^{-}Mtol^{+}$ phenotype. This amounts to no more than about 10 kb and no less than about 5 kb, consisting of one BamH1 fragment and two Hind III fragments, thus delineating very precisely the location of the *meta* pathway genes for the dissimilation of *m*-toluate, common to both plasmids. We have obtained a partial map of pWW53 from the digests of the various derivative plasmids and are in the process of refining the map by conventional mapping techniques. Preliminary results on the regulation of the pWW53 determined pathway have given no indications that its regulation is different from the model proposed for the isofunctional plasmids pWWO [56] and pWW20 [58]. Further investigations should indicate whether similarities exist in the structure and organization of the catabolic genes on pWWO and pWW53 and whether they share an evolutionary origin.

The Implications of Structural Instability to Plasmid Evolution

The results of Yen and Gunsalus [60] show that the naphthalene catabolic genes on *nah*7 are organized into two distinct operons each of which can be considered a metabolic module. The first operon encodes the conversion of naphthalene to salicylate, which is further metabolized by the *meta* pathway, determined by the second operon. The two operons are also physically separated on the plasmid. This structure mirrors almost exactly the *xyl* genes on pWWO, which are in two physically separate operons, the first involving the conversion of the hydrocarbons to the carboxylates (*m*-xylene to *m*-toluate) and the second the further metabolism of the carboxylates *via* the *meta* pathway [25,26,29,30]. A possible explanation of these results and the results of Kunz and Chapman [35] is that catabolic plasmids evolve by acquiring pre-evolved metabolic modules from locations on the chromosome or on other plasmids. A limited number of such translocatable gene clusters might give rise to a greater number of pathways. A corollary of their formation by the acquisition of DNA sequences should be that the plasmids formed in this way should be readily able to undergo further structural changes. Where those changes are associated with catabolic genes, the host strains would be expected to exhibit instability of catabolic phenotype when subjected to selection pressures which favor those changes.

One area of microbial metabolism which has not yet been explained was first described by Audus [1]. His work related to the metabolism of the chlorinated phenoxyacetate herbicides, but almost certainly his description would adequately fit the metabolism of a wide variety of other molecules which are not easily biodegraded. The most interesting feature of the system is that when a soil sample is selectively enriched in the laboratory by exposure to a low concentration of the herbicide as sole carbon source, there is a remarkably long delay before any biodegradation can be detected. For MCPA (2-methyl-4-chlorophenoxyacetate) in particular, there is often a period of 100 days with no detectable breakdown. Once degradation has started, however, the population becomes adapted and is able to degrade higher concentrations at a faster rate. Only during these later periods can strains capable of degrading the compound be isolated. This laboratory system is very similar to what occurs when herbicides are applied to soil in agricultural practice. The length of the lag phase indicates that no cells capable of the complete catabolism are present at the start of the enrichment, since one would expect a more rapid selection of a competent population. An additional feature of the system mentioned by Audus [1] is that degraders, once isolated show a remarkable instability in their capacity to degrade MCPA when removed from selective media and grown through cycles in nutrient broth. It seems possible that the lag phase could be the result of the assembly of genetic information originally present in different cells in the original population into one strain. The genetic instability of the resultant 'recombinant' pathway would be a direct reflection of its formation in this way. So far only one phenoxyacetic acid herbicide degrading strain has been subjected to genetic analysis. Alcaligenes paradoxus is capable of degrading 2,4D (2,4-dichlorophenoxyacetate) and has been shown to contain a plasmid which encodes for at least part of the pathway [24].

Although the data represent a moderately consistent scenario for the acquisition of the more esoteric catabolic activities by soil microbes, we believe that the situation may be even more complex. We have worked with a strain NCIB9061, originally isolated by Gaunt [27] using selective enrichment on MCPA, which is probably a Flavobacterium sp. It was the organism in which the catabolic pathway for MCPA utilization was first elucidated [27]. If this strain is subcultured through nonselective media, it segregates clones which have lost the ability to utilize MCPA (Jeenes and Williams, unpublished results). These clones have all the characteristics of derivatives which have lost a catabolic plasmid and are nonrevertible by all the usual microbial procedures for testing reversion. When these studies were undertaken we could find no procedure which would reproducibly isolate plasmid DNA from NC1B9061, so although occasional plasmid bands were detected, we could not be certain whether there were consistent differences in plasmid content between the $MCPA^+$ and the $MCPA^-$ strains. However, we did find that some of the $MCPA^-$ strains would eventually revert to $MCPA^+$ if inoculated into liquid MCPA- minimal medium and left for a period of weeks. This time period corresponded to the original lag period which occurred during the isolation of NC1B9061 from soil [27]. It may be that this switching-on and switching-off shares some genetic features in common with the variation of flagellar protein produced in Salmonella [48]. Further investigation of this, and other examples of the genetic instability of catabolic phenotypes in saprophytic bacteria should prove to be a fertile area of investigation for some years.

REFERENCES

1. Audus, L.J. 1960. In Herbicides and the Soil (Woodford, E.K. and Sagar, G.R. eds.), Blackwell Scientific Publications, Oxford, pp. 1-19.

2. Barnsley, E.A. 1976., Role and regulation of the ortho and meta pathways of catechol metabolism in Pseudomonads metabolising naphthalene and salicylate. J. Bacteriol. 125:404-408.

3. Bayley, S.A., C.J. Duggleby, M.J. Worsey, P.A. Williams, K.G. Hardy, and P. Broda. 1977. Two modes of loss of the Tol function from *Pseudomonas putida* mt-2. Molec. Gen. Genet. 154:203-204.

4. Bayly, R.C. and G.J. Wigmore, 1973. Metabolism of phenol and cresols by mutants of *Pseudomonas putida* J. Bacteriol. 113: 1112-1120.

5. Benson, S. and J. Shapiro. 1978. TOL is a broad-host range plasmid. J. Bacteriol. 135:278-280.

6. Boronin, A.M., V.V. Kochetkov, and G.K. Skryabin. 1980. Incompatibility groups of naphthalene degradative plasmids in *Pseudomonas*. FEMS Micribiol. lett. 7:249-252.

7. Boronin, A.M., V.V. Kochetov, I.I. Starovoitov, and G.K. Skryabin. 1977. Plasmids pBS2 and pBS3, controlling the oxidation of naphthalene in bacteria of the genus *Pseudomonas*. Doklady Nauk. S.S.S.R. 237:1205-1208.

8. Bradley, D.A. and P.A. Williams. 1982. TOL determines flexible pili and is naturally depressed for transfer. J. Gen. Microbiol. (submitted for publication).

9. Cane, P.A. and P.A. Williams. 1982. The plasmid coded metabolism of naphthalene and 2-methylnaphthalene in *Pseudomonas* strains: phenotypic changes correlated with structural modification of the plasmid pWW60-1. J. Gen. Microbiol, (in press).

10. Chakrabarty, A.M. 1972. Genetic basis of the biodegradation of salicylate in *Pseudomonas*. J. Bacteriol. 112:815-828.

11. Chakrabarty, A.M., G. Chou, and I.C. Gunsalus. 1973. Genetic regulation of octane dissimilation plasmid in Pseudomonas. Proc. Natl. Acad. Sci. U.S.A. 70:1137-1140.

12. Chakrabarty, A.M., D.A. Friello, and L.H. Bopp. 1978. Transposition of plasmid DNA segments specifying hydrocarbon degradation and their expression in various microorganisns. Proc. Natl. Acad. Sci. U.S.A. 75:3109-3112.

13. Cohen, S.N. 1976. Transposable genetic elements and plasmid evolution. Nature (London) 263:731-738.

14. Connors, M.A. and E.A. Barnsley. 1982. Naphthalene plasmids in Pseudomonads. J. Bacteriol. 149:1096-1101.

15. Davies, J.I. and W.C. Evans. 1964. Oxidative metabolism of naphthalene by soil Pseudomonads. Biochem. J. 91:251-261.

16. Doolittle, W.F. and C. Sapienza. 1980. Selfish genes, the phenotype paradigm and gene evolution. Nature (London) 284:601-603.

17. Dorn, E., M. Hellwig, W. Reineke, and H-J. Knackmuss. 1974. Isolation and characterization of a 3-chlorobenzoate-grown pseudomonad. Arch. Microbiol. 99:61-70.

18. Downing, R.G. and P. Broda. 1979. A cleavage map of the TOL plasmid of Pseudomonas putida mt-2. Molec. Gen. Genet. 168:189-191.

19. Downing, R.G., C.J. Duggleby, R. Villems, and P. Broda. 1979. An endonuclease cleavage map of the plasmid pWWO-8, a derivative of the TOL plasmid of Pseudomonas putida mt-2. Molec. Gen Genet.168:97-99.

20. Duggleby, C.J., S.A. Bayley, M.J. Worsey, P.A. Williams, and P. Broda. 1977. Molecular sizes and relationships of TOL plasmids in Pseudomonas. J. Bacteriol. 130:1274-1280.

21. Dunn, N.W., H.M. Dunn, and R.A. Austen. 1980. Evidence for the existence of two catabolic plasmids coding for the degradation of naphthalene. J. Gen. Microbiol. 117:529-533.

22. Dunn, N.W. and I.C. Gunsalus. 1973. Transmissible plasmid

coding early enzymes of naphthalene oxidation in Pseudomonas putida. J. Bacteriol. 114:974-979.

23. Falkow, S. 1972. Infectious multiple drug resistance, Pion Limited, London. 300p.

24. Fisher, P.A., J. Appleton, and J.M. Pemberton. 1978. Isolation and characterisation of the pesticide degrading plasmid pJP1 from Alcaligenes paradoxus. J. Bacteriol. 135:798-804.

25. Franklin, F.C.H., M. Bagdasarian, and K.N. Timmis. 1981. Manipulation of degradative genes of soil bacteria. In Microbial Degradation of Xenobiotics and Recalcitrant Compounds (Th. Leisinger, A.M. Cook, R. Hutter and J. Nuesch, eds.), Academic Press, London, pp. 109-130.

26. Franklin, F.C.H., M. Bagdasarian, M.M. Bagdasarian, and K.N. Timmis. 1981. Molecular and functional analysis of the TOL plasmid pWWO from Pseudomonas putida and cloning of genes for the entire regulated aromatic ring meta pathway Proc. Natl. Acad. Sci. U.S.A. 78:7458-7462.

27. Gaunt, J.K. and W.C. Evans. 1971. Metabolism of 4-chloro-2-methylphenoxyacetate by a soil pseudomonad. Biochem. J. 122:519-526.

28. Hartmann, J., W. Reineke, and H-J. Knackmuss. 1979. Metabolism of 3-chloro, 4-chloro-, and 3,5-dichloro-benzoate by a pseudomonad. App. Environ. Microbiol. 37:421-428.

29. Inouye, S., A. Nakazawa, and T. Nakazawa. 1981. Molecular cloning of TOL genes xylB and xylE in Escherichia coli. J. Bacteriol. 145:1137-1143.

30. Inouye, S., A. Nakazawa, and T. Nakazawa. 1981. Molecular cloning of gene xylS of the TOL plasmid: evidence for the positive regulation of the xylDEGF operon by xylS. J. Bacteriol. 148:413-418.

31. Jacoby, G.A., J.E. Rogers, A.E. Jacob, and R.W. Hedges. 1978. Transposition of Pseudomonas toluene-degrading genes and expression in Escherichia coli. Nature (London) 274:179-180.

32. Jeenes, D.J., W. Reineke, H-J. Reineke, and P. A. Williams. 1982. The TOL plasmid pWWO in constructed halobenzoate degrading Pseudomonas strains: enzyme regulation and DNA structure. J. Bacteriol. 150:180-187.

33. Jeenes, D.J. and Williams, P.A. 1982. Excision and integration of the degradative pathway genes from the TOL plasmid pWWO. J. Bacteriol. 150:188-194.

34. Kunz, D.A. and P.J. Chapman. 1981a. Catabolism of pseudocumene and 3-ethyltoluene by Pseudomonas putida (arvilla) mt-2: evidence for new functions of the TOL (pWWO) plasmid. J. Bacteriol. 146:179-191.

35. Kunz, D.A. and P.J. Chapman. 1981b. Isolation and characterisation of spontaneously occurring TOL plasmid mutants of Pseudomonas putida HS1. J. Bacteriol. 146:952-964.

36. Meulien, P., R.G. Downing, and P. Broda. 1981. Excision of the 40 kb segment of the TOL plasmid from Pseudomonas putida mt-2 involves direct repeats. Molec. Gen. Genet. 184:97-101.

37. Nakazawa, T., E. Hayashi, T. Yokota, Y. Ebina, and A. Nakazawa. 1978. Isolation of TOL and RP4 recombinant by integrative suppression. J. Bacteriol. 134:270-277.

38. Nakazawa, T., S. Inouye, and A. Nakazawa. 1980. Physical and functional mapping of RP4-TOL plasmid recombinants: analysis of insertion and deletion mutants. J. Bacteriol. 144:222-231.

39. Nakazawa, T., and T. Yokota. 1973. Conjugal transfer of benzoate pathway genes in Pseudomonas arvilla mt-2. Jap. J. Bacteriol. 28:46.

40. Orgel, L.E. and F.H.C. Crick. 1980. Selfish DNA: the ultimate parasite. Nature (London) 284:604-607.

41. Ornston, L.N. 1971. Regulation of catabolic pathways in Pseudomonas. Bacteriol. Rev. 35:87-116.

42. Ornston, L.N. and R.Y. Stanier, 1966. The conversion of catechol and protocatechuate to β-ketoadipate by Pseudomonas putida I. Biochemistry. J. Biol. Chem. 241:3776-3786.

43. Pickup, R.W., and P.A. Williams. 1982. Spontaneous deletions in the TOL plasmid pWW20 which give rise to the B3 regulatory mutants of Pseudomonas putida MT20. J. Gen. Microbiol, (in press).

44. Reineke, W. and H-J. Knackmuss. 1978. Chemical structure and biodegradability of halogenated aromatic compounds. Substituent effects on 1,2-dioxygenation. Biochim. Biophys. Acta. 542:412-423.

45. Reineke, W. and H-J. Knackmuss. 1979. Construction of haloaromatics degrading bacteria. Nature (London) 277:385-386.

46. Reineke, W., D.J. Jeenes, P.A. Williams, and H-J. Knackmuss. 1982. The TOL plasmid pWWO in constructed halobenzoate degrading Pseudomonas strains: prevention of meta pathway. J. Bacteriol. 150:195-201.

47. Rheinwald, J.G., A.M. Chakrabarty, and I.C. Gunsalus. 1973. A transmissible plasmid controlling camphor oxidation in Pseudomonas putida. Proc. Natl. Acad. Sci. U.S.A. 70:885-889.

48. Silverman, M., J. Zieg, G. Mandel, and M. Simon. 1981. Analysis of the functional components of the phase variation system. Cold Spring Harbor Symp. Quant. Biol. Vol. XV, Part 1. pp. 17-26.

49. Starlinger, P. 1980. IS elements and transposons. Plasmid. 3:241-259.

50. Wheatcroft, R.G. and P.A. Williams. 1981. Rapid methods for the study of both stable and unstable plasmids in Pseudomonas. J. Gen. Microbiol. 124:433-437.

51. Williams, P.A., F.A. Catterall, and K. Murray. 1975. Metabolism of naphthalene, 2-methylnaphthalene, salicylate and benzoate by Pseudomonas P_G: regulation of tangential pathways. J. Bacteriol. 124:679-685.

52. Williams, P.A. and K. Murray. 1974. Metabolism of benzoate and the methylbenzoates by Pseudomonas putida (arvilla) mt-2: evidence for the existence of a TOL plasmid. J. Bacteriol. 120:416-423.

53. Williams, P.A. and M.J. Worsey., 1976a. Plasmids and catabolism. Biochem. Soc. Trans. 4:466-468.

54. Williams, P.A. and M.J. Worsey. 1976b. Ubiquity of plasmids in coding for toluene and xylene metabolism in soil bacteria: evidence for the existence of new TOL plasmids. J. Bacteriol. 125:818-828.

55. Wong, C.L. and N.W. Dunn. 1974. Transmissible plasmid coding for the degradation of benzoate and m-toluate in Pseudomonas arvilla mt-2. Genet. Res. 23:227-232.

56. Worsey, M.J., F.C.H. Franklin, and P.A. Williams. 1978. Regulation of the degradative pathway enzymes coded for by the TOL plasmid(pWWO) from Pseudomonas putida mt-2. J. Bacteriol. 134: 757-764.

57. Worsey, M.J. and P.A. Williams. 1975. Metabolism of toluene and xylenes by Pseudomonas putida (arvilla) mt-2: evidence for a new function of the TOL plasmid. J. Bacteriol. 124:7-13.

58. Worsey, M.J. and P.A. Williams. 1977. Caracterisation of a spontaneously occurring mutant of the TOL20 plasmid in Pseudomonas putida MT20: possible regulatory implications. J. Bacteriol. 130:1149-1158.

59. Yano, K. and T. Nishi. 1980. pKJ1, a naturally occurring conjugative plasmid coding for toluene degradation and resistance to streptomycin and sulphonamides. J. Bacteriol. 143:552-560.

60. Yen, K-M., and I.C. Gunsalus. 1982. Plasmid gene organisation: naphthalene/salicylate oxidation. Proc. Natl. Acad. Sci. U.S.A. 79:874-878.

61. Zuniga, M.C., D.R. Durham, and R.A. Welch. 1981. Plasmid- and chromosome-mediated dissimilation of naphthalene and salicylate in Pseudomonas putida PMD-1. J. Bacteriol. 147:836-843.

DISCUSSION

Q. G. WALKER (MIT): Was it the presence of benzoate in some active sense that was stimulating the deletion and transposition-like events or was it simply the absence of a substrate that required the meta-pathway?

A. WILLIAMS: I believe the reason for the selection of the strains is purely biochemical, that you are selecting something that is using the other pathway and which is growing faster, thus outgrowing the wild type. The reason the 39 kilobases are deleted from pWWO is because there is a 1.4 kilobase direct repeat at either end of that 39 kilobase section. So I believe that it is a straight recombinational loss.

Q. WALKER: I was wondering whether you had some function that was induced by benzoate. You had this other instance later on where growth on benzoate was causing some other deletion that did not seem to make metabolic sense at that point.

A. WILLIAMS: What I think is happening with the two plasmid strain MT 14 is that there may be some mechanism which is acting on, or is part of, the Tol plasmid which is causing its deletion which may be acting in trans, if you like, on the other plasmid causing its deletion. But this is total speculation.

Q. WALKER: Doesn't mercury have some effect on the transposition of some of the mercury transposons? I am looking for some sort of a parellel in that sort of sense.

A. WILLIAMS: I don't know. In the Ti plasmid, transfer is induced by the opines, but we found nothing similar. It would be nice to think about a specific inducing role by chemicals in transposition, but there is no evidence.

Q. P. ROGERS (Minnesota): I just want to get one thing a little clearer on the question that Dr. Walker asked. If you grew these cells on succinate instead of benzoate, would you still get losses of pieces of plasmid?

A. WILLIAMS: No.

Q. ROGERS: So it's a benzoate-directed loss?

A. WILLIAMS: It is a benzoate-directed loss.

Q. ROGERS: And it's specific to benzoate? Nothing else will work?

A. WILLIAMS: Nothing that we have found. But I don't think that benzoate is doing anything genetically; I think that benzoate is simply selecting the strains that spontaneously do this at low frequency. I think that you can explain it almost all in those terms.

Q. S. HAYES (Univ. of Sasatchewan): Do these two plasmids in MT14 recombine with each other; do you get dimerization and essentially recombination and deletion of genetic material?

A. WILLIAMS: We get our sizes from restriction analyses. Adding up the fragments rather than looking at the plasmids (because they are just right at the top of the plasmid gel) is explicable in terms of two plasmids and we have never picked up a recombinant plasmid.

Q. J. WESTPHELING (Harvard): This may be a different aspect of the same question that was asked before, but do you think that all of the plasmid rearrangements are occurring by the same mechanism? And do you think that plasmid rearrangement in general is increased by catabolic selection?

A. WILLIAMS: No, I don't think that they are the same mechanism. I think that the 39 kb loss out of the pWWO is straight recombination because there are 1.4 kb direct repeats at the termination. I think that the 56 kb region is a transposon although we don't have a rec$^-$ Pseudomonas to do the proper experiments. So there are at least two different mechanisms involved there.

As regards your second question, no, I think that the overall frequency of rearrangement is higher than the overall frequency of point mutation; hence we pick up these rather than point mutants. All we are doing is selecting by biochemical means for strains carrying these changes. Or else occasionally we are picking up rare unselected events that have happened such as the three kilobase insertion in xylR in the chlorobenzenate strain WR211 for which I think there is no apparent chemical reasons; we have repeated the formation of WR211 a number of times and strains with the Mxy^{-} phenotype don't always appear.

Q. D. KUNZ (E.I. Dupont de Nemours Co.): On the MT-20, Peter, do you think that is just a deletion of the regulatory element, i.e., that that is all that has happened?

A. WILLIAMS: There are two different types of deletions found in B3 mutants of MT20 depending whether the core deletion extends to the right end or to the left end. All of the catabolic genes must remain in the residual plasmid because the strains grown on the hydrocarbon by the whole catabolic pathway. It may not be just a inside regulatory element; I think that there may be more than one element involved because we got the two different classes that are not only structurally different, but are also biochemically different. One expresses higher levels of enzymes than the other.

Q. KUNG: In other words, have you looked for a possible insertion, such as a 3 kb or a 17 kb insertion?

A. WILLIAMS: No, the 17 kb insertion is only going to occur in strains that had the original Tol plasmid pWWO and MT20 is a totally different isolate. There are no apparent insertions, just deletions.

CLOSING REMARKS

Alexander Hollaender
Council for Research Planning in Biological Sciences
Washington, DC 20036-2077

When Palmer Rogers spent a few months in Washington at the Department of Energy during 1980, we had many opportunities to discuss the developments of basic biology and its application to practical problems. He mentioned the annual colloquia and the visit of Allen Laskin to the University of Minnesota. He was also influential in the symposium on "Trends in the Biology of Fermentations" which was held at the Brookhaven National Laboratory in December of 1980 and assisted with the speedy appearance of the proceedings volume just a few months later. We agreed that a meeting and publication of this type should also be done with the upcoming colloquia planned in Minneapolis for 1982.

As with all symposia, it is important to have the right mix of topics, speakers, and local arrangements, not the least significant of which is the financial support.

As we have seen, the organizers wisely chose a set of five topics which fairly illustrate the biological basis of a variety of new developments in biotechnology. It is this mix of basic studies and their application to important technological problems that is so impressive at this meeting.

Some of the topics particularly appeal to my experience working on these problems when they were first developed. I am referring here especially to the refinement of antibiotics that became widely practical only 40 years ago.

A few years ago, the application of these new techniques to agriculture was a relatively virgin field. At a recent meeting in Beltsville, Maryland, the U.S. Department of Agriculture's symposium on the "Application of Genetic Engineering to Agriculture," there were more than 600 scientists in attendance. Also, the University of California at Davis plans a symposium on the application of "Genetic Engineering of Plants" during August, 1982 and it has already reached near capacity registration. This symposium in Davis will be somewhat different because it will also offer demonstrations of practical applications illustrated in field trips.

I, unfortunately, missed our session on the application of medicine. The subject of "Fuels and Chemicals from Biomass" is right now in the forefront since important sources of energy are introduced by these strong papers. As always, Harry Peck gave an elegant report on pyrophosphate. Graham Walker gave a very stimulating discussion. Linden's presentation on the anaerobic production of chemicals gave me new ideas for further work, while Bull's discussion of continuous culture techniques illustrated very well the many new developments in this area.

The earlier discussion on monoclonal antibodies illustrated the tremendous development in this field which started out in 1975. Both lecturers made very clear the steps necessary to apply monoclonal antibody techniques to practical problems. Dr. Sadowski illustrated the successful application of this relatively new technique to practical agricultural problems. This concluded a very full and interesting day.

Other discussions concentrated on biodegradation and special enzyme technology. Dr. Chibata's paper showed the tremendous development in enzyme chemistry (immobilized catalysts). Dr. Klibanov's paper on unconventional biotechniques stimulated all kinds of interesting ideas, and finally, Dr. Williams' very interesting paper showed that plasmids can have very great importance especially for soil bacteria.

I hardly have to tell you how much we appreciate the work of Dr. Rogers and Dr. Laskin in organizing this conference, but a symposium of such interest is not complete until its proceeding appear in print. We have a very good record for producing these volumes within three to five months. To accomplish this, the cooperation of all the speakers and discussants is needed. As you know, it takes an average of 15 months to get a paper published in a journal. But with your cooperation, we can do very much better with these volumes.

Finally, I want to thank all of the administration staff of the University of Minnesota, including Ms. Darla Eckroth who headed our front desk and Mr. Douglas Fenderson of the Office of Continuing Medical Education, as well as the very pleasant and efficient food service people who provided our meals. For their efforts under the direction of Drs. Rogers and Laskin, I offer an earnest "Thank you".

LIST OF SPEAKERS AND PARTICIPANTS

ABELES, Robert H.	Grad. Dept. of Biochemistry, Brandeis University, Waltham, MA 02254
ANDERSSON, Kristoffer	250 Bioscience, Genetics & Cell Biology, St. Paul, MN 55108
BAIN, Murray	University of Maine, Microbiology, Orono, ME 04469
BARDER, Michael J.	Economics Lab. Inc., Osborn Bldg., Chem. Eng., St. Paul, MN 55102
BARTON, Ken	Cetos Madison Corp., 2208 Parview Rd., Middleton, WI 53562
BENJAMIN, Jerry C.	4 Temple Street, Framingham, MA 01701
BEZANSON, G.D.	Lab for Disease Control, Health & Welfare, Ottawa, Ontario, CANADA - A1A0L2
BISWAS, B.B.	Biochemistry Dept., Bose Institute, Calcutta, West Bengal, INDIA
BLOOMFIELD, Victor	1479 Gortner Ave., Univ. of Minnesota, St. Paul, MN 55108
BOPP, Lawrence	General Electric, Box 8, Bldg. K-1, Rm. 7B46, Schnectady, N.Y. 12301
BOWIE, J.	1516 Grand Ave., St. Paul, MN 55105
BRINTZENHOFE, Karen	HS Unit A 17-226, Univ. of Minnesota, Minneapolis, MN 55455
BULL, Alan T.	Univ. of Kent at Canterbury, Canterbury Kent, ENGLAND - CT27NJ
BURNS, Richard	Glasgow Site 300 Dupont Development Division, Wilmington, DE 19898
CALDECOTT, R.S.	College of Biological Sciences, Univ. of Minnesota, St. Paul, MN 55108
CARR, Charles W.	Biochemistry Dept., Univ. of Minnesota, Minneapolis, MN 55455
CHAPMAN, Peter J.	170 Gortner Lab, Univ. of Minnesota - St. Paul Campus, St. Paul, MN 55108
CHIBATA, Ichiro	Tanabe Seiyaku Company, Kashima-3-chome, Osaka, JAPAN - 532
CHING, David	2300 Berkshire Ln. Plymouth, MN 55441
CLARIDGE, Charles	Bristol-Myers Corp., P.O. Box 657, Syracuse, N.Y. 13201
CLEARY, Patrick	790 6th Ave. NW, New Brighton, MN 55112

CLINE, Martin J.	Univ. of California, Health Sci. Ctr., Div. of Oncology, Los Angeles, 90024
COONEY, Charles L.	Massachusetts Institute of Technology, Biochem. Engineering, Cambridge 02139
CRAWFORD, Ronald L.	Grey Freshwater Bio. Institute, Box 100, Navarre, MN 55392
DAGLEY, Stanley	Dept. of Biochemistry, Univ. of Minnesota, St. Paul, MN 55108
DAVIS, H. Ted	Chem. Eng., 235A Amundsen Hall, Univ. of Minnesota, Minneapolis, MN 55455
DELOGGIO, Ted	Biochem. Technology, Inc., 66 Great Valley Pkwy., Malvern, PA 19355
DIRKSEN, Joe	Cargill, Inc., P.O. Box 9300, Minneapolis, MN 55440
DOREMUS, Michael	Colorado State Univ., Agri. & Chem. Eng., Ft. Collins, CO 80523
DOUTHART, Richard J.	Batelle Northwest Lab., Box 999, Richland, WA 99352
DWORKIN, Marty	Microbiology, Box 196 Mayo, Univ. of Minnesota, Minneapolis, MN 55455
FREDRICKSON, Arnold G.	Univ. of Minnesota, Chem. Engineering, Minneapolis, MN 55455
FUSEE, Murray C.	7379 Route 32, W.R. Grace & Co., Columbia, MO 21044
GERMAINE, Greg R.	Dept. of Oral Biology, Univ. of Minnesota, Minneapolis, MN 55455
GINSBURG, Hershel	Box 511 Mayo Bldg., Univ. of Minnesota,Minneapolis, MN 55455
GOLDSTEIN, Jack	N.Y. Blood Center, 310 E. 67th St., New York, N.Y. 10021
GRAY, Patrick	460 Point San Bruno Blvd., Genentech, Inc., San Francisco, CA 94080
GREEN, Charles E.	903 Agronomy Bldg., Univ. of Minnesota, St. Paul, MN 55108
GUIRE, Patrick	6741 Tartan Curve, Eden Prairie, MN 55344
HANG, Yong D.	Cornell Univ., Geneva, N.Y. 14456
HANSON, Richard	Gray Freshwater Biol. Institute, Country Rd., Navarre, MN 55392
HATCHER, Herbert J.	Economics Lab. Inc., Osborn Bldg., Chem. Eng., St. Paul, MN 55102
HAYES, Sidney	Univ. of Saskatchewan, Microbiology, Saskatoon, CANADA S7NOWO
HELLER, Steve	9000 Plymouth Ave. No., Minneapolis, MN 55447
HOGENKAMP, Harry H.	Biochem. Dept., 4-225 Millard Hall, Univ. of Minnesota, Minneapolis 55455
HOLLAENDER, Alexander	Council for Research Planning, 1717 Mass. Ave. NW, Washington, D.C. 20036
HUNTER, Meredith M.	Harvard Medical School, Mass. General Hosp., Boston, MA 02114

JACOBS, Grace E.	Northwestern College of Chiro., 1834 So. Mississippi, St. Paul, MN 55116
JARFLE, Allen	980 American Center Bldg., 150 E. Kellogg, St. Paul, MN 55101
JENSEN, K.E.	30 Thumbull Rd., Waterford, CT 06385
JONES, Frank H.	Cargill Inc., P.O. Box 9300, Minneapolis, MN 55440
JONES, Lester T.	3M Center, Bldg., 201-15-12, St. Paul, MN 55144
JOO, P. Kim	P.O. Box 959, Minneapolis, MN 55440
KELLER, Kenneth,	Academic Affairs, Univ. of Minnesota, Minneapolis, MN 55455
KLEESE, Roger	Molecular Genetics, 10320 Bren Rd. East, Minnetonka, MN 55343
KLIBANOV, Alexander	Mass. Institute of Technology, Nutrition, Cambridge, MA 02139
KOERNER, James F.	4-225 Millard Hall, Univ. of Minnesota, Minneapolis, MN 55455
KOLANKO, Bill	6301 Lincoln Ave., Travenol Labs, Morton Grove, IL 60053
KRIVIT, William	Pediatrics, Univ. of Minnesota, Box 391 Mayo, Minneapolis, MN 55455
KUNZ, Daniel A.	E.I. du Pont de Nemours, Exp. Station E328/B40, Wilmington, DE 19898
KVETKAS, Marilyn	515 Greenview Dr., Wauconda, IL 60084
LAHTI, Carol	148 W. George St., St. Paul, MN 55107
LAIBLE, Nancy	Microbiology, Univ. of Minnesota, Minneapolis, MN 55455
LASKIN, Allen I.	Exxon Research & Engineering, Box 45, Linden, N.J. 07036
LINDEN, James C.	Agri. & Chem. Eng., Colorado State Univ., Ft. Collins, CO 80523
LIVINGSTON, Dennis	Biochemistry, Univ. of Minnesota, Minneapolis, MN 55455
LOHMAR, Patricia	2620 Dupont Ave. So., #1, Minneapolis, MN 55408
LOVRIEN, Rex	Biochemistry, 270 Gortner Lab, Univ. of Minnesota, St. Paul, MN 55108
LU, Deru	4853 Cordell Ave., Bethesda, MD 20814
MAC FARLANE, Gordon	HS Unit A17-226, Univ. of Minnesota, Minneapolis, MN 55455
MAGEE, Walter L.	Stauffer Chemical Co., Eastern Res. Ctr., Dobbs Ferry, N.Y. 10522
MAJDE, Jeannine A.	Offic of Naval Research, 800 N. Quincy St., Arlington, VA 22217
MALEWICZ, Barbara	801 16th Ave., N.E., Austin, MN 55912
MARKOVETZ, A.J.	Univ. of Iowa, Microbiology, Iowa City, IA 52240
MARTINIS, Joanne	Hybritech Inc., 11085 Torreyana Rd., San Diego, CA 92121

MATTES, Ralf	Boehringer Mannheim GMBH, Biothemica Werk Tutzing, W. GERMANY
MC CORMACK, Robert T.	3532 46th Ave. So., Minneapolis, MN 55406
MC IVER, Robert	111 Food Science & Nutrition, Univ. of Minnesota, St. Paul, MN 55108
MC KAY, Larry L.	248 Food Science & Nutrition, Univ. of Minnesota, St. Paul, MN 55108
MEHTA, Nikhil	Colorado State Univ., Agri. & Chem. Eng., Ft. Collins, CO 80523
MESSING, Joachim	Biochemistry, Univ. of Minnesota, St. Paul, MN 55108
MILLER, Daniel G.	3M Center, Bldg. 201-2W-17, St. Paul, MN 55144
MILLER, Larry	Univ. of Minnesota, Minneapolis, MN 55455
MODELEVSKY, Joseph L.	Eli Lilly & Co., MC963, Indianapolis, IN 46285
MULLEN, Joe	General Mills, 9000 Plymouth Ave. No., Minneapolis, MN 55427
MURAKAMI, Seishi	2647 Emerson Ave. So. #22, Minneap-olis, MN 55408
NASH, III, Claude H.	Sterling-Winthrop Res. Inst., Rens-selaer, N.Y. 12144
NELSON, Thomas C.	Univ. of Wisconsin Botany Dept., Box 413, Milwaukee, WI 53201
NEWELL, Nanette	U.S. Congress Office of Tech. Human Resources, Washington, D.C. 20510
ORMAN, Bruce	7354 No. 72nd, Brooklyn Pk., MN 55428
PARSON, Kathleen	Macalester College, 1600 Grand Ave., St. Paul, MN 55105
PASS, Franklin	10320 Bren Rd. East, Minnetonka, MN 55343
PECK, Jr., Harry D.	Biochemistry, Univ. of Georgia, Athens, GA 30602
PEDERSEN, Daniel E.	Economics Lab. Inc., Osborn Bldg., St. Chem. Eng. Ctr., Paul, MN 55102
POLANSKI, M.	2968 West River Parkway, Minneapolis, MN 55406
PRETAYKO, A.W.	1500 Spring Garden St., Philadelphia, PA 19101
RABSON, Robert	U.S. Dept. of Energy, ER-17 GTN, Washington, D.C. 20545
RAJAMANNAN, A.H.J.	Agro-K-Corp., 5750 Main St., Minneap-olis, MN 55432
REESE, Laure L.	Economics Lab., Inc., Osborn Bldg., Chem. Eng. Ctr., St. Paul, MN 55102
RENN, Don	5 Maple Street, Rockland, ME 04841
RHEINBERGER, Mary Ann	818 W. Olive Street, Stillwater, MN 55082

ROBINSON, James R.	7070 Commerce Circle, Pleasanton, CA 94583
ROGERS, Palmer	1973 Sheridan Ave. So., Minneapolis, MN 55405
ROSS, Laurie A.	7080 Glenross Rd., Woodbury, MN 55125
RUBINOVITZ, Chalm	National Institutes of Health, Bldg. 6, Rm. B1-31 Bethesda, MD 20205
RUIZ, Leonard P.	Land O'Lakes Inc., P.O. Box 116, Minneapolis, MN 55440
RUSSELL, Martha G.	220 Coffey Hall, Univ. of Minnesota, St. Paul, MN 55108
SADOWSKI, Peter	Molecular Genetics, Inc., 10320 Bren Rd. East, Minnetonka, MN 55343
SAUER, Richard J.	280 Coffey Hall, Univ. of Minnesota, St. Paul, MN 55108
SAUERBIER, Walter	442 Biological Sciences, Univ. of Minnesota, St. Paul, MN 55108
SCHRODER, Joe	Max Plank Institute for Plant Breeding Research, Koln, WEST GERMANY - D-5000
SHERMAN, Mary M.	425 No. Charter St., Univ. of Wisconsin Pharm. Dept., Madison, WI 53706
SIH, Charles J.	Univ. of Wisconsin, 425 No. Charter St., Madison, WI 53706
SKATRUD, Thomas J.	Bio-Technical Resources Inc., 7th & Marshall, Manitowoc, WI 54220
SPERBER, William H.	311 Second St. SE, Minneapolis, MN 55414
STABA, E. John	Unit F 9-106 Coll. of Pharm., Univ. of Minnesota, Minneapolis, MN 55455
STAEHLE, Roger W.	105 Lind Hall, I.T. Dept., Univ. of Minnesota, Minneapolis, MN 55455
STAMER, John R.	N.Y. State Agri. Expt. Station, Cornell University, Geneva, N.Y. 14456
STARLINGER, Peter	Institute for Genetic Research, Univ. of Koln, Koln, WEST GERMANY - D-5000
SUBDEN, Ronald	Dept. of Genetics, Univ. of Guelph, Ontario, CANADA N1G2W1
SULLIVAN, Mary A.	Box 672, Univ. of Rochester Med. Ctr., Rochester, N.Y. 14642
SYU, Wan-Jr	706 H Eagle Heights, Madison, WI 53706
TARSIO, Joe	17-226 HS Unit A, Oral Biology, Univ. of Minnesota, Minneapolis, MN 55455
TELLEFSON, Lois	17-246 Helath Science Unit A, Univ. of Minnesota, Minneapolis, MN 55455
THOMPSON, Phillip G.	Patent Adm., 333 Morrill Hall, Univ. of Minnesota, Minneapolis, MN 55455
TOMASEK, Paul H.	Gray Freshwater Biol. Inst., Box 100, Shadywood Rd., Navarre, MN 55392

TREND, J.E.	3M Company, 3M Center 201-3E, St. Paul, MN 55144
TSUCHIYA, H.M.	Dept. of Chem. Eng., Univ. of Minnesota, MN 55455
TUOMINEN, F.W.	Henkel Corporation, 2010 E. Hennepin Ave., Minneapolis, MN 55413
UY, Rosa	3M Center, 201-1W, St. Paul, MN 55101
VAN HULLE, Glenn	General Mills, 9000 Plymouth Ave. No., Minneapolis, MN 55427
VERMEULEN, Mary W.	351 Chester St., Minneapolis, MN 55419
WALKER, David	934 W. 3rd St., Maryville, MO 64468
WALKER, Graham C.	Massachusetts Institute of Technology, Biology, Cambridge, MA 02139
WATSON, Dennis W.	Microbiology, Box 196 Mayo, Univ. of Minnesota, Minneapolis, MN 55455
WEBER, Mark	526 W. Washington Ave. #3B, Madison, WI 53703
WESTPHELING, Janet	Biological Laboratories, Harvard University, Cambridge, MA 02139
WHITTENBURY, Roger	Biological Sciences, Univ. of Warwick, Coventry, ENGLAND - CV47AL
WIERMAN, Constance	425 No. Charter St., Univ. of Wisconsin, Pharm. Dept., Madison, WI 53706
WILLIAMS, Peter A.	Univ. College of North Wales, Bangor, Gwynedd, UNITED KINGDOM - L572UW
WILSON, Claire M.	Council for Research Planning, 1717 Mass. Ave. NW, Washington, D.C. 20036
WORKMAN, Wesley R.	3M Center, Bldg. 201-1S-12, St. Paul, MN 55144
WRIGHT, Clifford D.	Box 124 Mayo Bldg., Univ. of Minnesota, Minneapolis, MN 55455
ZABORSKY, Oskar	National Science Foundation, 1800 G St., NW, Washington, D.C. 20550

INDEX